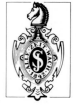

Surgery of Female Incontinence

Second Edition

Edited by

Stuart L. Stanton and Emil A. Tanagho

Foreword by Frank Hinman, Jr.

With 229 Figures

Springer-Verlag
Berlin Heidelberg New York Tokyo

Stuart L. Stanton, FRCS, MRCOG
Consultant Gynaecologist,
St. James and St. George's Hospitals,
London, England; and Honorary Senior Lecturer,
Department of Obstetrics and Gynaecology,
St. George's Hospital Medical School,
London SW17 ORE, England

Emil A. Tanagho, MD
Professor and Chairman
Department of Urology, School of Medicine,
University of California, San Francisco, CA 94143,
U.S.A

ISBN 3-540-15821-9 2nd Edition Springer-Verlag Berlin Heidelberg New York Tokyo
ISBN 0-387-15821-9 2nd Edition Springer-Verlag Berlin Heidelberg New York Tokyo

ISBN 3-540-10155-1 1st Edition Springer-Verlag Berlin Heidelberg New York Tokyo
ISBN 0-387-10155-1 1st Edition Springer-Verlag Berlin Heidelberg New York Tokyo

Library of Congress Cataloging in Publication Data
Main entry under title:
Surgery of female incontinence.
Includes bibliographies and index.
1. Urinary stress incontinence—Surgery. I. Stanton, Stuart L. II. Tanagho, Emil A., 1929–   . [DNLM: 1. Urinary
Incontinence—surgery. WJ 146 S961] RG485.S7S87 1986 617'.462 85-22065
ISBN 0-387-15821-9 (U.S.)

© Springer-Verlag Berlin Heidelberg 1980, 1986
Printed in Great Britain

The use of registered names, trademarks etc. in this publication does not imply, even in the absence of a specific
statement, that such names are exempt from the relevant laws and regulations and therefore free for general
use.

Product Liability: The publisher can give no guarantee for information about drug dosage and application thereof
contained in this book. In every individual case the respective user must check its accuracy by consulting other
pharmaceutical literature.

Filmset and printed in Great Britain by BAS Printers Limited, Over Wallop, Hampshire

2128/3916 543210

Dedication

To our friend and colleague C. Paul Hodgkinson, gynaecologist and scientist, whose pioneering work on bladder pressure measurement and detrusor instability forms one of the corner-stones of modern urodynamics

Foreword

In this book we have expert urologists and gynaecologists on the two sides of the Atlantic working together with a common interest, the inadequate female urethra. What makes this volume so valuable is that it is not restricted to one speciality or one cult, but bravely (and systematically) presents established principles and practice.

Not only is the current knowledge of the anatomy and function of the continence mechanisms defined by experts carefully selected by the two authorities in the field, but this information is directly applied to clinical problems for the reader to use in the care of patients.

Because the basics are presented first, and followed by the methods of diagnosis, the sections describing each form of treatment, whether medical or surgical, are set on rational bases. These are not cookbook directions. This background is especially valuable because the incontinent female usually has a complicated disorder, each case being different, so that the responsible gynaecologists or urologists must apply as much understanding as technique if their efforts are to achieve dryness. The clear descriptions and illustrations in this book, then, act as guides as much as directives.

This second edition builds on the success of the first. All of us trying to help these unfortunate women will do more for them from having this new edition at hand.

Frank Hinman, Jr., MD,
Clinical Professor of Urology,
University of California, San Francisco

Preface to Second Edition

In the six years since the first edition, many advances have occurred in medical practice. It is too soon to see whether the surgical cure of incontinence has improved, but the main ideas in the first edition, namely that suprapubic surgery is likely to result in a higher rate of cure than vaginal surgery, and the importance of the interrelationship of urethral and bladder pressures in the genesis of incontinence, are still held.

Disappointingly few practical advances have taken place in urodynamic investigation; some investigations have been rejected and others now have a more defined role. Ultrasound and studies involving electromyography and electric conductance are likely to become increasingly relevant.

There are five new contributors to the book and six new chapters. We believe that adequate attention needed to be given to the correct management of incontinence in childhood. It also seemed right to include a chapter on Bob Zacharin's "abdominoperineal urethral suspension procedure", based on his elegant studies of the female pelvic anatomy. Voiding difficulties are frequently encountered after bladder neck surgery, and two new chapters have been added in which this is discussed.

In a book contributed to and edited by gynaecologists and urologists, with nine different surgical procedures (excluding repair of fistula) to correct incontinence, it seemed sensible to have "a consumer guide" written by the editors, putting forward their management of the incontinent patient. The editors, however, do caution that they have not yet discovered the infallible operation.

We thank the many artists who have helped prepare the illustrations and in particular, Robert Lane, London, who has illustrated Chapters 3, 6 and 8.

Once again we acknowledge the skill and enthusiasm of Michael Jackson of Springer-Verlag and thank him for his valued professional guidance.

Finally, to our respective wives, Ann and Mona, and to our children, we thank them for their continued understanding, patience and support during the preparation of this second edition.

London and San Francisco   Stuart L. Stanton
February 1986   Emil A. Tanagho

Preface to First Edition

Urinary incontinence in the female has begun to attract wide interest as an increasingly common condition which needs investigation and treatment. For instance, there are an estimated 2 million women suffering from incontinence in the United Kingdom (which is 7% of the total female population) and there are reported post-operative recurrence rates up to 45%. There can be little place now for the acceptance of conventional views on the management of urinary incontinence.

The controversy over the mechanism of continence control, the bewildering array of electronic gadgetry available for the urodynamic investigations and the choice of over 100 varieties of surgical procedures seemed adequate reasons to the editors that there was scope and demand for this book. That the book is edited by a gynaecologist and a urologist is an indication of the interdisciplinary nature of this condition.

To be able to adequately treat urinary incontinence it is necessary to understand the anatomy, physiology and pathophysiology of the bladder and urethra and supporting structures. The investigation of incontinence has become more complex and although many patients can be diagnosed on history taking and clinical examination, twin-channel subtracted cystometry and measurement of bladder pressure and urine flow recordings with or without radiology, and urethral pressure measurements are necessary in dealing with complicated histories, recurrent incontinence or a voiding difficulty and incontinence.

Nineteen internationally known gynaecologists and urologists have contributed their views and described procedures with which they are familiar, with indications, contraindications, post-operative management including their results. Whilst we may not always agree with the views stated here, we feel that this is a developing area and that conventional as well as controversial latter day opinions need to be expressed. Our views may be summarised as follows: modern interpretation of bladder and urethral function recognises that the bladder has a filling and an emptying phase. The main parameters of function are bladder and urethral pressure measurements, their relationships to each other and to abdominal pressure and the transmission of abdominal pressure to bladder and urethra. The work carried out by the bladder during voiding can be measured by the voiding pressure or the pressure rise on isometric detrusor contraction, the urine flow rate and urethral pressure. The role of radiology is less important but valuable in assessing bladder neck function, descent of the bladder neck and bladder base, ureteric reflux, and the ability to empty completely. Less emphasis is placed nowadays on the posterior urethrovesical angle.

The trend in incontinence surgery for urethral sphincter incompetence is towards suprapubic methods of control. The vaginal repair is included because it undoubtedly cures some patients of incontinence and prolapse and is used and taught by most gynaecologists throughout the world. We believe that the first operation has the best chance of cure and for this reason prefer a suprapubic procedure which we believe is more effective. Reconstructive surgery and the artificial sphincter are included as these are now techniques which have been evaluated and have a real role in the management of recurrent incontinence. Diversion procedures are described because some patients are so handicapped by incontinence that they have a right to be dry, by whatever means.

Detrusor instability as a cause of incontinence remains enigmatic. Cystodistension and vaginal denervation procedures should be used cautiously and not until pharmacological or bladder retraining methods have been tried and failed.

Incontinence due to overflow retention is becoming a more readily recognised condition in the female, although its cause is often difficult to ascertain. Urethrotomy and drug therapy are the mainstays of treatment.

During the last stage of this book we learnt of the sad death of Thomas H. Green. His early work on incontinence was part of the foundation of our understanding of this subject. His surgical skills both in correction of incontinence and in the more general sphere of gynaecology were renowned. We were fortunate that he had agreed to be a contributor and hope that the final book would have met with his approval.

We acknowledge and thank Michael Jackson of Springer-Verlag for his help and enthusiasm in this project. We thank the many different artists who have contributed illustrations and would especially mention Mr. Alan Jones of the Educational Technology Unit at St. George's Hospital Medical School, whose illustrations are contained in Chapters 1, 2, 3, 4 and 5. The brunt of collating and typing the final manuscript has fallen on Mrs. Daphne Penfold, Urodynamic Unit, St. George's Hospital Medical School. Without her energies, attention to detail and humour this task would not have been completed.

Finally we humbly acknowledge the patience and forebearance of our wives, Ann and Mona, and our respective children, and hope that the book will be sufficient justification for some of the time spent away from them.

London and San Francisco   Stuart L. Stanton
August 1980   Emil A. Tanagho

Contents

Contributors

William L. Furlow MD FACS
Professor of Urology, Department of Urology, Mayo Medical School, Mayo Clinic, Rochester, MN 55901, U.S.A.

Paul Hilton MD MRCOG
Senior Lecturer and Honorary Consultant, Department of Obstetrics and Gynaecology, Princess Mary Maternity Hospital, Newcastle upon Tyne, NE2 3BD, England

Rudolph Hohenfellner MD
Urologische Klinik, Johannes Gutenberg-Universitat, D-6500 Mainz, Federal Republic of Germany

Christopher N. Hudson MCnir FRCS FRCOG FRACOG
Consultant Obstetrician and Gynaecologist, St. Bartholomew's Hospital, London EC1A 7BE

Kermit E. Krantz MD
Chairman and Professor of Obstetrics and Gynecology, College of Health Sciences and Hospital, University of Kansas Medical Center, Kansas 66103, U.S.A.

John B. Lawson FRCOG
Consultant Obstetrician and Gynaecologist, Newcastle General Hospital, Newcastle upon Tyne, NE4 6BE and Clinical Lecturer in Obstetrics and Gynaecology, University of Newcastle upon Tyne, NE4 6BE, England

Eckhard Petri MD
Klinik für Geburtschilfe und Frauenkrankheiten, Johannes Gutenberg Universitat, D-6500 Mainz, Federal Republic of Germany

A. M. K. Rickwood FRCS
Consultant Urological Surgeon, Alder Hey Children's Hospital, Liverpool L12 2AP, England

Peter R. Riddle FRCS
Consultant Urologist, St. Peter's Hospitals, London, England

Richard A. Schmidt MD
Department of Urology, School of Medicine, University of California, San Francisco, CA 94143, U.S.A.

Thomas A. Stamey MD
Professor of Surgery, Chairman, Division of Urology, Stanford University Medical Center, Stanford, California 94305, U.S.A.

Stuart L. Stanton FRCS MRCOG
Consultant Gynaecologist, St. James and St. George's Hospitals, London, England and Honorary Senior Lecturer, Department of Obstetrics and Gynaecology, St. George's Hospital Medical School, London SW17 ORE

Emil A. Tanagho MD
Professor and Chairman, Department of Urology, School of Medicine, University of California, San Francisco, CA 94143, U.S.A.

David Warrell MD FRCOG
Consultant Obstetrician and Gynaecologist, St. Mary's Hospital, Manchester, England

Alan J. Wein MD
Professor and Chairman, Division of Urology, School of Medicine, Hospital of the University of Pennsylvania, 5 Silverstein, Philadelphia, Pennsylvania 19104, U.S.A.

Peter H. L. Worth FRCS
Consultant Urologist, St. Peter's Hospitals and University College Hospitals, London, WC1E 6AU, England

W. Keith Yeates MD MS FRCS FRCSEd
Honorary Consultant Urologist, Newcastle University Hospitals, Newcastle upon Tyne, England

Robert F. Zacharin FRCS FRCOG FRACS FRACOG
Department of Gynaecology, Alfred Hospital and Royal Children's Hospital, Melbourne, Australia

1 The Mechanism of Continence

Paul Hilton

Introduction

Urinary incontinence may be defined as "a condition in which involuntary loss of urine is a social or hygienic problem, and is objectively demonstrable" (Bates et al. 1983). Continence then, by inference, might be considered as the ability to retain urine within the bladder, between episodes of voluntary micturition. In order to comprehend fully the pathological processes which lead to the development of urinary incontinence, a clear understanding of the normal mechanisms for the maintenance of continence is of course fundamental; this in turn must be based on a knowledge of the development, anatomy, and physiology of the bladder and urethra, and their supporting structures. This chapter aims to provide this background information.

Embryology of the Lower Urinary Tract

Development of the Embryonic Plate

In the earliest stages of human development the embryonic plate is a bilaminar structure made up of ectoderm above and endoderm below. At approximately 15 days following fertilisation these layers become separated by a layer of intra-embryonic mesoderm, spreading out from the primitive streak to produce a trilaminar disc. The ingrowth of mesoderm is, however, incomplete, leaving areas where the bilaminar structure persists cranially (the buccopharyngeal membrane) and caudally, in the region of the connecting stalk (the cloacal membrane) (Fig. 1.1a).

Formation of the Cloaca

An endodermal outgrowth in the region of the cloacal membrane, the allantois, extends into the connecting stalk at around 16–17 days after fertilisation. With subsequent increasing growth of the embryonic plate, folding occurs both in the coronal plane, along the whole length of the plate, and in the sagittal plane, in the head and tail regions, with the incorporation of fore and hind gut from the endodermal lining of the yolk sac (Fig. 1.1b). Further folding of the embryo brings both the connecting stalk and the cloacal membrane onto the ventral surface, and leads to the development of the cloaca, being that part of the hind gut lying caudal to the attachment of the allantois (Fig. 1.1c).

Partitioning of the Cloaca

At around 28 days after fertilisation the shelf of mesoderm at the base of the allantois begins to grow and migrate along the curvature of the embryo towards the cloacal membrane. It thus forms a septum, the urorectal septum, partitioning the cloaca into a ventral urogenital sinus and a dorsal rectum, which are isolated from one another by the final closure of the cloacal duct when the septum meets the cloacal membrane at approximately 38 days after fertilisation (Fig. 1.1d).

Development of Nephrogenic Mesoderm

Whilst growth and folding of the embryo lead to the development of the cloaca from the endoderm of the yolk sac, developing within the intra-embryonic mesoderm is the pronephros. The pronephric duct (ultimately to become the mesonephric duct) grows caudally, and at around 28 days after fertilisation reaches the lateral aspect of the cloaca. This effectively divides the urogenital sinus into two regions: that between the mesonephric ducts and the allantois being called the vesicourethral canal, and that below the mesonephric ducts the definitive urogenital sinus. At around the same time, a proliferation of cells in the region of the genu produces the ureteric bud, and it is the growth of the latter towards the caudal end of the nephrogenic ridge which initiates the development of the definitive kidney, or metanephros, between 30 and 37 days after fertilisation.

Formation of the Bladder, Urethra and Trigone

The subsequent formation of the bladder and urethra from the vesicourethral canal is dependent on two events which proceed simultaneously. Derotation of the tailfold brings the cloacal membrane more caudally, and with growth of the anterior abdominal wall the ventral surface of the canal increases considerably in size. Simultaneously, positional changes between the mesonephric duct and the ureteric bud occur such that the ureter, initially a posteromedial outgrowth, comes to lie posterolaterally with respect to the duct. Whilst this migration is going on the common excretory duct shortens and is incorporated into the bladder base. This has the effect of giving the endodermal wall of the vesicourethral canal a mesodermal contribution derived from the nephrogenic ridge; by 42 days following fertilisation the trigone may be defined as that region of the vesicourethral canal lying between the ureteric orifices and the termination of the mesonephric ducts (Fig. 1.1e). Concomitant with the development of the trigone, changes within the vesicourethral canal lead to a dilatation of its cranial portion to produce the definitive bladder, whereas the caudal or phallic portion remains narrow and represents the urethra. In the female this region gives rise to the whole urethra; in the male it produces the proximal, prostatic urethra only, the membranous and spongy urethra being derived

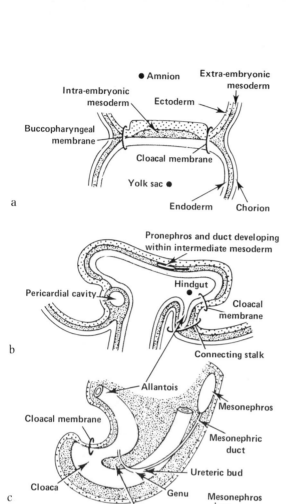

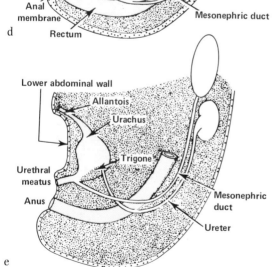

from urogenital sinus. Anal and urogenital openings are formed by the breakdown of the respective membranes at around 42 days after fertilisation (Fig. 1.1e).

Epithelium of the Bladder Base and Urethra

Although the trigone and proximal urethra are undoubtedly derived from nephrogenic mesoderm, the origin of their epithelial linings is unclear. Some have suggested that they too are mesodermally derived; others hold that endodermal epithelium from the vesicourethral canal migrates to cover the region derived from mesonephric duct. Certainly the epithelium in this area retains some differences from that over the rest of the bladder, and some similarities to that of the lower genital tract, being oestrogen sensitive (Smith 1972).

Anatomy of the Lower Urinary Tract

The Bladder

Detrusor

The bladder muscle or detrusor is often described as consisting of three distinct smooth muscle layers, the outer being orientated longitudinally, the middle circularly, and the inner longitudinally. More recent studies, however, suggest that there is frequent interchange of fibres between bundles, and separate layers are not easily defined. Indeed, from a functional point of view the detrusor appears constructed to contract as a single syncytial mass. With the exception of the muscle fibres of the superficial trigone, all areas of the detrusor show similar histological and histochemical characteristics. In distinc-

---

Fig. 1.1a–e. Schematic drawings to show stages in development of the lower urinary tract. **a** 15 days after fertilisation or 4 weeks gestational age (presomitic embryo); **b** 22 days after fertilisation or 5 weeks gestation (2 mm crown–rump length, 6–8 somite embryo); **c** 28 days after fertilisation or 6 weeks gestation (4.5 mm crown–rump length, 30 somite embryo); **d** 38 days after fertilisation or 7–8 weeks gestation (12 mm crown–rump length, 42 somite embryo); **e** 42 days after fertilisation or 8 weeks gestation (16 mm crown–rump length).

tion from other smooth muscle cells in the urinary tract, those of the detrusor are shown to contain significant amounts of acetylcholinesterase, in keeping with their abundant cholinergic parasympathetic nerve supply (Gosling 1979).

Trigone

The smooth muscle of the trigone, in contrast to that of the rest of the bladder, is easily distinguished into two layers (Fig. 1.2a). The deep trigonal muscle is in all respects similar to the detrusor; the superficial muscle in this region has, however, several distinguishing features. It is relatively thin and consists of small muscle bundles; the cells themselves are devoid of acetylcholinesterase and have a more sparse cholinergic nerve supply. It may be traced distally where it fades out in the proximal urethra, forming a low crest on the posterior wall (Tanagho and Smith 1966), and proximally, where it is continuous with the ureteric smooth muscle (Donker et al. 1976). Indeed, it has been suggested that whilst the bulk of this muscle is too small for it to be of relevance in bladder neck or urethral function, it may have significance in control of the ureterovesical junction during voiding, thereby preventing ureteric reflux (Tanagho and Pugh 1963; Gosling 1979).

Bladder Neck

The smooth muscle of the bladder neck is also distinct from that of the detrusor. In the male a well-defined preprostatic smooth muscle sphincter is present, consisting of small-diameter muscle bundles. In the female, however, whilst the smooth muscle in the bladder neck is similarly distinct from the detrusor in terms of muscle bundle size, the orientation of bundles is largely oblique or longitudinal and they appear to have little or no sphincter action (Kluck 1980).

Urothelium

The mucosal lining of the bladder is consistent in appearance in all regions in the distended state and is made up of two or three layers of transitional cells. When empty, however, except over the trigone, the bladder is thrown into extensive rugae and the urothelium may be up to six cells thick.

The Urethra

The normal female urethra is between 30 and 50 mm in length from internal to external meatus.

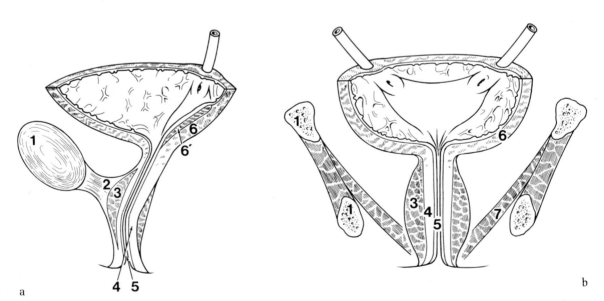

Fig. 1.2. Schematic diagrams of female bladder and urethra in **a** sagittal section and **b** coronal section. *1*, pubic symphysis/rami; *2*, posterior pubourethral ligaments; *3*, intrinsic striated muscle (rhabdosphincter urethrae); *4*, intrinsic smooth muscle; *5*, mucosa and submucosal vascular tissues; *6*, smooth muscle of detrusor/deep trigone; *6'*, smooth muscle of superficial trigone; *7*, extrinsic striated muscle/levator ani. (Hilton 1981, modified after Gosling 1979)

Its structure, in particular that of the smooth and striated muscle components, has been the subject of considerable debate.

Urethral Smooth Muscle

It was previously held by many workers that the smooth muscle of the bladder and that of the urethra are distinct (Hutch 1971; Donker et al. 1976); others, however, have suggested that they are in direct continuity, inner longitudinal and outer oblique layers of urethral muscle being continuous with the inner and outer longitudinal layers of the detrusor (Tanagho and Smith 1966). More recently Gosling (1979) has advocated a return to the concept of bladder and urethral smooth muscle being separate entities. Whilst morphologically they may appear continuous, histochemically they are different in that the urethral smooth muscle cells are apparently devoid of acetylcholinesterase: however, Tanagho (1984) disputes this.

Urethral and Periurethral Striated Muscle

Controversy has also surrounded the striated muscle components of the urethra. Langreder (1956) considered that the external striated urethral sphincter and periurethral striated muscle of levator ani were in continuity. There is now increasing evidence that they are distinct (Donker et al. 1976; Gosling and Dixon 1979). The intrinsic (external or rhabdosphincter) striated portion of the urethral sphincter mechanism consists of bundles of circularly arranged fibres maximal in bulk at the mid-urethral level anteriorly, thinning laterally and being almost totally deficient posteriorly (Fig. 1.2). The extrinsic periurethral striated muscle of levator ani has no direct contiguity with the urethra, being separated from it by a connective tissue septum. Its muscle bundles lie in general terms lateral to the urethra, being inserted into the lateral vaginal walls, and their bulk is maximal at the junction of middle and lower thirds of the urethra, i.e. at a somewhat lower level than the intrinsic rhabdosphincter. Gosling et al. (1981) have also demonstrated that these muscles are histochemically distinct, and appear of different functional specialisation. The intrinsic striated muscle is made up of small diameter muscle fibres, rich in acid stable myosin ATPase, and possessing numerous mitochondria;

they are therefore classified as slow twitch fibres, and are thought to be responsible for the striated contribution to urethral closure at rest. By contrast, the extrinsic periurethral striated muscle fibres are mostly made up of large diameter fibres of a heterogeneous population, some of which show the above characteristics of slow twitch muscle, while others are rich in alkaline stable myosin ATPase, characteristic of fast twitch muscle. The latter are suspected to contribute an additional reflex component to aid urethral closure on stress.

Mucosa and Submucosa

The epithelial lining of the urethra is of two types; proximally it is continuous with that of the bladder and consists of pseudostratified transitional cells; distally it is continuous with the introital skin and consists of non-keratinised stratified squamous cells. The junction between the two varies with age and oestrogen status (Hilton and Varma 1984) and may be of significance with regard to the prevention of ascending infection.

Huisman (1979) studied the structure of the female urethra in different age groups. He identified two prominent venous plexi within the submucosa: a distal one whose structure varied little with age, and a proximal one beneath the bladder neck, where marked age-related changes were seen. In women of reproductive age the vessels were highly folded, thin walled, and with numerous arteriovenous anastomoses, giving a cavernous appearance to the submucosa not seen in postmenopausal women. His interpretation of these findings was that this vascular system played a major role in the closure of the urethra in young women. Gosling et al. (1983), however, whilst agreeing that the region has indeed a rich blood supply, find no specialised features in the vessels, and suggest that the vascular contribution to urethral resistance is negligible. Zinner et al. (1976) have emphasised the role of mucosal softness in the effective occlusion of the urethral lumen.

Pubourethral Ligaments

The pubourethral ligaments form an important suspensory mechanism for the female urethra. They are described as consisting of a single anterior and paired posterior ligaments, the latter being of much greater functional significance. Zacharin (1963) described three anatomical expansions of the posterior ligaments: posteriorly to the paraurethral tissues, laterally to the levator fascia, and recurrently, beneath the subpubic arch towards the anterior ligament, and forming the so-called intermediate ligament. From histological examination of cadaveric specimens Zacharin (1963) has described the ligaments as consisting of parallel collagen bundles and elastic connective tissue. Wilson et al. (1979), however, in operative and post mortem specimens, found the "ligaments" to contain large numbers of smooth muscle bundles. Gosling et al. (1983) have described these fibres as extending upwards towards the lower fibres of the bladder, and indeed have found them to be histochemically identical with the detrusor, possessing an abundant presumptive cholinergic nerve supply. But Wilson et al. failed to demonstrate tissue acetylcholinesterase activity in these fibres and therefore suggested that they were of different origin to the detrusor. Whatever their origin, it may well be that these ligaments provide both active and passive components to the maintenance of the normal spatial relationships of urethra, bladder and pelvis.

Neurological Control of Micturition

The main function of the bladder is to convert the continuous excretory function of the kidneys into a more convenient, intermittent process of evacuation. In order to achieve this the bladder must serve firstly as an efficient, i.e. continent, low pressure reservoir whose function interferes minimally with an individual's other activities, and secondly it must allow the intermittent voluntary relinquishment of that former function, within socially acceptable limits with respect to time and place, to allow voiding. These two requirements call for an extraordinarily complex neural control to co-ordinate sensory input from and motor output to bladder and urethra in reciprocal fashion (Fig. 1.3).

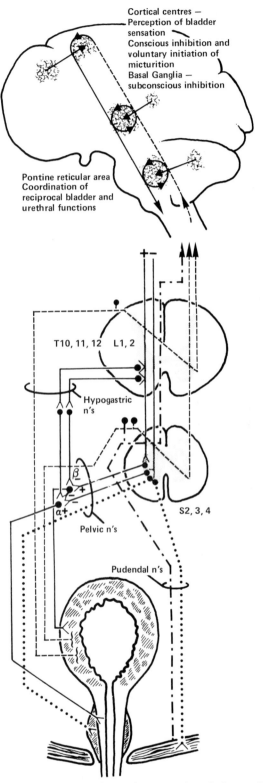

Fig. 1.3. Peripheral and central nerve supply to the lower urinary tract. ——— visceral efferents (parasympathetic and sympathetic); – – – visceral afferents; . . . . somatic efferents; –·–· somatic afferents. (Modified after Abrams et al. 1983)

Innervation of the Detrusor

Parasympathetic Supply

The bladder muscle is diffusely and richly supplied with cholinergic nerve fibres, to the extent that each individual muscle cell may be supplied by one or more cholinergic nerves (Gosling 1979). The cell bodies of these fibres lie either within the pelvic plexus, or within the bladder wall itself. These post-ganglionic fibres are supplied by pre-ganglionic fibres with cell bodies in the intermediolateral grey columns of the sacral segments S2 to S4.

Sympathetic Supply

Several authors have reported noradrenergic terminals to be present throughout the bladder in small numbers (Benson et al. 1979) and in greater concentration in the bladder neck (Ek et al. 1977). Gosling et al. (1977), however, found such terminals to be surprisingly sparse, and suggested that what fibres are present in the bladder wall are associated with blood vessels. It is suggested that sympathetically mediated inhibition of the bladder depends not on direct effects from noradrenergic fibres on the detrusor, but on indirect inhibition of the excitatory parasympathetic supply within the ganglia of the pelvic plexus. The pre-ganglionic fibres supplying these post-ganglionic noradrenergic fibres have cell bodies in the intermediolateral grey areas of the thoracic and lumbar segments T10 to L2. They travel in the sympathetic chain and then via the lumbar splanchnic nerves to the superior hypogastric plexus. From there the right and left hypogastric nerves ramify within the pelvic plexus.

There is clear evidence that acetylcholine acting as transmitter from parasympathetic efferents is responsible for detrusor contraction during micturition (Kuru 1965). Noradrenaline, however, may be excitatory or inhibitory depending on the predominant receptor type. In several mammalian species alpha receptor sites, producing contraction in response to noradrenaline binding, have been shown to predominate in the bladder base, whilst beta receptors, producing relaxation, are predominant in the vault (Fletcher and Bradley 1978).

Visceral Afferent Supply

Visceral afferent fibres may be identified travelling with both sacral and thoracolumbar visceral efferent nerves. Sacral afferents have been shown to be evenly distributed between muscle and submucosa throughout the bladder; they appear to convey touch, pain and bladder distension and are essential to complete micturition. Afferents in the thoracolumbar nerves become active only during marked bladder distension and their transection seems to have little effect on voiding (Fletcher and Bradley 1978).

All the above findings conform to the hypothesis that the sympathetic innervation of the bladder, along with the associated thoracolumbar visceral afferent supply, is concerned mainly with the filling and storage phases of micturition, whereas the parasympathetic supply and accompanying sacral afferent fibres are important for normal voiding.

Innervation of Urethral Smooth Muscle

Sympathetic and parasympathetic efferent and associated visceral afferent fibres from the vesical plexus also innervate the urethra. Parasympathetic efferents terminate in the urethral smooth muscle and cholinergic stimulation produces contraction. The functional significance of this muscle remains in some doubt. The orientation of its fibres suggests little sphincteric action, and its parasympathetic innervation suggests importance with respect to voiding function, contraction producing shortening and widening of the urethra along with detrusor contraction during micturition. Sympathetic efferents also innervate the intrinsic smooth muscle which possesses predominantly alpha adrenoreceptor sites. Whilst there are no sex differences in the adrenergic innervation of the bladder body, the sympathetic innervation of the bladder neck and urethra in the female is much less dense than in the male, where it has been suggested to have a genital rather than urinary function.

Innervation of Striated Muscle

Intrinsic Urethral Striated Muscle

It was long held that the rhabdosphincter urethrae was supplied by somatic efferent fibres via the pudendal nerves, but it has now been shown that this muscle is supplied via the pelvic splanchnic nerves travelling with the parasympathetic fibres to the intrinsic smooth muscle of the urethra.

Extrinsic Periurethral Striated Muscle

In contrast to the intrinsic striated muscle sphincter, the levator ani is innervated by motor fibres from the pudendal nerves. The above findings have clinical significance, in that firstly pudendal blockade might not reduce urethral resistance to a major degree, since the intrinsic striated sphincter will be unaffected, and secondly in that EMG activity recorded from the pelvic floor does not necessarily correlate with the activity of the external sphincter.

Associated somatic afferent fibres also travel in the pudendal nerves; they ascend via the dorsal columns to convey proprioception from the pelvic floor.

Central Nervous Connections of the Lower Urinary Tract

The connections of the lower urinary tract within the central nervous system are extraordinarily complex. Several micturition centres have been identified within the pontine reticular formation, the basal ganglia and the cerebral cortex, although their full function and interactions are incompletely understood (Fig. 1.3).

Within the pontine reticular formation are two closely related areas with inhibitory and excitatory effects on the sacral micturition centre in the conus medullaris. Lesions of the cord below this always lead to incoordinate voiding, with failure of synchronous urethral relaxation during detrusor contraction; lesions above this level may be associated with normal, though involuntary micturition.

The basal ganglia may also influence the final integration of bladder and urethral activity in pontine and sacral centres, and appear to be important with respect to the subconscious inhibition of detrusor activity.

Centres in the cerebral cortex on the medial aspect of the parietal lobe, and on the superior frontal gyrus, are important in the perception of bladder sensation and in the conscious inhibition and subsequent initiation of voiding. These areas both connect via the pontine reticular formation to the sacral centre, their interaction being modulated by influences from other cortical areas, the cerebellum, the limbic system and the hypothalamus. The central nervous control of micturition is reviewed in greater detail by Torrens (1984).

Physiology of the Lower Urinary Tract

From the definitions given in the introductory section of this chapter it is self-evident that continence is dependent on "the powers of urethral resistance exceeding the forces of urinary expulsion", a concept first expressed by Barnes (1940). The first proof of this concept came from Enhorning (1961), who showed that continence was maintained when the maximum urethral pressure exceeded the bladder pressure, or when the urethral closure pressure was positive. As a corollary, normal micturition may be said to result from the controlled reversal of that equilibrium, and incontinence from its uncontrolled reversal.

The Behaviour of the Bladder

The behaviour of the bladder at extreme filling rates has been investigated experimentally by van Mastrigt et al. (1978). During rapid stepwise filling the detrusor pressure rises rapidly, and afterwards decays exponentially with time; this time dependence is similar to that expected of a passive viscoelastic solid. However, under the near static conditions of physiological filling, the detrusor's behaviour is more accurately described as elastic (Griffiths 1980). That is to say, the detrusor pressure rises little as the bladder volume increases from zero to functional capacity.

The Urethra

In order to maintain continence it is vital not only that the intravesical pressure remains low during the storage phase of the micturition cycle, but also that the urethral lumen should seal completely. Zinner et al. (1976) described three components of urethral function necessary to achieve this hermetic property:

1. Urethral inner wall softness
2. Inner urethral compression
3. Outer wall tension

Whilst the closure of any elastic tube can be obtained if sufficient compression is applied to it, the efficiency of closure is dramatically increased if its lining possesses the property of plasticity, or the ability to mould into a watertight seal.

There has been much debate over the morphological components of the functional characteristics of softness, compression and tension in the urethra. Several authors have commented on the vascularity of the urethra and have pointed out that the submucosal vascular plexi far exceed the requirements of a blood supply for the organ. Some have suggested a significant vascular contribution to urethral closure (Huisman 1979; Rud et al. 1980) though others have found no specific features to suggest an important occlusive role for the urethral vascular supply. Nevertheless, whatever the contribution of the urethral blood supply to the measured intraluminal pressure, it is likely to be of significance as regards the plasticity of the urothelium and submucosa. Although attempts have been made to quantify this latter parameter (Plevnik and Vrtacnik 1981), the technique has not yet found a place in clinical practice.

The structures leading to inner wall compression by virtue of their contribution to outer wall tension can and have been quantified in the form of the urethral pressure profile (Fig. 1.4). These structures may include the intramural elastic fibres, the intrinsic smooth and striated muscle, and the extrinsic or periurethral striated muscle. Tanagho et al. (1969a,b), extrapolating from urethral pressure studies in dogs, suggested that approximately 50% of the resting pressure was due to striated muscle components. In contrast Lapides et al. (1957) demonstrated that it is possible to remain continent following striated muscle blockade. Rud et al. (1980), following a series of per-operative studies during radical pelvic surgery, showed that approximately one-third of the resting urethral pressure is due to striated muscle effects, one-third to smooth muscle effects, and one-third to its vascular supply.

Whatever the relative importance of the above factors to active wall tension, it should be remembered that these same structures also contribute a passive or elastic tension, along with the supporting elements of collagen and elastin. The usual level of continence in the female is not as one might expect in mid-urethra, at the region of maximum resting pressure, but at the bladder neck. This region in the female has no sphincteric circular smooth muscle, and is virtually devoid of striated muscle (see p. 5 and Fig. 1.2); it would seem that passive elastic tension is the most important factor leading to closure of the bladder neck and proximal urethra. In mid-urethra the most prominent structural feature is the

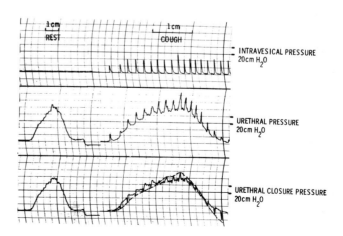

Fig. 1.4. Example of resting and stress urethral pressure profiles in a symptom-free woman. (Hilton and Stanton 1983a)

rhabdosphincter, and electronmicroscopic and histochemical evidence of Gosling and Dixon (1979) suggests that this may be responsible for the bulk of active urethral tone at rest. Electromyographic studies (Anderson et al. 1976), histochemical evidence (Gosling et al. 1981) and urethral pressure measurements (Hilton and Stanton 1983a) all suggest that the periurethral striated muscles have their maximum effect at a level slightly distal to that of the resting profile peak (Fig. 1.4), and do not contribute greatly to the maintenance of continence at rest. It is likely, however, that these muscles have a significant role in the maintenance of urethral closure in the face of stress, a factor considered in greater detail on p. 12.

The Normal Micturition Cycle

From the background information contained in the previous sections of this chapter it is now possible to discuss the mechanisms whereby urine is retained within the bladder during filling and storage phases, and is evacuated during the voiding phase of the normal micturition cycle.

Filling and Storage Phase

The bladder normally fills with urine by a series of peristaltic ureteric contractions, at a rate between 0.5 and 5 ml/min; under these conditions the bladder pressure increases only minimally (see p. 8), and in normal symptom-free individuals by no more than 15 cm water even at functional capacity.

Urethral closure, meanwhile, is maintained by the combined passive and active effects of its smooth and striated muscle components, its elastic content, and its blood supply. The hermetic efficiency is accentuated by the softness of its mucosa.

During the early stages of bladder filling, proprioceptive afferent impulses from stretch receptors within the bladder wall pass via the pelvic nerves to sacral roots S2–S4. These impulses ascend in the cord via the lateral spinothalamic tracts and a detrusor motor response is subconsciously inhibited by descending impulses from the basal ganglia (Fig. 1.5a).

As the bladder volume increases, further afferent impulses ascend to the cerebral cortex, and the sensation of bladder filling associated with the desire to micturate is first consciously appreciated, usually

at between 200 and 300 ml, or around half the functional bladder capacity. Inhibition of detrusor contraction is now cortically mediated, although the desire to void may be further suppressed to subconscious levels again, given sufficient distracting afferent stimuli. Whilst descending impulses inhibit the pre-ganglionic parasympathetic cell bodies in the sacral cord, there may also be excitatory effects on the sympathetic neurones in the thoracolumbar region, causing increased efferent discharge to the beta adrenoreceptors within the bladder (and/or further inhibition within the pelvic plexus of parasympathetic fibres to the bladder), leading to its relaxation, and to alpha adrenoreceptors in the proximal urethra (and/or further excitation within the pelvic plexus of post-ganglionic parasympathetic fibres to the urethra), leading to a slight increase in urethral pressure (Figs. 1.3, 1.5b).

With further filling, afferent impulses within the visceral afferent fibres accompanying the sympathetic efferents to thoracolumbar roots T10 to L2 ascend to the cerebral cortex, and a reinforced desire to void will be appreciated; reinforced conscious inhibition of micturition occurs whilst a suitable site and posture for micturition are sought (Yeates 1972). During this time, in addition to the cortical inhibition of detrusor activity, there may also be a voluntary pelvic floor contraction in an attempt to maintain urethral closure. This may be evidenced by further marked variations in urethral pressure (Asmussen and Ulmsten 1976) as the sensation of urgency becomes increasingly severe (Fig. 1.5c).

Initiation Phase

When a suitable time, site and posture for micturition are selected the process of voiding commences. This may be considered in two phases: the initiation or transition from the non-voiding state, and micturition itself. Several theories have been suggested to explain the transition phase. Denny-Brown and Robertson (1933) proposed a reciprocal functional relationship between bladder neck and detrusor, the former undergoing active relaxation as the latter contracts. Bradley et al. (1974) suggested that smooth muscle relaxation alone was not sufficient to account for the initiation of voiding, and that the muscles of the pelvic floor relax in concert with the urethral smooth muscle in response to detrusor contraction. Lapides (1958) proposed that transition to the voiding state occurred not by relaxation of urethral smooth muscle fibres, but rather by an increase in their tension, consequent upon detrusor contraction, and resulting in shortening and widening of the urethra. This is, of course, not incompatible with the "relaxation theories", since relaxation of the urethral and periurethral striated muscle may occur coincident with detrusor and urethral smooth muscle contraction.

Hutch (1965) developed a new concept of the structure of the muscle bundles of the bladder base, and a new theory regarding the initiation of micturition, which he called the "base-plate theory". Other workers have been unable to confirm the proposed configuration of muscle bundles suggested by Hutch, and there seems little to support this concept. Tanagho and Miller (1970) put forward the "funnelling theory" suggesting that by virtue of the continuity of the longitudinal smooth muscle fibres of the detrusor and urethra, funnelling of the bladder neck was encouraged as the detrusor contracts; in addition the insertion of circular detrusor fibres into the deep trigone enhances this effect (Tanagho 1984).

The process of initiation is perhaps best looked on as combining features of each of the above theories.

Relaxation of the pelvic floor may be shown to occur early in the process, both radiologically and electromyographically; it is likely that simultaneous relaxation of the intrinsic striated muscle also occurs, since a marked fall in urethral pressure is seen before the intravesical pressure rises, during both voluntary and provoked voiding (Karlson 1953), and the same has been shown in response to sacral nerve stimulation (Torrens 1976) (Fig. 1.5d).

A few seconds later the descending inhibitory impulses from the cortex acting on the sacral micturition centre are suppressed, allowing a rapid discharge of efferent parasympathetic impulses via the pelvic nerves to cause contraction of the detrusor, and probably also to pull open the bladder neck and shorten the urethra; simultaneous inhibition of the efferent sympathetic discharges via the thoracolumbar outflow to the pelvic plexus probably also occurs, encouraging detrusor contraction and urethral relaxation. Depending on the relationship between the force of detrusor contraction and the residual urethral resistance, the intravesical pressure may rise to a variable extent (usually less than 60 cm water). When the falling urethral pressure and increasing intravesical pressure equate, urine flow will commence (Fig. 1.5e).

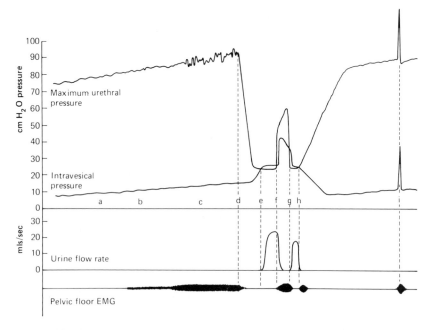

Fig. 1.5. The normal micturition cycle showing changes in urethral and intravesical pressure, urine flow rate and pelvic floor electromyogram. *a*, phase of subconscious inhibition; *b*, phase of conscious (suppressible) inhibition; *c*, phase of reinforced (unsuppressible) inhibition; *d*, initiation or transition; *e*, voiding; *f*, interruption of voiding; *g*, resumption of micturition; *h*, end of void; *i*, cough.

Voiding Phase

The application of physical laws to explain the mechanism of continence is often considered inappropriate and misleading. In considering the bladder during micturition, however, the law of Laplace may be useful. It states that the pressure (P) in a vessel varies directly with the mural tension (T), and inversely with the radius (R). Since the bladder at the initiation of micturition takes on a nearly spherical shape, and has walls which are thin in comparison to its radius, its behaviour may be usefully expressed in the basic formula of the law as applied to a sphere: $P = 2T/R$. As the mural tension rises in the absence of voiding, the intravesical pressure also rises. When a critical opening pressure is achieved, urine will start to flow and the bladder radius fall. The pressure, however, usually remains constant during voiding (Bottaccini et al. 1973), and the mural tension therefore must fall. Once initiated, therefore, the process of micturition requires little to sustain it. Whilst active tension is required throughout, the effectiveness of detrusor contraction increases as the muscle fibres shorten and therefore decreasing forces are required as micturition proceeds (Zinner et al. 1976).

If micturition is voluntarily interrupted midstream, this is usually achieved by a contraction of the extrinsic striated muscle of the pelvic floor. In association with this contraction the urethral pressure rises rapidly to exceed the intravesical pressure and therefore urine flow stops. The detrusor, being a smooth muscle, is much slower to relax, and therefore goes on contracting against a closed sphincter. That is to say an isometric contraction occurs, and again applying the law of Laplace, the intravesical pressure rises (Fig. 1.5f). If micturition is resumed by relaxation of the pelvic floor, both urethral and intravesical pressures will return to their previous voiding state (Fig. 1.5g).

At the end of micturition the intravesical pressure gradually falls as urinary flow diminishes (Fig. 1.5h). The pelvic floor and intrinsic striated muscle are contracted and flow is interrupted in mid-urethra; the few drops of urine left in the proximal urethra are milked back into the bladder by the intrinsic mechanisms discussed above which contribute to the hermetic closure of the urethra and bladder neck competence. Simultaneously the subconscious inhibition of the sacral micturition centre is reapplied as the filling phase of the cycle recurs.

The Mechanism of Stress Continence

The above discussion of the normal micturition cycle relates to the events occurring in a patient essentially at rest, and assumes the intravesical pressure is unaffected by extravesical influences. Acute intra-abdominal pressure rises due to coughing, or more sustained pressure variations due to straining or movement, bring other influences to bear on the mechanism of continence.

The factors which maintain the positive urethral closure at rest (i.e. which ensure that urethral pressure exceeds bladder pressure) have been considered above. This positive closure pressure is also maintained in symptom-free women in the face of intra-abdominal pressure rises (Fig. 1.5i) by at least two mechanisms.

Firstly there is a passive or direct mechanical transmission of the intra-abdominal pressure change to the proximal urethra (Fig. 1.6b). This effect is dependent upon the maintenance of the normal relationships between bladder and urethra, and on their fixation in a retropubic position by the posterior pubo-urethral ligaments. The extent of this transmission of intra-abdominal pressure rises to the urethra may be determined by urethral pressure profiles recorded during stress (Henriksson et al. 1977; Hilton 1983). The pressure transmission ratio is defined as the increment of urethral pressure on coughing as a percentage of the simultaneously recorded increment of intravesical pressure; this parameter may be recorded for several points along the urethra, and a pressure transmission profile constructed which details the transmission of intra-abdominal pressure rises from bladder neck to external urethral meatus (Hilton and Stanton 1983a). Using this technique it has been shown that in normal women transmission of intra-abdominal pressure rises is effective throughout the proximal three-quarters of the urethral length, i.e. throughout that portion of the urethral lying above the urogenital diaphragm (Fig. 1.9b).

It may also be shown by simultaneous bladder and urethral pressure measurements that in a region around the third quarter of the urethral length, pressure transmission ratios often exceed 100% (Figs. 1.4, 1.9b). It has been suggested that this may reflect a reflex pelvic floor contraction in response to stress, augmenting urethral closure (Fig. 1.6c). Certainly the observed pressure changes do fit closely with the current concepts of the anatomy of the region (p. 5 and Fig. 1.2b) and an

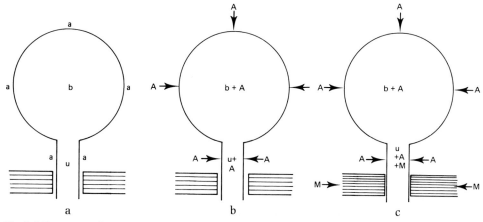

Fig. 1.6. Diagram to show the relationship between bladder, urethra and pelvic floor in the resting state **a** and on stress to illustrate the passive **b** and active **c** components of pressure transmission to the proximal urethra aiding stress continence. *a*, resting intra-abdominal pressure; *b*, resting bladder pressure; *u*, resting urethral pressure; *A*, abdominal pressure rise on coughing; *M*, pelvic floor muscle response on coughing.

active element to stress continence is accepted by many authors. However Rud (1981) has demonstrated that this accentuated pressure transmission is maintained after curarisation, thus throwing doubt on its origin in a striated muscle effect. It is possible that some other as yet undefined, passive mechanical defect may account for this augmentation in urethral closure in the distal urethra.

Pathophysiology of Urinary Incontinence

General Considerations

Assuming an intact lower urinary tract, urine flow only occurs when the intravesical pressure exceeds the maximal urethral pressure or when the maximum urethral closure pressure becomes zero or negative (Enhorning 1961). In general terms this may occur as a result of:

1. A fall in urethral pressure associated with an increase in intravesical pressure—as in normal voiding or in many cases of detrusor instability, primarily those of psychosomatic origin, or those resulting from neurological lesions above the level of the pontine micturition centre.

2. An increase in intravesical pressure associated with an increase in urethral pressure, the latter being insufficient to maintain a positive closure pressure—as in detrusor instability with associated detrusor sphincter dyssynergia, resulting from neurological lesions below the pontine micturition centre.

3. An abnormally high increase in detrusor pressure during bladder filling—a condition considered by some workers to be equivalent to detrusor instability, but perhaps better termed impaired bladder compliance; a similar situation probably also accounts for the incontinence in chronic urine retention where the bladder pressure may rise acutely at the end of bladder filling.

4. Loss in urethral closure pressure alone—as in urethral instability.

5. Where on stress the intravesical pressure rises to a greater extent than the intraurethral pressure—as in genuine stress incontinence.

These various mechanisms are shown diagrammatically in Fig. 1.7. Since this book is concerned mainly with the surgical treatment of genuine stress incontinence in the female, the pathophysiology of this condition is considered in greater detail.

Genuine Stress Incontinence

In the past many theories have been proposed to explain the pathophysiology of genuine stress incontinence and these have been fully reviewed

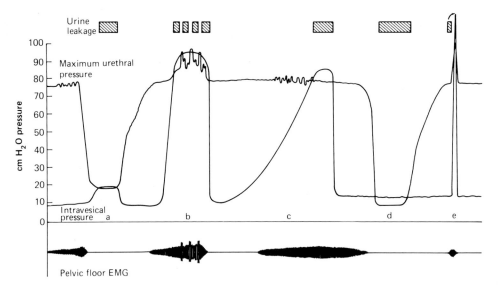

Fig. 1.7. Mechanisms of urinary incontinence showing changes in urethral and intravesical pressure and pelvic floor electromyogram at various stages of bladder filling in different types of incontinence. *a*, normal voiding pattern or detrusor instability; *b*, detrusor sphincter dyssynergia; *c*, impaired bladder compliance; *d*, urethral instability; *e*, genuine stress incontinence.

elsewhere (Hilton 1981); the author's personal view regarding the cause of this condition is presented below.

By simultaneous recording of intravesical and urethral pressure by a microtransducer technique (see Chap. 2) urethral pressure profiles may be recorded at rest and on stress, from which multiple parameters of urethral function may be determined (Fig. 1.8). By an analysis of these parameters in symptom-free women, and in those with genuine stress incontinence of varying severity, several aspects of urethral function of possible relevance to the development of stress incontinence have been defined (Hilton and Stanton 1983a).

The Maximum Urethral Closure Pressure at Rest (Fig. 1.8d). This was significantly lower in stress incontinent women than in continent women, and showed a consistent trend from mild to severe grades of incontinence (Fig. 1.9a). Furthermore, it has previously been shown that urethral pressure falls, and intravesical pressure rises, with increasing age in both continent (Rud 1980) and stress incontinent women (Hilton 1981). This trend appears to be continuous, throughout the age ranges studied (Fig. 1.10) with no obvious effect of the menopause. Whilst 95% of the continent women in our study had a maximum urethral closure pressure greater than 24 cm of water, this range also included all

the mildly stress incontinent women, and 80% of all stress incontinent women. This parameter could not therefore be considered a major determinant of stress incontinence as suggested by Bunne and Obrink (1978a), though it may be important with respect to the severity of symptoms in patients otherwise predisposed to urinary leakage.

Intrinsic Variation in Maximal Urethral Closure Pressure (Fig. 1.8k). If the maximal urethral closure pressure is observed continuously it can be seen to vary considerably over time. In part this variability is due to cyclical vascular and respiratory effects but other less regular variations in urethral pressure are seen, the origin of which could presumably lie in the central neurological control of urethral closure or in the smooth or striated muscle components. The extent of variation in urethral closure pressure differs between individuals, and occurs to a greater degree in those patients with more severe stress incontinence. It was also shown that this intrinsic variability in urethral pressure reduces dramatically with advancing age, suggesting that this parameter may be a feature of the oestrogen sensitivity of the urethra.

Intra-abdominal Pressure Variations (Fig. 1.8i). The increments in intra-abdominal pressure generated during stress profiles are significantly higher in

MRS J.H.   1.2.81

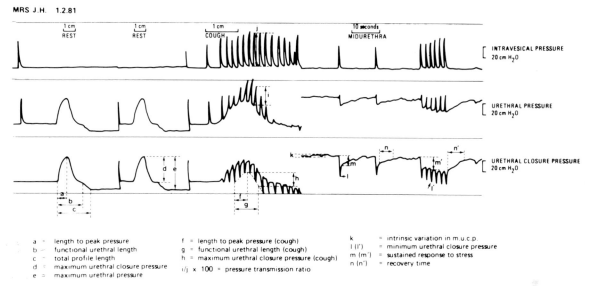

a =	length to peak pressure	f = length to peak pressure (cough)
b =	functional urethral length	g = functional urethral length (cough)
c =	total profile length	h = maximum urethral closure pressure (cough)
d =	maximum urethral closure pressure	i/j × 100 = pressure transmission ratio
e =	maximum urethral pressure	

k	= intrinsic variation in m.u.c.p.
l (l')	= minimum urethral closure pressure
m (m')	= sustained response to stress
n (n')	= recovery time

Fig. 1.8. Example of resting and stress urethral pressure profiles in a stress incontinent patient recorded using a microtransducer technique, showing the parameters recorded. (Hilton and Stanton 1983a)

stress incontinent women than in controls. Although this is a rather crude assessment, it suggests that the extent of intra-abdominal pressure variation during a patient's accustomed activities may be of some relevance in determining the severity of her symptoms.

Sustained Response to Stress (Fig. 1.8m). Following the acute intra-abdominal pressure rise on coughing there is a reduction in urethral pressure which is sustained for a variable period of time. If further stresses are applied within that recovery time a further loss in closure pressure may occur which plateaus out after four or five stresses. This loss in closure pressure occurs to a similar extent in all incontinent women (averaging 49%, and recovering over 10.7 s) but was significantly less marked in controls (averaging 14.3% and recovering over 5.2 s). The underlying cause for this phenomenon is uncertain but several possibilities exist: it is possible that the intra-abdominal pressure rise generated by the cough may cause expulsion of blood from submucosal vascular plexuses thereby reducing their contribution to urethral pressure; relaxation of intrinsic urethral smooth or striated muscle in response to stress could have a similar effect. Rud et al. (1980) suggested that one-third of resting urethral pressure was due to vascular tone, one-third to smooth muscle, and one-third to striated muscle effects. This sustained response to stress

leads to an average loss of closure pressure of 45%, and in individual cases pressure losses approaching 100% have been observed. It would seem, therefore, that either the coincidence of all the above factors or the active distraction of the urethral wall by contraction of its longitudinally arranged fibres must be considered. Whatever the underlying cause of this phenomenon, its extent in individual patients may be of relevance to the severity of symptoms in patients already predisposed to urinary leakage, and in occasional patients may be of sufficient degree to cause incontinence where all other aspects of urethral function are normal.

Pressure Transmission Ratio (Fig. 1.8i,j). Pressure transmission ratios were shown to be of a similar order in all groups of stress incontinent women showing a near linear decrease from bladder neck to external urethral meatus (Fig. 1.9b). Continent women on the other hand show greater maintenance of transmission in the proximal urethra to values approaching and often exceeding 100%. Of the 120 stress incontinent women studied, only three showed pressure transmission ratios exceeding 95% whereas all the 20 controls had ratios above this value at some point in the urethra (Hilton and Stanton 1983a). It appears, therefore, that the pressure transmission ratio has an all-or-none effect in the determination of continence. The exact cause of the impairment of transmission in stress incon-

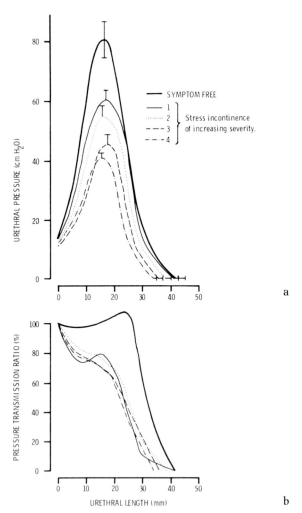

that the greater the degree of urethral softness the greater the efficiency of urethral closure, and that the loss of urethral vascular tone seen post-menopausally may account for the increase in genuine stress incontinence seen in older age groups.

From these observations it would seem that under normal circumstances continence is maintained at the bladder neck level as a result of efficient transmission of intra-abdominal pressure rises to the proximal three-quarters of the functional urethral length. The efficiency of this mechanism is improved by the softness of the urethral mucosa and submucosa in this region. On rare occasions a profound loss in closure pressure occurring after stress or stresses may overcome an efficient pressure transmission mechanism. The remaining features of urethral function, rather than distinguishing the continent from the incontinent state, are of greater relevance to the determination of the severity of incontinence in a patient already predisposed to urinary leakage by virtue of impaired transmission. This predisposition may be converted to symptoms, or looked at another way, the maximum urethral closure pressure on coughing may be brought to zero by a low resting urethral closure pressure, marked intrinsic variation in urethral closure pressure, extreme intra-abdominal pressure variations, an excessive sustained response to stress, impaired urethral softness, or, of course, by any combination

Fig. 1.9. a Average resting urethral pressure profiles and **b** pressure transmission profiles in a group of symptom-free women and four groups with stress incontinence of varying severity. (Hilton and Stanton 1983a)

tinent women is difficult to define. Certainly it is often associated with hypermobility of the proximal urethra, and may result from deficiency of the pubourethral ligaments or pelvic floor muscle as a consequence of aging or obstetric trauma. Anderson (1984) has shown evidence of anal sphincter denervation in stress incontinent women, and it may be that the effects of aging and parity are not directly on the muscle but on its peripheral nerve supply.

Urethral Softness. The measurement of urethral softness is as yet not a practical proposition, and its contribution to urethral closure mechanisms is therefore difficult to assess. It would seem, however,

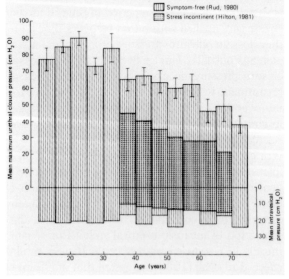

Fig. 1.10. Average maximum urethral closure pressure and intravesical pressure with age in continent and stress incontinent women.

of these factors. It would seem logical, therefore, to look at genuine stress incontinence not as a single defect in urethral physiology but as the summation of these several functional characteristics whose interaction determines an individual's residual closure pressure on stress, or their margin to continence. A diagrammatic representation of this concept is shown in Fig. 1.11. The exact relationship between these functional characteristics and the morphological components of the urethra can at present be only speculative, but it is considered to some extent in the section "Physiology of the Lower Urinary Tract".

The Effects of Incontinence Surgery on Urethral Function

Over 100 different operations have been devised for the treatment of genuine stress incontinence (Stanton 1978), reflecting not merely the inadequacy of any single procedure to deal satisfactorily with all cases, but also uncertainties about the nature of the problem and the mechanism of its cure. The aims of incontinence surgery have been variously defined as: tightening of the pubocervical fascia; elevation

of the bladder neck; restoration of the posterior urethrovesical angle; increasing urethral pressure; increasing functional urethral length; and increasing urethral resistance. There is, however, little information as to the extent to which these aims are achieved by the various operative techniques. Cure rates of between 40 and 97% have been reported (Green 1980) but what aspects of the procedures, or of urethral function determine success or failure is still poorly understood.

Obrink et al. (1978) recorded urethral pressure profiles at rest before, during and after a pubococcygeal repair operation. Whilst marked changes were noted during the course of the operation, there were no significant changes at 3 months post-operatively even though 15 of their 16 patients were symptomatically cured. In a subsequent study extended to include urethral profiles under stress the same authors found improvement in mid-urethral pressure transmission from 65% pre-operatively to 80% post-operatively (Bunne and Obrink 1978b). Similar findings have been made in relation to suprapublic incontinence surgery. Studies of the Marshall–Marchetti–Krantz urethrocystopexy, Burch colposuspension, suburethral sling and bladder neck suspensory procedures, have failed to demonstrate any significant change in the resting urethral pressure profile but have shown improvements in urethral closure on stress resulting from

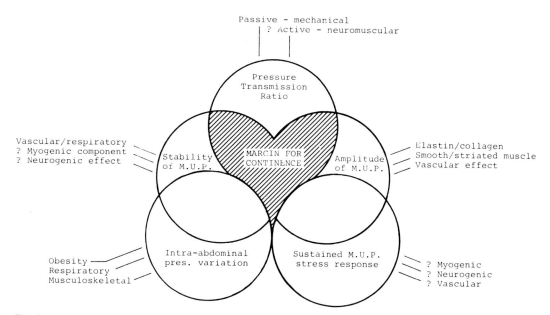

Fig. 1.11. Diagrammatic representation of the interaction of morphological and functional components of the urethra and their role in determining stress continence. (Hilton and Stanton 1983a)

increased pressure transmission (Henriksson and
Ulmsten 1978; Obrink and Bunne 1978; Constantinou et al. 1980; Hilton and Stanton 1983b,c; Weil
et al. 1984) (Figs. 1.12, 1.13). Whilst qualitatively
the results of these various studies are similar, there
are considerable quantitative differences, improvements in pressure transmission varying from only
a few per cent (Weil et al. 1984) to well over 100%
(Constantinou et al. 1980; Hilton and Stanton
1983b,c).

The nature of the improvement in urethral pressure transmission following surgery is uncertain. It
has previously been suggested that it is due to elevation of the bladder neck and proximal urethra which
allows improved passive transmission to the region
(Enhorning 1976). Whilst this would explain transmission ratios approaching 100%, it clearly could
not explain ratios over 100% as cited above. It is
possible that the bladder neck elevation not only
allows improved pressure transmission but also promotes greater efficiency of the pelvic floor reflex with
accentuation of urethral closure by active means
(Heidler et al. 1979). The distribution of pressure
transmission along the urethra following successful
colposuspension is quite different from that seen in
healthy women (Hilton and Stanton 1983b) (compare Figs. 1.9b and 1.13b) and the delay between
intravesical and urethral pressure rises on coughing, around 10 ms, is too short to involve a
neuromuscular reflex (Hertogs and Stanton 1983).
It would seem likely that the improvement in pressure transmission post-operatively therefore has a
mechanical rather than neuromuscular basis. The
most obvious anatomic change seen following successful suprapubic incontinence surgery is the relo-
cation of the urethra in a retropubic position, and
it is possible that downward pressure from abdominal viscera on coughing compresses the urethra
against the posterior surface of the symphysis accen-
tuating urethral closure.

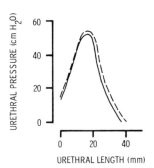

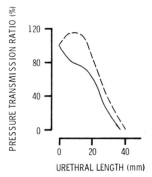

Fig. 1.13. Average pre-operative (——) and post-operative (----)
resting urethral pressure profiles (*above*) and pressure transmission profiles (*below*) in patients undergoing successful Burch
colposuspension.

On the basis of standard urodynamic measurements the commonest effect of incontinence surgery
appears to be an increase in urethral resistance as
evidenced by a reduction in peak urine flow rate,
often accompanied by an increase in voiding
detrusor pressure. This effect is more obvious following suprapubic surgery than vaginal surgery (Stanton and Cardozo 1979). Whether the element of
obstruction induced by suprapubic procedures is a
necessary accompaniment of successful surgery
remains in doubt, although it seems much more
likely that the repositioning is the critical factor, and
obstruction an undesirable side-effect (Hilton and

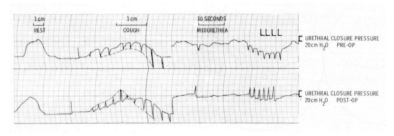

Fig. 1.12. Example of pre- and post-operative urethral closure pressure recordings in a patient undergoing successful Burch colposuspension. L, demonstrated urinary leakage during pre-operative trace. (Hilton and Stanton 1983b)

Stanton 1981). It has been suggested that incontinence operations may be divided into those which are urodynamically pure repositioning procedures (anterior colporrhaphy and vagino-obturator shelf procedure) and those with an element of urethral fixation or compression (Marshall–Marchetti–Krantz procedure, Burch colposuspension, suburethral slings and bladder neck suspensions) (Turner-Warwick 1984). It seems, however, that those operations which give the best results in terms of cure of stress incontinence are those which produce maximum urethral and bladder neck elevation and fixation, and also those with the greatest risk of increasing urethral resistance; operations which produce lesser degrees of elevation may cause less post-operative voiding difficulties, but also are less likely to cure the stress incontinence. This principle has been proven for the Burch colposuspension in particular (Dundas et al. 1981), and probably applies also to incontinence surgery as a whole.

Little research has been done into the effects of unsuccessful incontinence surgery on bladder and urethral function. It has, however, been shown that the improvements in pressure transmission noted above following successful surgery are not found following unsuccessful surgery. It has also been shown that following some failed procedures a reduction in urethral closure pressure may ensue (Hilton and Stanton 1983c; Weil et al. 1984), and that the more unsuccessful procedures a patient has undergone, the less efficient her urethral closure is likely to be (Fig. 1.14) and the poorer the prognosis for future surgical cure.

Conclusions

If urinary incontinence is to be effectively treated then the choice of treatment employed must be optimal. This choice must be based on a firm knowledge of the normal mechanisms of continence, and of the mechanisms whereby this normal control may break down. Only in the light of this knowledge can the meaningful investigation of the individual incontinent patient be carried out. The results of this investigation, taken in conjunction with a knowledge of the effects of various treatment modalities, should allow the surgeon to offer a rational and specific therapy for each patient.

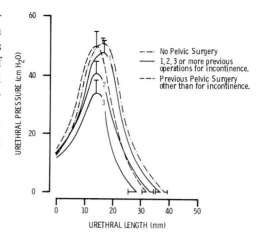

Fig. 1.14. Average resting urethral pressure profiles for stress incontinent patients according to previous surgical history. $-\cdot-\cdot$ no pelvic surgery ($n = 58$); ——1 ($n = 25$), 2 ($n = 14$) or $\geqslant 3$ ($n = 7$) previous unsuccessful incontinence operations; ----previous pelvic surgery other than for incontinence ($n = 16$).

References

Anderson JT, Bradley WE, Timm GW (1976) The urethral electromyographic and gas pressure profile. Scand J Urol Nephrol 10:185–188

Anderson RS (1984) A neurogenic element to urinary genuine stress incontinence. Br J Obstet Gynaecol 91:41–46

Asmussen M, Ulmsten U (1976) Simultaneous urethrocystometry by a new technique. Scand J Urol Nephrol 10:7–11

Barnes AC (1940) A method for evaluating the stress of urinary incontinence. Am J Obstet Gynecol 40:381–390

Bates CP, Bradley WE, Glen E et al. (1983) Standardisation of terminology of lower urinary tract function. Collation of the first 4 reports by the Standardisation Committee of the International Continence Society

Benson GS, McConnell JA, Wood JG (1979) Adrenergic innervation of the human bladder body. J Urol 122:189–191

Bottaccini MR, Gleason DM, Byrne JC (1973) Resistance measurement in the human urethra. In: Lutzeyer, Melchior (eds) Urodynamics. Springer, Berlin Heidelberg New York, pp 302–316

Bradley WE, Timm TW, Scott FB (1974) Innervation of the detrusor muscle and urethra. Urol Clin North Am 1:3–27

Bunne G, Obrink A (1978a) Urethral closure pressure with stress. A comparison between stress incontinent and continent women. Urol Res 6:127–134

Bunne G, Obrink A (1978b) The influence of pubococcygeal repair on urethral closure pressure at stress. Acta Obstet Gynecol Scand 57:355–359

Constantinou CE, Faysal MH, Govan DE (1980) The impact of bladder neck suspension on the mode of distribution of abdominal pressure along the female urethra. In: Proceedings of 10th International Continence Society Meeting, Los Angeles

Denny-Brown D, Robertson EG (1933) On the physiology of micturition. Brain 56:149–190

Donker PJ, Droes JThPM, van Ulden BM (1976) Anatomy of the musculature and innervation of the bladder and urethra. In: Williams DI, Chisholm GD (eds) Scientific foundations of urology. Heinemann, London, p 32

Dundas D, Hilton P, Williams JE, Stanton SL (1982) Aetiology of voiding difficulties following colposuspension. 12th International Continence Society Meeting, Leiden, p 132

Ek A, Alm P, Anderson KE, Persson CGA (1977) Adrenergic and cholinergic nerves in the human urethra and urinary bladder. A histochemical study. Acta Physiol Scand 90:345–352

Enhorning G (1961) Simultaneous recording of the intravesical and intraurethral pressure. Acta Chir Scand [Suppl] 276:1–68

Enhorning G (1976) A concept of urinary continence. Urol Int 31:3–5

Fletcher TF, Bradley WE (1978) Neuroanatomy of the bladder-urethra. J Urol 119:153–160

Gosling JA (1979) The structure of the bladder and urethra in relation to function. Urol Clin North Am 6:31–38

Gosling JA, Dixon J (1979) Light and electronmicroscopic observations on the human external urethral sphincter. J Anat 129:216

Gosling JA, Dixon JS, Critchley HOD, Thompson SA (1981) A comparative study of human external sphincter and periurethral levator ani muscle. Br J Urol 53:35–41

Gosling JA, Dixon JS, Humpherson JR (1983) Functional anatomy of the urinary tract. Churchill Livingstone, London

Gosling JA, Dixon JS, Lendon RG (1977) The autonomic innervation of the human male and female bladder neck and proximal urethra. J Urol 118:302–305

Green TH (1980) Vaginal repair. In: Stanton SL, Tanagho EA (eds) Surgery of female incontinence. Springer, Berlin Heidelberg New York, pp 31–46

Griffiths DJ (1980) Urodynamics. Adam Hilger, Bristol

Heidler H, Wolk H, Jonas U (1979) Urethral closure mechanism under stress conditions. Eur Urol 5:110–112

Henriksson L, Ulmsten U (1978) A urodynamic evaluation of the effects of abdominal urethrocystopexy and vaginal sling urethroplasty in women with stress incontinence. Am J Obstet Gynecol 113:78–82

Henriksson L, Ulmsten U, Anderson KE (1977) The effects of posture on the urethral closure pressure in healthy women. Scand J Urol Nephrol 11:201–206

Hertogs K, Stanton SL (1983) The mechanism of successful colposuspension: a new model. In: Proceedings of the 13th International Continence Society Meeting, Aachen

Hilton P (1981) Urethral pressure measurement by microtransducer: observations on methodology, the pathophysiology of genuine stress incontinence, and the effects of its treatment in the female. MD Thesis, Newcastle upon Tyne

Hilton P (1983) Urethral pressure measurement on stress: a comparison on profiles on coughing and straining. Neurourol Urodynamics 2:55–62

Hilton P, Stanton SL (1981) The urodynamic effects of successful and failed incontinence surgery. In: Proceedings of the International Urogynaecologists' Association Meeting, Stockholm

Hilton P, Stanton SL (1983a) Urethral pressure measurement by microtransducer: the results in symptom-free women and in those with genuine stress incontinence. Br J Obstet Gynaecol 90:919–934

Hilton P, Stanton SL (1983b) A clinical and urodynamic assessment of the Burch colposuspension for genuine stress incontinence. Br J Obstet Gynaecol 90:934–939

Hilton P, Stanton SL (1983c) A clinical and urodynamic evaluation of the polypropylene (Marlex) sling for genuine stress incontinence. Neurourol Urodynamics 2:145–153

Hilton P, Varma TR (1984) The menopause. In: Stanton SL (ed) Clinical gynecologic urology. C. V. Mosby, St. Louis, Missouri

Huisman AB (1979) Morphologie van de Vrouwelijke Urethra. MD Thesis, Groningen, Netherlands

Hutch JA (1965) A new theory of the anatomy of the internal urethral sphincter and physiology of micturition. Invest Urol 3:36–58

Hutch JA (1971) The internal urethral urinary sphincter. A double loop system. J Urol 105:375–383

Karlson S (1953) Experimental studies on the functioning of the female urinary bladder and urethra. Acta Obstet Gynecol Scand 32:285–307

Kluck P (1980) The autonomic innervation of the human urinary bladder, bladder neck and urethra. A histochemical study. Anat Rec 198:439–447

Kuru M (1965) Nervous control of micturition. Physiol Review 44:425

Langreder W (1956) Die weibliche Urethra; funktionelle Anatomie Pathologie und Therapie des Verschlussmechanismus. Zentralbl fur Gynakol 78:651–759

Lapides J (1958) Structure and function of the internal vesical sphincter. J Urol 80:341–353

Lapides J, Sweet R, Lewis LW (1957) Role of striated muscle in urination. J Urol 77:247–250

Obrink A, Bunne G (1978) The margin to incontinence after three types of operation for stress incontinence. Scand J Urol Nephrol 12:209–214

Obrink A, Bunne G, Ulmsten U, Ingleman-Sundberg A (1978) The urethral pressure profile before, during and after the pubococcygeal repair for stress incontinence. Acta Obstet Gynecol Scand 57:49–61

Plevnik S, Vrtacnik P (1981) How to measure urethral softness? In: Zinner N, Sterling A (eds) Female incontinence. Alan R. Liss, New York, pp 253–258

Rud T (1980) The urethral pressure profile in continent women from childhood to old age. Acta Obstet Gynecol Scand 59:331–335

Rud T (1981) The striated pelvic floor muscles and their importance in maintaining urinary continence. In: Zinner N, Sterling A (eds) Female incontinence. Alan R. Liss, New York, pp 105–112

Rud T, Anderson KE, Asmussen M, Hunting A, Ulmsten U (1980) Factors maintaining intraurethral pressure in women. Invest Urol 17:343–347

Smith P (1972) Age changes in the female urethra. Br J Urol 44:667–676

Stanton SL (1978) Surgery for urinary incontinence. Clin Obstet Gynaecol 5.1:83–108

Stanton SL, Cardozo LD (1979) A comparison of vaginal and suprapubic surgery for the correction of incontinence due to urethral sphincter incompetence. Br J Urol 50:497–499

Tanagho EA (1984) Thoughts on the neurophysiology of micturition. Today's Therapeutic Trends 2:65–70

Tanagho EA, Pugh RCB (1963) Anatomy and function of the ureterovesical junction. Br J Urol 35:151–165

Tanagho EA, Smith DR (1966) Anatomy and function of the bladder neck. Br J Urol 38:54–71

Tanagho EA, Myers FH, Smith DR (1969a) Urethral resistance. Its components and implications. I. Smooth muscle components. Invest Urol 7:136–149

Tanagho EA, Myers FH, Smith DR (1969b) Urethral resistance. Its components and implications. II. Striated muscle components. Invest Urol 7:195–205

Tanagho EA, Miller ER (1970) Initiation of voiding. Br J Urol 42:175–183

Torrens M (1976) Urethral sphincter responses to stimulation of sacral nerves in the human female. Proceedings of the 6th International Continence Society Meeting, Antwerp

Torrens M (1984) Neurophysiology. In: Stanton SL (ed) Clinical gynecologic urology. C. V. Mosby, St. Louis, Missouri

Turner-Warwick R (1984) A urodynamic view of the principles of female urinary incontinence procedures. In: Proceedings of the Royal College of Surgeons in Ireland Bicentenary

Symposium, Dublin

van Mastrigt R, Coolsaet BLRA, van Duyl WA (1978) Passive properties of the urinary bladder in the collection phase. Med Biol Eng Comput 16:471–482

Weil A, Reyes, H, Bischoff P, Rottenberg RD, Krauer F (1984) Modifications of the urethral resting and stress profiles after different types of surgery for urinary stress incontinence. Br Obstet Gynaecol 91:46–55

Wilson PD, Dixon JS, Brown ADG, Gosling JA (1979) A study of the pubourethral ligament in normal and incontinent women. Proceedings of the 9th International Continence Society Meeting, Rome

Yeates WK (1972) Disorders of bladder function. Ann R Coll Surg Engl 50:335–353

Zacharin RF (1963) The suspensory mechanism of the female urethra. J Anat 97:423–427

Zinner NR, Ritter RC, Sterling AM (1976) The mechanism of micturition. In: Williams DI, Chisholm GD (eds) Scientific foundations of urology. Heinemann, London, pp 39–51

2 Investigation of Incontinence

Stuart L. Stanton

Introduction

Surgical procedures to correct incontinence may fail. In addition, they may have side-effects and be accompanied by mortality and morbidity. In assessing a patient for incontinence surgery, the following questions require an answer.

—What is the diagnosis?

—Is surgery the best mode of treatment?

—Which operation should be performed?

—What are the risk factors associated with this patient?

Establishment of the correct diagnosis may require a series of invasive investigations. Strict asepsis is always necessary to avoid urinary tract infection and sensible control of investigations is important to ensure that only those likely to benefit the patient are performed.

Being continent is desirable, but not essential to life. Continence operations (save urinary diversion, which may be performed to prevent further upper urinary tract deterioration and renal failure) are not life saving and therefore the patient ultimately must determine for herself, after consideration of medical advice, whether she undergoes surgery.

The multiplicity of corrective procedures for incontinence reflects the uncertainty of their mode of action. It indicates our need to monitor the patient closely at follow-up, to decide which procedures are effective and why. Follow-up should be both subjective and objective and continue for at least 2, and preferably for 5 years.

Classification of Incontinence

Incontinence may occur through the urethra or outside the urethra:

Urethral
— Urethral sphincter incompetence (genuine stress incontinence)
— Detrusor instability
— neuropathic (hyperreflexia)
— non-neuropathic (idiopathic)
— Retention with overflow
— Congenital, e.g. epispadias
— Urethral diverticulum
— Miscellaneous, e.g. drugs, urinary tract infection
— Functional—psychosomatic

Extra-urethral
— Congenital—ectopic ureter
— bladder exstrophy
— Fistula — ureteric
— vesical
— urethral

It is important to appreciate that there are several factors responsible for the condition known as urethral sphincter incompetence:

1. Failure of elevation of the bladder neck.

2. Bladder neck elevated, but inadequate transmission of intra-abdominal pressure to the proximal urethra.

3. Loss of intra-urethral pressure or resistance: a functionless scarred urethra resulting from previous bladder neck surgery.

Miscellaneous conditions include transient incontinence due to urinary tract infection (especially in the elderly) or drug therapy, such as a-adrenergic blocking agents. A functional cause should only be diagnosed after other causes have been excluded.

Adverse Factors

The following may adversely affect normal bladder and urethral anatomy and physiology.

Neuropathy
— Supra- or infrasacral lesions affecting the innervation of the bladder, urethra and pelvic floor.

"Pelvic" lesion
— Genital prolapse
— Mass, e.g. impacted fibroids
— Inflammation of bladder, urethra, vulva or vagina
— Faecal impaction
Menstrual cycle
Medical disorders, e.g. diabetes mellitus
Side-effects of drugs, e.g. a-adrenergic blocking agents
Psychological disorders
Previous bladder neck surgery
Previous childbearing (Snooks et al. 1984).

Continence is the ability to void voluntarily at a socially convenient time and place. As there is a significant cortical and conscious component to being continent, the patient's mental state and her ability to co-operate must be considered in her assessment.

The patient should be as physically fit as possible prior to surgery. Patients with respiratory disease should not be operated on during the winter months (as bronchitis etc. may be aggravated and the resultant coughing will adversely affect wound healing). Epidural anaesthesia is helpful in these circumstances.

Obesity is not a factor in the recurrence of incontinence (Stanton et al. 1978). However, some women state that after losing weight, their incontinence improves. Surgery is undoubtedly more difficult to perform and there are increased risks of deep venous thrombosis in the obese during the post-operative period.

Age on its own should not debar a patient from surgery (Gillon and Stanton 1984). The same medical and mental desiderata apply. Additional precautions need to be taken however; the programme for her recovery should be explained to her relatives and nursing staff and as far as possible to the patient herself, so that all are aware of her expected progress. Early mobilisation in the post-operative period with attention to pressure areas and the use of low beds (so that the patient can get out easily) and easy access to toilet facilities or the use of a bedside commode are important. Over-sedation at night should be avoided. Small and frequent doses of analgesia are required. Finally, the nursing and medical staff must anticipate the special needs and problems of the elderly and should be aware of the development of confusional states.

Indications for Urodynamic Studies

The prime indication is to confirm a clinical diagnosis with objective and measurable data:

1. To diagnose the cause of incontinence, especially when one procedure to correct urethral sphincter incompetence has already failed.
2. To detect detrusor instability.
3. To detect voiding difficulties in a patient who may be asymptomatic or prior to bladder neck surgery.
4. In a patient with bladder symptoms and a neuropathy.
5. Prior to radical pelvic surgery.

A lesser indication is the need nowadays for objective assessment of lower urinary tract function for medicolegal purposes.

Clinical Assessment

History

Discrepancy between the patient's history and the clinical or objective findings is sometimes found. This is due either to the patient wishing to minimise her symptoms of incontinence (because she is improved rather than cured following treatment or does not want further surgery) or to the investigations having been too strenuous and having produced an artificially positive response. It is important to accept that if a patient says she is dry (despite investigations indicating the contrary) this may be an acceptable state for her and further treatment should not be imposed upon her. This, however, does lead to difficulty in assessing the results of surgery, which should in this case be regarded as "failure" or "improvement" but not "cure". If a patient's only symptom is incontinence and, despite exhaustive clinical and objective testing, this cannot be demonstrated, it would be wrong to proceed with surgery (with all its potential complications) because of the difficulty thereafter of assessing her claims.

The patient may emphasise that her incontinence dates from a recent operation, such as a total abdominal hysterectomy, yet a carefully taken history prior to this operation may have failed to disclose this. In attempting to assess symptoms which are present at follow-up and the benefits or otherwise of a procedure, it is important to obtain a full history prior to surgery. The original urodynamic questionnaire of Cardozo et al. (1978) has been enlarged by Hilton (1985, personal communication) and is reproduced here (Figs. 2.1, 2.2). It is administered by the doctor and is designed to code the response for computerisation. It is divided into the following sections:

1. *Current*
—Main complaint, where there is a succinct and chronological statement of the patient's presenting symptoms and their order of importance
—Urological symptoms—duration and severity
—Neurological symptoms
—Gynaecological symptoms and their relationship to urological complaint
—Obstetrical history
—Medical history
—Current drug regimen

2. *Past urological history*
—Enuresis, retention and episodes of proven or unproven urinary tract infection over the last 2 years
—Drug regimes
—Pelvic surgery

The diagnosis may sometimes be inferred from the history alone. The sole complaint of stress incontinence is likely to suggest incontinence due to urethral sphincter incompetence (Cardozo and Stanton 1980). On the other hand, nocturia and urge incontinence suggest detrusor instability (Farrar et al. 1975). In between, combinations of stress incontinence, urgency, urge incontinence,, frequency and enuresis are less likely to be helpful diagnostic features, but will indicate the extent of the disability.

Neurological symptoms (weakness and sensory change in the lower limbs, lack of awareness of bladder sensation, sweating, postural hypotension and rectal soiling) may indicate the presence of a neuropathy which will require a neurological opinion. Bladder outflow obstruction may be indicated by the symptoms of poor stream, straining to void, retention of urine and incomplete emptying (Stanton et al. 1983).

URODYNAMIC DATA 1

Hospital No. ....   Surname ....

Source of referral ....   Forename ....

Date of 1st consultation ....   Age .... Code as D.O.B.(6–11)

Unit No. 2

6

1 1

PRESENTING COMPLAINTS   Duration

1.   12

2.   15

3.   18

    Duration 1 = <1/12; 2 = 1–6/12; 3 = 7–12/12; 4 = 13/12–2 yrs; 5 = 3–5 yrs;
              6 = 6–10 yrs; 7 = >10 yrs

OTHER SYMPTOMS

Frequency 1 = ≦4; 2 = 5–7; 3 = 8–10; 4 = 11–14; 5 = 15–19; 6 = ≧20   21

Nocturia 0 = 0; 1 = 1–2; 2 = 3–4; 3 = ≧5   22

Urgency (23)	Hesitancy (29)	23 29
Impaired sensation (24)	Stains to void (30)	24 30
Bladder pain (25)	Poor flow (31)	25 32
Dysuria (26)	Intermittent flow (32)	26 32
Haematuria (27)	Incomplete emptying (33)	27 33
Unable to interrupt steam (28)	Post-mict. dribble (34)	28 34

0 = no; 1 = occasional; 2 = frequent

URINARY INCONTINENCE

Stress Incontinence (35)	Urge Incontinence (43)	
cough (36)	"key in door" (44)	35 43
laugh (37)	running water (45)	36 44
sneeze (38)	cold (46)	37 45
walk (39)	other (47)	38 46
run (40)	specify	39 47
bend (42)		40
other (42)		41
specify		42

Nocturnal Enuresis (48)   **Incontinence on Intercourse (49)**   48 49

  Code as No. 50   0 = none

                     1 = penetration

                     2 = orgasm

Frequency of Urinary Leakage (50)   50

0 = none; 1 = <monthly; 2 = weekly–monthly; 3 = q 3–7 days; 4 = q 1–3 days
5 = daily; 6 = >daily

Severity of Urinary Leakage (51)   51

0 = none; 1 = minimal; 2 = change pants 1 × /day; 3 = change 2–3 × /day;
4 = sanitary protection

No of Pads Per Day (52)   52

  Type ....

Social Restrictions (53)   53

0 = none; 1 = restricted; 2 = housebound

UTEROVAGINAL PROLAPSE (54)   54

0 = none; 1 = dragging or discomfort; 2 = lump of vulva

Fig. 2.1a

Fig. 2.1a–c. Urodynamic questionnaire (Hilton 1985, personal communication) modified from Cardozo et al. (1978). The question-naire is completed by the doctor at the first visit. The *right-hand column* is for computerisation.

URODYNAMIC DATA 2

Hospital No. .... Surname ....

Source of referral .... Forename ....

Date of 1st consultation .... Age ....

Unit No. 2

	1	2

NON-URINARY SYMPTOMS

Dyspareunia (6)   Constipation (9)   6 ☐   9 ☐

Chronic cough (7)   Rectal soiling (10)   7 ☐   10 ☐

Neurological symptoms (8)   Other (11)   8 ☐   11 ☐

  specify ....   specify ....

0 = no; 1 = occasional; 2 = frequent

OBSTETRIC HISTORY

Parity   No. of pregnancies of 28 weeks or more (12)   12 ☐

                    No. of pregnancies terminating before 28 weeks (13)   13 ☐

Birthweights: <1·5 Kg No. ...... Deliveries: SVD   No. ......   14 ☐ 18 ☐

                    1.6–2.5 Kg No. ......   Forceps No. ......   15 ☐ 19 ☐

                    2.6–4 Kg No. ......   Breech   No. ......   16 ☐ 20 ☐

                    >4 Kg   No. ......   LSCS   No. ......   17 ☐ 21 ☐

GYNAECOLOGICAL HISTORY

Menstrual Status (22)   22 ☐

1 = premenarchal; 2 = menstrual; 3 = perimenopausal; 4 = post-menopausal (or TAH + BSO);
5 = TAH with ovaries conserved; 6 = TAH with ovaries conserved + menopausal symptoms

O/C (23) 0 = no; 1 = yes   specify ....   23 ☐

HRT (24) 0 = no; 1 = yes   specify ....   24 ☐

Cycle ....   LMP ....

Effect of Menstruation on Urinary Symptoms (25)   25 ☐

0 = unaffected; 1 = aggravated premensturally/menstrually;
2 = improved premenstrually/menstrually; 3 = only symptomatic with menses

PAST MEDICAL HISTORY

Diabetes mellitus (26) specify: type I, type II ....   26 ☐

Neurological disease (27) specify: ....   27 ☐

Psychological disease (28) specify: ....   28 ☐

Other (29) specify: ....   29 ☐

0 = no; 1 = yes

DRUG HISTORY

                                         code of drugs affecting bladder (30–33)

1. ....   1 = anticholinergic   30 ☐

2. ....   2 = cholinergic   31 ☐

3. ....   3 = sympatholytic   32 ☐

4. ....   4 = sympathomimetic   33 ☐

                                              5 = diuretic

                                              6 = sedative

                                              7 = other

Fig. 2.1b

URODYNAMIC DATA 3

Hospital No. ....   Surname ....   Unit No. 2

Source of referral ....   Forename ....

Date of 1st consultation ....   Age ....

1 | 3

PAST UROLOGICAL HISTORY

Nocturnal Enuresis (6–8)
0 = no; 1 = yes; specify age of control .... years

6

Urinary Infections (9–11)
0 = no; 1 = yes; specify no. of infections in last 2 years ....

9

Retention (12)
0 = none; 1 = spont.; 2 = post-partum; 3 = post-op.

12

Drug Treatment of Urinary Symptoms (13–24)

specify   effect   duration of improvement

1. ....
2. ....
3. ....

13
17
21

Drug code as per 2:30
Effect 0 = none; 1 = improved; 2 = cured; 3 = worse
Duration code in months improvement

Surgery for Urinary Symptoms (25–44)

specify   effect   duration of improvement

1. ....
2. ....
3. ....
4. ....
5. ....

25
29
33
37
41

Operation 0 = none; 1 = urethal diln.; 2 = urethrotomy; 3 = vag. repairs;
4 = vag. hyst. & repair; 5 = colposuspension; 6 = MMK; 7 = sling;
8 = other, unspecified; 9 = no data

Effect   0 = no success; 1 = improved; 2 = cured; 3 = worse

Duration   Code in months improvement

OTHER SURGERY

Pelvic Surgery (45)
0 = none; 1 = TAH(+ / −); 2 = TAH + BSO; 3 = MRH; 4 = RHND;
5 = large bowel surgery; 6 = other, specify ....

45

Effect on Urinary Symptoms (46)
0 = none; 1 = aggravated; 2 = improved; 3 = initiated

46

Other Surgical History
1. ....
2. ....
3. ....

Fig. 2.1c

URODYNAMIC DATA 4

Hospital No. ....   Surname ....

Source of referral ....   Forename ....

Date of 1st consultation ....   Age ....

Unit No. 2

		1	4

PHYSICAL EXAMINATION

Height (6–8) ....m   Weight (9–11) ....Kg

Breasts

Other Systemic Findings

   specify ....

6

9

Abdomen: Bladder palpable (12)

        0 = no; 1 = yes

        Other sign. findings

           specify ....

12

Vaginal Examination

Mucosa (13)

1 = healthy; 2 = atrophic changes

Anterior wall: cystocoele (14)

              cystourethrocoele (15)

Posterior wall: rectocoele (16)

              enterocoele (17)

Cervical vault descent (18)

0 = none; 1 = slight; 2 = marked

Bladder neck (19)

1 = normal mobility; 2 = excess mobility; 3 = rigid

Vaginal capacity (20)

1 = normal; 2 = restricted

13

14

15

16

17

18

19

20

Uterus (21)

0 = absent; 1 = normal; 2 = <12/52; 3 = >12/52

21

Stress incontinence

Extent (22)

0 = none; 1 = slight (only after series of coughs); 2 = marked (after single cough)

Posture (23)

1 = supine; 2 = L. lateral; 3 = standing; 4 = standing at capacity

(code) lowest number appropriate)

22

23

Other Pelvic Pathology

   specify ....

Anal Spincter Tone (24)

1 = normal; 2 = decreased

S_{234} **Sensation** (25)

Anal Reflex (26)

1 = normal; 2 = decreased

Neuropathy (27)

o = no; 1 = yes

   specify ....

24

25

26

27

Clinical Diagnosis (28–33)

Code up to 3 diagnoses as per 6:71

28

30

32

Fig. 2.2a

Fig. 2.2a–c. Urodynamic questionnaire for physical examination and investigation (Hilton 1985, personal communication).

URODYNAMIC DATA 5

Hospital No. ....   Surname ....

Source of referral ....   Forename ....

Date of 1st consultation ....   Age ....

Unit No.   3 | 1 | 5 |

INVESTIGATIONS

M.S.U. (7)

1 = sterile; 2 = insign. growth; 3 = sign. growth ($\geq 10^5$/ml) specify org. ....

7 ☐

Free Flow Rate (date (8–13) ....)

8 ☐☐☐☐☐☐

Peak flow rate (mls/sec) (14–15)

Vol. voided (mls) (16–18)

16 ☐☐ (14)
☐☐☐ (19)

Pattern (19)

1 = normal; 2 = all strain; 3 = strain element; 4 = obstructed;
5 = unsustained contraction

Cystometry/Videocystourethrography (date (20–25) ....)

20 ☐☐☐☐☐☐

Residual (mls) (26–29)

First sensation (mls) (30–33)

Vol. at first contraction (mls) (34–37) – 999 if stable

Capacity (mls) (38–41)

26 ☐☐☐☐
30 ☐☐☐☐
34 ☐☐☐☐
38 ☐☐☐☐

Pressure rise on filling   PR$_{500}$ (42–43)
                            PR$_{cap}$ (44–45)

42 ☐☐
44 ☐☐

Pressure rise on provocation   PR .... (46–47)

46 ☐☐

Maximum voiding pressure (cm H$_2$O) (48–50)

48 ☐☐☐

Peak flow rate (with catheter) (mls/sec) (51–52)

51 ☐☐

Interrupt quickly (53)
0 = no; 1 = yes

53 ☐

Vol. at interrupt (54–62)   (a)   (b)   (c)

Pres. at interruption (63–68)   (a)   (b)   (c)

P$_{Iso}$ (69–74)   (a)   (b)   (c)

54 ☐☐☐ ☐☐☐ ☐☐☐
63 ☐☐ ☐☐ ☐☐
69 ☐☐ ☐☐ ☐☐

Residual volume (mls) (75–78)

75 ☐☐☐☐

Stress Incontinence (79)

0 = none; 1 = slight (only with series of coughs); 2 = marked (with single cough)

79 ☐

VIDEO FINDINGS

Bladder Contour (80)

1 = normal; 2 = trabeculated; 3 = sacculated; 4 = diverticulum

80 ☐

Bladder Base (81)

1 = normal; 2 = moderate mobility; 3 = marked excess mobility; 4 = rigid

81 ☐

Bladder Neck (82)

1 = competent at all times; 2 = open on jumping; 3 = open on cough/strain
4 = open on filling

82 ☐

Reflux (83)

0 = none;; 1 = left; 2 = right; 3 = bilateral

83 ☐

Fistula (84)

0 = no; 1 = yes   specify site ....

84 ☐

Fig. 2.2b

URODYNAMIC DATA 5

Hospital No. ....   Surname ....
Source of referral ....   Forename ....   Unit No.   3 [ ][ ][1][6]
Date of 1st consultation ....   Age ....

URETHRAL PRESSURE PROFILES (date (7–12 ....)   7 [ ][ ][ ][ ][ ][ ]

Total profile length (mm) (13–14)   13 [ ][ ]
Functional profile length (mm) (15–16)   15 [ ][ ]
Length to peak pressure (mm) (17–18)   17 [ ][ ]
Maximim urethal pressure (cm H_2O) (19–21)   19 [ ][ ][ ]
Maximum urethral closure pressure (cm H_2O) (22–24)   22 [ ][ ][ ]

Cough Profile

Functional profile length (mm) (25–26)   25 [ ][ ]
Length to peak pressure (mm) (27–28)   27 [ ][ ]
Maximum urethral closure pressure (cm H_2O) (29–31)   29 [ ][ ][ ]
Mean cough amplitude (cm H_2O (32–34)^2 32 [ ][ ][ ]
PTR Q_1 (%) (35–37)   35 [ ][ ][ ]
       Q_2 (%) (38–40)   38 [ ][ ][ ]
       Q_3 (%) (41–43)   41 [ ][ ][ ]
       Q_4 (%) (44–46)   44 [ ][ ][ ]

Mid Urethral Responses

Intrinsic variability (% of mcup) (47–48)   47 [ ][ ]
"Sustained response" (% of mucp loss with cough series) (49–50)   49 [ ][ ]
No. of coughs to min. mucp (51–52)   51 [ ][ ]
Minimum ucp (mid-urethal) (cm H_2O) (53–55)   53 [ ][ ][ ]
Recovery time (secs) (56–57)   56 [ ][ ]

Urilos (date (58–63) ....)   58 [ ][ ][ ][ ][ ][ ]

1 = standard stress test)
2 = standard time test) (64) specify duration ....   64 [ ]

Meter Reading (mls) (65–67)   65 [ ][ ][ ]

Pad Wgt. Change (gms) (68–70)   68 [ ][ ][ ]

Urodynamic Diagnosis (71–76) Code up to 3 diagnoses

0 = no significant abnormality
1 = urinary tract infection   71 [ ][ ]
2 = urethral syndrome   73 [ ][ ]
3 = hypersensitive bladder   75 [ ][ ]
4 = genuine stress incontinence
5 = detrusor instability
6 = urethral instability
7 = voiding difficulty – detrusor hypotonia
8 = voiding difficulty – outflow obstruction
9 = vesico or urethro vaginal fistula
10 = urethral diverticulum
11 = congenital abnormality
12 = other
     specify ....

Fig. 2.2c

The patient's mental state may be indicated by her demeanour, and the manner in which she responds to questions. Psychiatric questionnaires have been used to determine the psychiatric state of patients with disorders of bladder function (Hafner et al. 1977). Studies by Macaulay et al. (1985) have pointed towards differentiation between patients with detrusor instability (who are chronic worriers and have guilt feelings), those with sensory urgency (who have low self-esteem) and those with urethral sphincter incompetence (who are unlikely to have these complaints).

The use of protective underwear is a guide to the severity of incontinence.

Urinary diary (Fig. 2.3)—Additional information about the patient's habits will be obtained by using a urinary diary, which will record the time and volume of each void, together with the daily fluid intake. It can also be used to record the time of each "urge", the precipitating event and whether it has led to urge incontinence. When recording urological symptoms, it is important to note their frequency and severity and the precipitating events, if any.

There is often a close relationship between gynaecological and urological symptoms. The presence of a dragging feeling in the vagina may indicate anterior vaginal wall prolapse, which is present in about 50% of women with urethral sphincter incompetence. Incontinence may be aggravated during the second half of the menstrual cycle, which is progesterone dominated.

A record of drug therapy is relevant because (a) the patient may already be taking drugs acting specifically on the bladder and urethra and (b) some drugs exert potent side-effects on micturition (Stanton 1978).

The past surgical history should include details of any operation likely to affect bladder and urethral function or further surgical access. These include neurological operations, upper urinary tract operations, and abdominal or pelvic operations, including Caesarean section, hysterectomy, vaginal repair and bladder neck surgery. Where relevant, the indication for and success of the operation should be noted.

Examination

General

The examination should include a brief assessment of the patient's fitness for anaesthesia, including respiratory and cardiological systems, measurement of blood pressure and pulse and note of the patient's weight and height.

If elderly or disabled, a dementia score (Fig. 2.4) or a mobility score (Fig. 2.5) should be completed.

Neurological

The eyes should be examined for the pupillary reaction and to exclude nystagmus. The limbs (particularly lower limbs) are examined for tone, power, reflexes and sensation with special reference to dermatomes S2, S3 and S4 (Fig. 2.6). The anal sphincter tone and perineal sensation are noted. The patient is positioned upright with her eyes closed and examined to exclude defective balance. Her back is examined for stigmata of any underlying vertebral column lesion.

Special Tests. It is also necessary to confirm the activity and continuity of the sacral reflex centres. These tests include the bulbocavernosus reflex, which is elicited by lightly touching or tapping the clitoris. This will produce a contraction of the external anal sphincter. It will also be observed that

DAY: *TUESDAY MAY 20*

TIME	INTAKE (ml)	OUTPUT (ml)	LEAKAGE			
			ACTIVITY	Amount	Urge	Wet Bed
07.10		300				
08.15			WASHING	2	YES	
08.30	150					
09.45		150				

Fig. 2.3. Urinary diary, completed by the patient over 7 days.

Dementia score

1. Age.
2. Time (to nearest hour).
3. Address for recall at end of test – this should be repeated by patient to ensure it has been heard correctly: 42, West Street.
4. Year.
5. Name of hospital.
6. Recognition of two persons (doctor, nurse etc.).
7. Date of birth (day and month sufficient).
8. Year of first World War.
9. Name of present Monarch.
10. Count backwards 20 – 1.

3b. Recall of address.

Dementia score = /10

Fig. 2.4. Dementia score completed by the doctor or nurse at the first visit. It is used for patients with suspected dementia and those aged over 65 years.

Mobility score

1. Mobile.
2. Walks with stick/frame.
3. Confined to chair, but can stand.
4. Cannot stand, but in chair.
5. Bed bound.

Mobility score =

Fig. 2.5. Mobility score, completed by the doctor or nurse on the first visit.

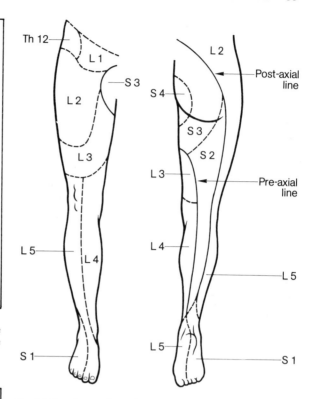

Fig. 2.6. Lumbosacral root dermatomes. (Last 1977)

the external anal sphincter will contract visibly in response to pinprick stimulation of the perineal skin.

Carefully performed, these tests will exclude a neuropathy. If a lesion is suspected, either from the history or clinical examination, the patient should be referred to a neurologist.

Gynaecological and Urological

The abdomen is palpated to exclude a full bladder and the loins examined to detect any renal enlargement. Vulval excoriation may be present if incontinence is continuous. Congenital lesions such as epispadias should be recognised, but the opening of an ectopic ureter may be difficult to detect. The urethra is examined for discharge, tenderness, undue rigidity and fixity. The latter may be sequelae of repeated surgery or infection. The vagina is examined for capacity and mobility (which may be compromised by previous pelvic surgery). Adequate mobility is necessary for some urethrovesical suspension procedures. The anterior and posterior vaginal walls and vault are examined to detect prolapse, and if the uterus is present, its size, mobility and descent are noted. Stress incontinence is detected by coughing, either in the supine left lateral position (using a Sim's speculum) or standing up. The bladder should contain some urine. Bonney's test (prevention of incontinence by digital elevation of the bladder neck) may stop leakage by compression, without regard to aetiology, and is therefore not recommended.

The pelvic examination will also exclude any pelvic pathology (e.g. ovarian masses). The presence of a loaded rectum will be noted on rectal examination.

Investigations

As many investigations of the lower urinary tract are invasive, it is necessary that the patient's interests are placed first. Only those investigations which are directly helpful should be performed. A full blood count, chest X-ray and ECG should be carried out before major pelvic surgery. An intravenous urogram (pyelogram) is indicated when there is recurrent urinary tract infection, continuous incontinence, congenital anomaly or outflow obstruction. With the latter, serum creatinine, urea and glomerular filtration rate are relevant. Culture and sensitivity of a mid-stream specimen of urine should be performed in all patients. Any urinary tract infections should be treated before further investigations and certainly before surgery is performed. Urinalysis for glucose and protein should also be performed.

It is reassuring to know that careful sterile urethral instrumentation for investigation carries a very low risk of urinary tract infection (Walter and Vejlsgaard 1978).

Urethrocystoscopy

Urethrocystoscopy should be regarded as a sterile procedure and carried out under local or light general anaesthesia. With the former it may be difficult to determine full bladder capacity if this is in doubt. Either water or carbon dioxide may be employed as a filling medium. Interchangeable telescopes of 0°, 30° fore-oblique or 70° side-viewing can be used with a single sheath, and a fibre optic light-source is recommended.

Ideally urethrocystoscopy should be performed prior to all surgery on the bladder or urethra. Specific indications include the following:

—Haematuria
—Persistent urgency and frequency
—Retention or difficulty in voiding
—Continuous urinary incontinence
—Urethral tenderness and fixity
—Suspected urethral diverticulum
—Neuropathic bladder disorder
—Suspected urethral/bladder/ureteric injury
—Assessment of pelvic malignancy

The following observations can be made:

—Residual urine
—Bladder capacity (normal is 400–500 ml)
—Bladder mucosa
  —neoplasia
  —injection
  —ureteric orifices (normal or ectopic)
—Bladder wall
  —presence of trabeculation, diverticulum or sacculation
—Internal meatus
  —well formed, or patulous and funnelled
—Presence of calculi or foreign bodies

Trabeculation is consistent with either mechanical obstruction or neuropathic disorder. No pertinent observations can be made about the function of the internal urethral meatus.

Uroflowmetry

Measurement of the urine flow rate provides an objective assessment of voiding ability and disability. It is indicated when a patient complains of difficulty or hesitancy in voiding, incomplete bladder emptying, poor stream or retention of urine, and in the assessment of patients for incontinence surgery (Stanton et al. 1978).

The measurements obtained from a flow rate are shown in Fig. 2.7: the *voided volume* is the total volume expelled via the urethra. *The maximum flow rate* is the maximum measured volume of the flow rate. *The average flow rate* is the voided volume divided by the flow time. *The flow time* is the time over which measurable flow rate actually occurs. *The time to maximum void* is the elapsed time from onset of flow to maximum flow.

Various methods are used. The three commonly available are:

1. Recording the volume of fluid voided using a strain-gauge weighing transducer placed at the bottom of a cylinder. The volume is electronically converted to a flow rate and a simultaneous record of urine volume and flow rate is produced.

2. Voiding onto a disc rotating at a constant speed will reduce the rotational speed of the disc. The flow rate can be deduced from the power needed to main-

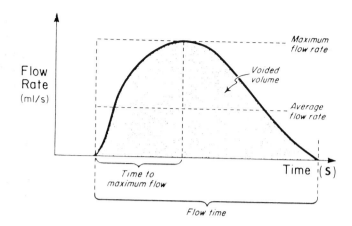

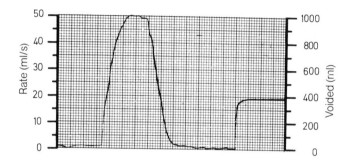

Fig. 2.7. Uroflow data measured on a stylised flow pattern.

Fig. 2.8. Normal uroflow on the *left* with volume voided on the *right*. The traces are made consecutively rather than synchronously. (Dantec Limited)

tain the disc at its original speed. The volume is calculated at the end of voiding, so the record is not simultaneous. A normal trace is shown in Fig. 2.8.

3. Capacitance flow meter—the transducer is a plastic dipstick coated in metal, which dips into the vessel containing the voided urine. The rate and volume are deduced by a change in electrical conductance. The advantages of this method are accuracy, absence of moving parts and cheapness. A decreased flow rate measured by this method is shown in Fig. 2.9.

For a flow rate to be significant at least 150 ml of fluid should be voided. Whilst there is no upper limit of normality, a repeated flow rate below 15 ml/s indicates outflow obstruction or impaired voiding ability.

This test has the advantage of being rapid, non-invasive and practical to use in a hospital clinic or consulting room/office. Further information may be obtained by simultaneously measuring the detrusor pressure, which will be the maximum voiding pressure.

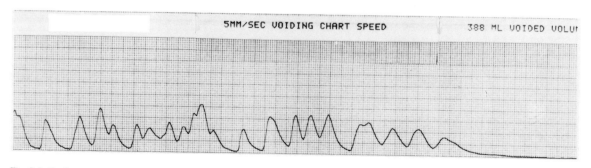

Fig. 2.9. Uroflow in a patient with detrusor sphincter dyssynergia. (Ormed Limited)

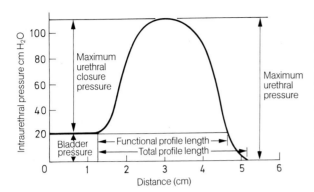

Fig. 2.10. Schematic representation of urethral closure pressure profile. (Static)

Urethral Function Tests

Urethral Pressure

Measurement of static urethral pressure gives little practical guide to urethral function, because of overlap between measurements found in healthy asymptomatic patients and those in patients with urethral sphincter incompetence. The parameters of the urethral pressure profile are indicated in Fig. 2.10. Some refinement is achieved by the use of a twin microtip transducer catheter (Fig. 2.11). By slowly withdrawing the catheter, a dynamic urethral profile can be constructed of urethral and intravesical pressures during coughing and straining, so providing a more accurate assessment of intra-urethral forces. Resting and cough profiles are

shown in a continent female (Fig. 2.12) and in a female with urethral sphincter incompetence (Fig. 2.13). Because of rotational artefacts due to catheter stiffness, the method is unreliable for the patient who has had past bladder neck surgery (when there is urethral fixity and curvature) and the direction of the sensing transducers must be consistent and controlled (Hertogs and Stanton 1983; Plevnik et al. 1983a).

Pressure Fluid Bridge Test

The first defence against incontinence is the bladder neck portion of the urethral sphincter mechanism. Fluid descending into the urethra will establish a fluid bridge between the bladder and test point in the proximal urethra, which can be detected with a double lumen fluid bridge catheter (Sutherst and Brown 1980). Bladder and urethral pressures are simultaneously displayed on a cathode ray screen.

Urethral Electric Conductance

Urethral electric conductance (UEC) represents a new parameter for evaluation of urethral and bladder function (Plevnik et al. 1983b). The equipment used to measure the UEC consists of a specially constructed 7F flexible probe bearing two ring electrodes separated by 1 mm (Fig. 2.14). A constant sinusoidal voltage is applied and the current, i.e. conductance between them is measured. As the catheter is withdrawn from the urethra at a con-

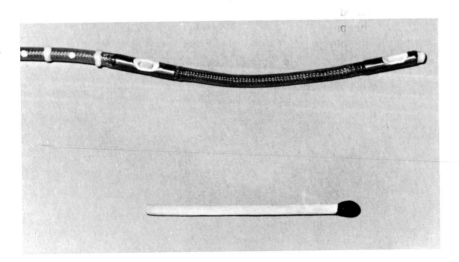

Fig. 2.11. Twin transducer catheter with a transducer separation of 6 cm. (Gaeltec Limited)

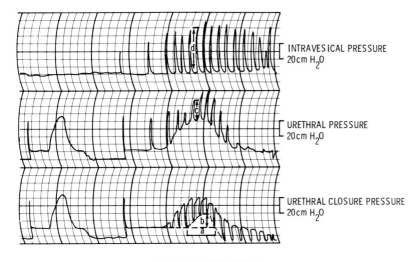

a = FUNCTIONAL LENGTH ON STRESS

b = MAXIMUM CLOSURE PRESSURE ON STRESS

$\frac{c}{d}$ x 100 = PRESSURE TRANSMISSION RATIO

Fig. 2.12. Dynamic urethral pressure profile in a patient who is continent. (Courtesy of P. Hilton)

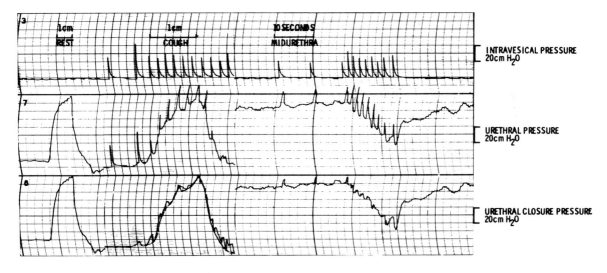

Fig. 2.13. Dynamic urethral pressure profile in a patient with stress incontinence due to urethral sphincter incompetence. *Left*, static profile; *middle*, normal dynamic profile; *right*, repeated coughing with transducer in mid-urethra demonstrates gradual loss of urethral closure pressure. (Courtesy of P. Hilton)

stant rate, the urethral electric conductance profile is obtained, which allows for an accurate identification of the bladder neck mechanism and external urethral meatus (Fig. 2.15). By measuring the time course of conductance, bladder neck activity and urethral closure mechanisms can be studied. Any urinary leakage is reflected by an increase in conductance.

Urethral electric conductance measurements are of clinical value in detecting and timing urine loss during provocative manoeuvres such as coughing, exercising and handwashing, at any point along the urethra. The distal UEC test involves placing the electrodes 1.5 cm from the external urethral meatus and has been shown to be rapid and accurate in identifying incontinence, with a pick up rate of 75%

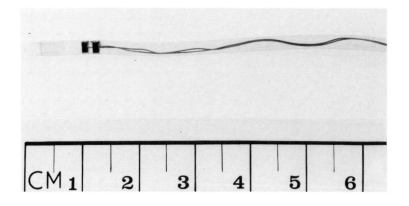

Fig. 2.14. Urethral electric conductance profile catheter showing two measuring electrodes.

U. E. C. P.

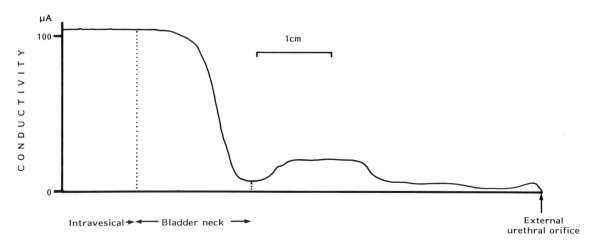

Fig. 2.15. Change in electric impedance on withdrawing measuring electrodes or UECP catheter from bladder to urethra. (Plevnik et al. 1983b). (Courtesy of D. Holmes)

and without false-positives or -negatives (Holmes et al. 1985). In addition, characteristic UEC tracings will allow differentiation between leakage due to urethral sphincter incompetence and that due to increased detrusor activity or urethral relaxation.

Cystometry

Bladder pressure measurements during the filling and voiding phases are probably the most widespread and useful test of bladder function. Zero reference for pressure is the level of the superior edge of the symphysis pubis. It is accepted that the patient is awake and neither sedated nor taking drugs

which will affect bladder function. Single channel cystometry is the simplest mode but lacks refinement and will not yield the information or provide the accuracy of the twin channel subtracted method. However, with some practice, the observer can tell the difference between abdominal pressure change and the detrusor contraction (Sutherst and Brown 1984).

It is important to specify the following:

1. Access—transurethral or percutaneous (suprapubic): The latter is considered unnecessarily invasive by most clinicians, but it has a role in the assessment of young children (when transurethral catheter measurements are unreliable) and in cases of infravesical obstruction.

2. Medium—water or carbon dioxide: The latter is less "messy", quicker and avoids the viscous drag effect of water, but it has the disadvantages of being unphysiological, not providing quantitatively reproducible data and being unable to allow measurement of peak flow rate during the voiding phase.

3. Temperature: All studies should be performed with the medium at room temperature.

4. The position of the patient during filling and voiding: Provocative tests for detrusor instability include filling with the patient in the erect position and heal bouncing.

5. Filling rate: Nowadays this is almost always continuous rather than incremental. Rates should be clearly defined. Slow fill cystometry is up to 10 ml/min and is preferred for suspect or overt neuropathy. Medium fill cystometry is between 10 and 100 ml/min and a rapid fill is over 100 ml/min. The latter is a further provocative test for detrusor instability.

Intravesical and abdominal pressures are measured by either fluid-filled catheters (1 or 2 mm external diameter flexible polyethylene tubing) or a catheter tip transducer.

The *intravesical pressure* is the pressure within the bladder. The *abdominal pressure* is the pressure surrounding the bladder and is usually measured by a 2-mm external diameter fluid-filled line protected by a finger cot and inserted into the rectum. Gastric, intra- and extra-peritoneal pressure measurements may be taken instead. *Detrusor pressure* is that component of intravesical pressure created by active or passive forces on the bladder wall. It is obtained by electronic subtraction of abdominal pressure from intravesical pressure.

Modern twin channel subtracted cystometry (Fig. 2.16) includes the following:

1. Intravesical and rectal pressure catheters (Fig. 2.17). The former is slotted into the side of the

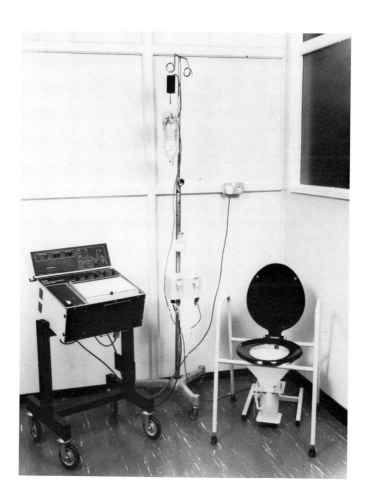

Fig. 2.16. Five channel cystometry apparatus (Ormed Limited) comprising recording machine, transducer stand and uroflowmeter. The five channels include intravesical pressure, abdominal (rectal) pressure, subtracted detrusor pressure, inflow volume and uroflow measurement and CMG recording.

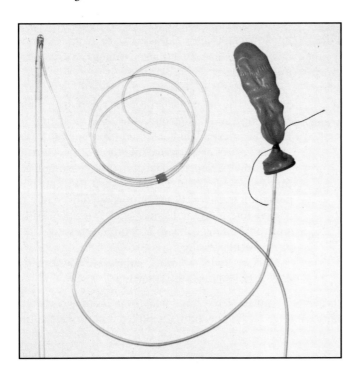

Fig. 2.17. *Left*, 12F filling catheter with a 1-mm E.D. flexible intravesical pressure measuring catheter slotted into the side for easy insertion into the bladder. The intravesical catheter is disengaged once the catheters are in the bladder. *Right*, 2-mm E.D. rectal pressure catheter, protected from faecal blockage by a finger cot.

12F filling catheter for easy access to the bladder. The rectal catheter is protected against faecal blockage by a finger cot and is commercially available.

2. A force transducer attached to the inflow fluid to measure the volume entering the bladder.

At the end of bladder filling, the filling catheter is removed and the patient stood erect and asked to cough. She then voids in privacy, sitting on a flow meter, with the pressure lines still in place, and is asked to voluntarily interrupt her stream.

Provocative testing for detrusor instability can be performed at this stage and include:

1. Fast filling in the erect position.
2. Heel bouncing with a full bladder.
3. Turning on the water taps with a full bladder.

The parameters of normal bladder function are:

1. A residual < 50 ml.
2. First sensation between 150 and 200 ml.
3. Strong desire to void at upwards of 400 ml.
4. Absence of detrusor contractions and a bladder compliance of < 15 cm of water. (This figure is arbitrary and more reliance is placed on the absence of any uninhibited detrusor contraction.)

5. No incontinence on coughing.
6. A rise of detrusor pressure on voiding (maximum voiding pressure) < 70 cm. H_2O with a peak flow rate greater than 15 ml/s for a volume voided of at least 150 ml.
7. The patient should be able to interrupt her urinary stream on command.

A normal trace is shown in Fig. 2.18 and detrusor instability is demonstrated in Fig. 2.19.

Cystometry, whilst detecting detrusor instability and voiding difficulties, cannot indicate bladder neck or urethral function or the presence of residual urine following voiding (except when using suprapubic access). Urethral sphincter incompetence is only diagnosed when fluid is seen exiting from the external urethral meatus: bladder neck incompetence cannot be defined more precisely than that. The technique, nevertheless, is simple, inexpensive and reliable.

Radiology

Plain

Plain radiography has a place in the identification of conditions which may cause incontinence or

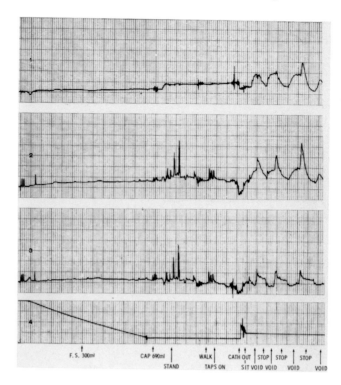

Fig. 2.18. Normal twin channel subtracted cystometric trace.

G. F. 10.12.79 RESIDUAL = 150 ml

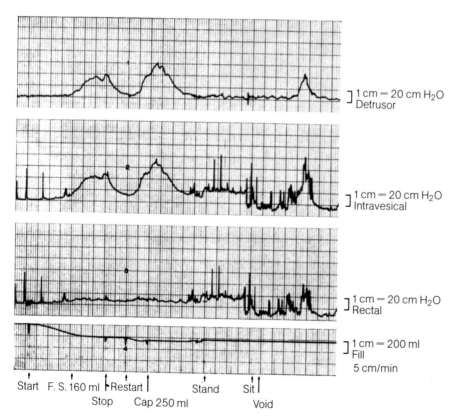

Fig. 2.19. Twin channel subtracted cystometric trace demonstrating detrusor instability.

compromise the results of surgery. Whilst bladder exstrophy is gross and an obvious diagnosis, the lesser variant of epispadias can occasionally fail to be detected in childhood and incontinence may persist into adult life. Separation of the symphysis is found, due to failure of fusion of midline somites which involves the vulva, symphysis and the bladder neck (Fig. 2.20). Diastasis of the symphysis pubis following blunt trauma (e.g. road traffic accident) will cause rupture of the posterior pubo-urethral ligaments and dislocation of the proximal urethra and bladder neck from the symphysis pubis (Fig. 2.21). Incontinence may not be suspected because of the greater concern about injury to other pelvic organs.

Failure of an artificial urinary sphincter may be due to loss of activating fluid (Fig. 2.22) or kinking of tubing (Fig. 2.23).

Urinary retention may masquerade as an ovarian cyst: Fig. 2.24 shows a patient with chronic urinary retention and a fluid level due to gas-forming organisms.

Vertebral column defects with underlying spinal cord anomalies are identified by lumbar spine radiography—e.g. spina bifida occulta (Fig. 2.25) and sacral agenesis (Fig. 2.26).

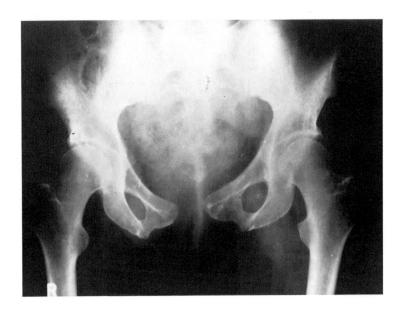

Fig. 2.20. Typical separation of symphysis pubis found in epispadias.

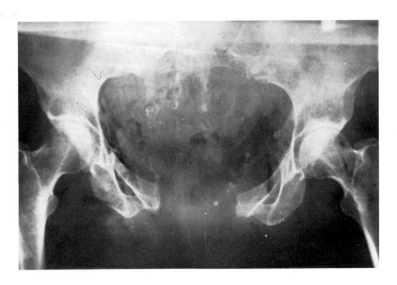

Fig. 2.21. Diastasis of the symphysis pubis following blunt trauma to the pelvis.

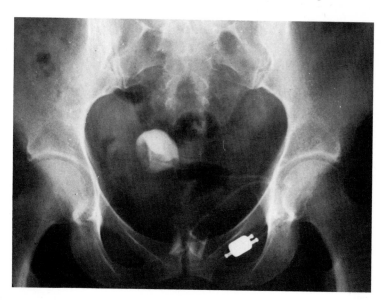

Fig. 2.22. Loss of activating fluid in an artificial urinary sphincter (AMS 792) due to leakage.

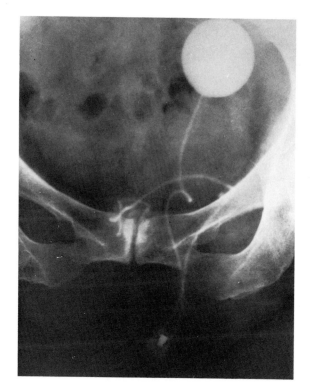

Fig. 2.23. Kinking of tubing found in a patient with an AMS 800 sphincter.

Videocystourethrography

Videocystourethrography (VCU) is the addition to micturition cystography of simultaneous bladder and abdominal pressure and uroflow measure-ments, which are recorded with sound commentary on video cassette (Fig. 2.27). Micturition cysto-graphy will show bladder outline during bladder fill-ing, loss of contrast on coughing, the ability to voluntarily interrupt the urinary stream during voiding, ureteric reflux and post-micturition residual. Unless simultaneous pressure measure-ment is taken, it will neither detect detrusor instability nor determine the cause of complex void-ing disorders.

VCU was developed by Enhorning, Earl Miller and Hinman (1964) at the University of California S.F. Medical School and is my preference for the investi-gation of complex disorders of lower urinary tract function.

The patient is prepared as for cystometry. She arrives with a comfortably full bladder and a uroflow measurement is carried out beforehand in privacy. The patient then lies supine on a tilting radiological table (Fig. 2.28); sterile urethral catheterisation using a 12F catheter is performed and the residual urine measured. The bladder is fil-led with 25% Diodone at a rate of 100 ml/min by gravity feed (a neuropathic bladder should be filled more slowly at between 5 and 10 ml/min).

At maximum cystometric capacity (strong desire to void), the filling catheter is removed (the bladder pressure line remaining in place) and the patient positioned upright. She is radiologically screened in the erect oblique position. She is asked to cough and leakage and movement of the urethrovesical junc-tion and bladder base are noted. She is next asked

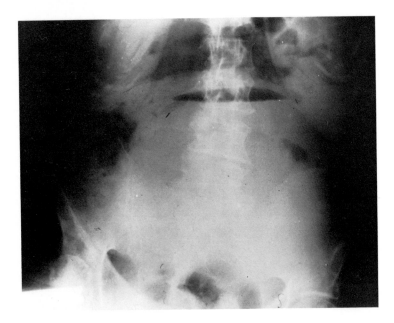

Fig. 2.24. Fluid level in the bladder, due to gas-forming organisms in chronic urinary retention.

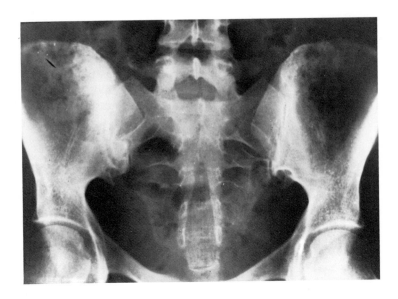

Fig. 2.25. Lumbosacral spine radiograph showing vertebral column lesion in spina bifida occulta.

to void and after voiding about 200 ml, is asked to voluntarily interrupt her stream. Peak flow rate and volume voided are recorded simultaneously with the detrusor pressure (maximum voiding pressure). The ability to milk-back is noted. Voiding is resumed and she is re-screened after emptying to detect any residual contrast. Any difficulty in voiding when erect (which is found in about 20% of women) may be overcome by moving the patient with pressure lines in situ, to an adjacent side room where she can

void in privacy seated on a commode above a uroflowmeter.

All pressure flow data are recorded on a six-channel recorder. During the voiding phase a television camera positioned above the recorder selects three channels (intravesical and detrusor pressures, and peak flow rate) and with the aid of a mixing device, a fused image is obtained of the radiological screening of bladder and urethra with the pressure flow data. This is displayed on a television monitor.

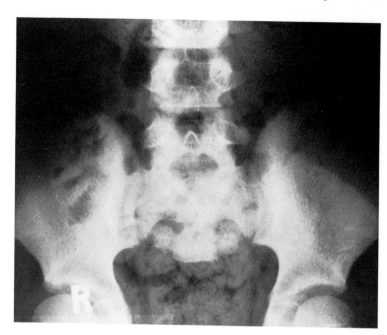

Fig. 2.26. Sacral agenesis.

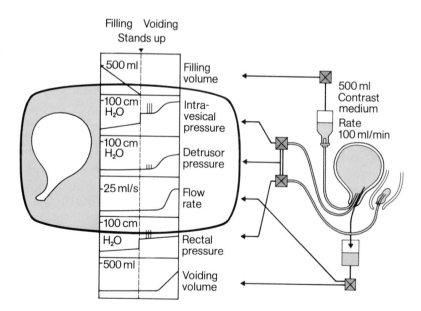

Fig. 2.27. Videocystourethrography schema. Simultaneous recording of bladder and rectal pressure changes during supine cystometry, combined with a display of bladder filling volume shown on the *left-hand side* of the polygraph trace. On voiding, the bladder and rectal pressures with the voiding rate of volume are recorded on the *right* of the trace. Television cameras select three parameters (intravesical pressure, detrusor pressure and voiding rate) which are added to the radiographic image of the bladder (shown on the *extreme left* of the diagram) and recorded with sound commentary on video cassette.

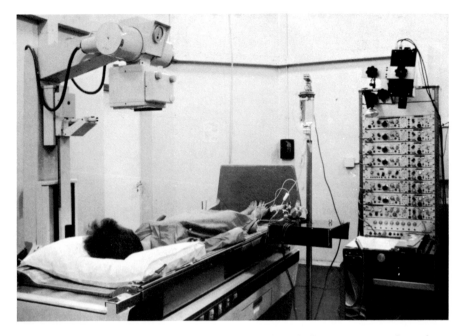

Fig. 2.28. Patient on a radiological tilting table, Grass recorder and television camera and transducer stand.

The combined picture is recorded on video cassette with simultaneous sound commentary and is used for instant or later replay.

The provocative tests for detrusor instability are employed. The total screening time is less than 1 min and each examination takes approximately 20 min. Six patients may be screened easily in a morning or afternoon. Using image itensification, the X-ray dose to the ovaries is approximately 2.7 mGy, which is the same as an intravenous urogram series.

Normal Bladder Function (Fig. 2.29). The parameters of normal bladder function have been referred to earlier under cystometry. Radiological screening demonstrates the presence of leakage, mobility of the bladder neck and voluntary interruption of voiding. With the latter, the urinary stream is interrupted in the mid-urethra and fluid proximal to this point is "milked" back into the bladder. The bladder neck gradually closes and the detrusor pressure falls to pre-micturition levels. Fluid distal to the mid-urethra is voided. No significant residual should remain on completion of voiding and there should be no ureteric reflux.

Indications for VCU. Causes of complicated urinary incontinence and voiding difficulties may be diag-

nosed with this technique:

1. *Urethral sphincter incompetence.* The bladder neck may be open at rest or on coughing without a detectable rise in detrusor pressure or a detrusor contraction. Stress incontinence is shown in Fig. 2.30.

2. *Detrusor instability.* This is characterised by either an uninhibitable systolic contraction or a low-complaint rise of detrusor pressure, produced in response to bladder filling or provocative testing. It is no longer believed that a numerical value of 15 cm H_2O represents a cut-off point for a rise in detrusor pressure. Leakage of contrast depends on the detrusor pressure rise exceeding the urethral pressure, so that a negative urethral closure pressure exists. If the urethral sphincter mechanism is competent, this may not happen. Raised detrusor pressure is shown during bladder filling (Fig. 2.31), standing erect (Fig. 2.32) and on coughing (Fig. 2.33).

3. *Retention with overflow.* This is characterised by a delay in first sensation, enlarged bladder capacity, and, in some cases, a normal detrusor pressure rise on filling or standing (despite the capacity sometimes exceeding 1–2 litres). Stress incontinence may be demonstrated. The flow rate may be < 15 ml/s: ureteric reflux, bladder trabeculation and sacculation and a significant residual may be present.

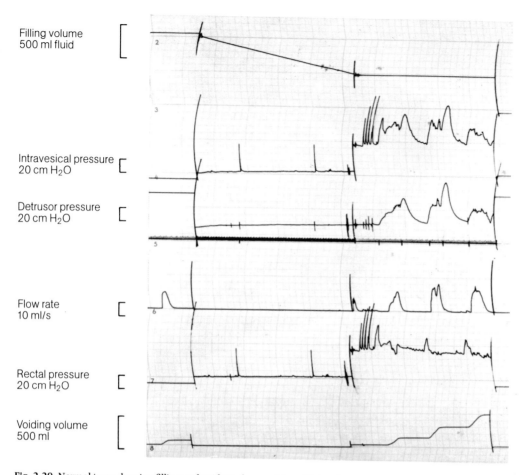

Filling volume
500 ml fluid

Intravesical pressure
20 cm H$_2$O

Detrusor pressure
20 cm H$_2$O

Flow rate
10 ml/s

Rectal pressure
20 cm H$_2$O

Voiding volume
500 ml

Fig. 2.29. Normal trace showing filling and voiding phases with multiple voluntary interruption of voiding.

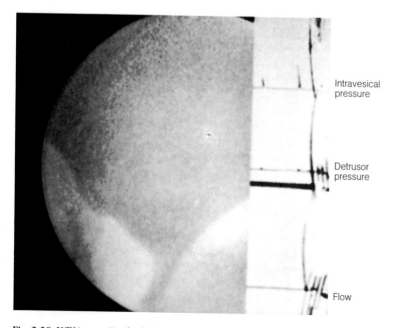

Intravesical
pressure

Detrusor
pressure

Flow

Fig. 2.30. VCU image. Urethral sphincter incompetence with evidence of stress incontinence.

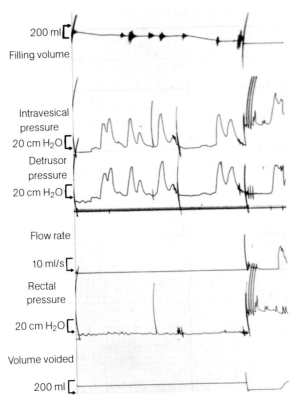

200 ml — Filling volume

Intravesical pressure 20 cm H₂O

Detrusor pressure 20 cm H₂O

Flow rate 10 ml/s

Rectal pressure 20 cm H₂O

Volume voided 200 ml

Fig. 2.31. Trace showing uninhibited detrusor contractions during bladder filling.

Bead Chain Urethrocystography

It is sometimes relevant to know the position of the bladder neck and its alignment with that of the proximal urethra to the symphysis pubis. The bead chain technique (originally described by Hodgkinson in 1953) will give this information. A sterile bead chain (Fig. 2.34) is introduced into the bladder with the aid of a 14F filling catheter, together with 250 ml of contrast medium. The filling catheter is then removed and the patient screened in the erect lateral position at rest and on straining (using a Valsalva manoeuvre or cough). Films are taken at rest and on straining. Simultaneous recording of intra-abdominal (rectal) pressure will allow precise measurement of the force of the Valsalva manoeuvre. A pre-operative bead chain urethrocystogram showing a poorly elevated bladder neck (Fig. 2.35) is compared to the well elevated and aligned bladder neck following successful colposuspension (Fig. 2.36).

Intravenous and Retrograde Urography

Intravenous urography, in this context, is indicated when there is:

— Continuous incontinence with otherwise normal micturition (especially following pelvic surgery)
— Diurnal incontinence
— Neuropathic bladder
— Obstructive uropathy (in conjunction with ultrasound)
— Persistent "vaginal discharge", e.g. ectopic ureter (Fig. 2.37).

Retrograde urography is used to diagnose a uretero-vaginal fistula (Fig. 15.10).

Electromyography

Striated muscle activity may be studied by measuring the bioelectric potentials generated by the depolarisation of muscle fibres secondary to an excitatory impulse from an anterior horn cell. The technique can be used to detect whether the muscle is contracted or relaxed and to test the integrity of the muscle and its nerve supply. The potentials may be detected either by surface electrodes applied to the skin overlying the muscle (which give a gross and imprecise recording) or by needle electrodes directly inserted into the muscle. The latter may be introduced into either a single fibre or several muscle fibres. The needle may be monopolar (which requires a second reference or ground electrode), bipolar or concentric; the latter is the most practical to use. Single fibre electromyography (EMG) is obtained with a very small recording surface (25 μm), requires a second reference electrode and allows extracellular recording from a single muscle fibre during voluntary activity (Anderson 1984). It is a very precise technique and can be used in clinical practice.

Surface electrode sampling is relatively inaccurate. The innervation of the external urethral sphincter and external anal sphincter are separate and different (Gosling et al. 1983), and this is confirmed by clinical evidence (Blaivas et al. 1977; Nordling and Meyhoff 1979) (Fig. 2.38). Therefore, genuine urethral sphincter activity requires measurements of either external urethral sphincter EMG (Fig. 2.39) or the pubococcygeal portion of the pelvic floor.

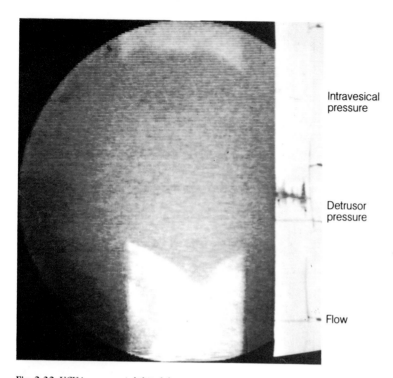

Fig. 2.32. VCU image: uninhibited detrusor contraction to 30 cmH$_2$O water on standing erect. The bladder neck is open.

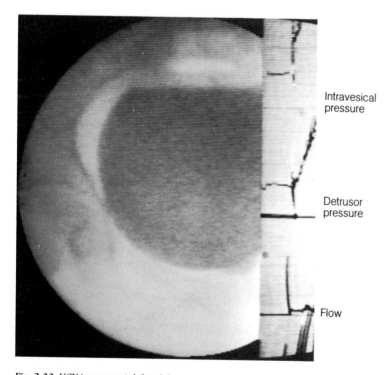

Fig. 2.33. VCU image: uninhibited detrusor contraction to 60 cmH$_2$O on coughing whilst erect. The bladder neck is open.

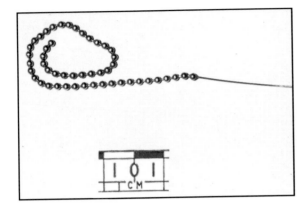

Fig. 2.34. Bead chain, as used in urethrocystogram.

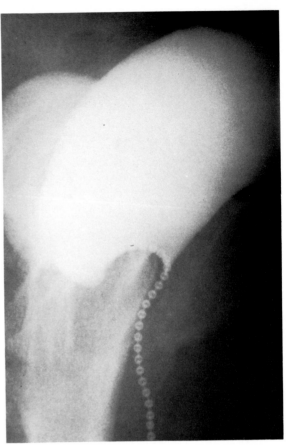

Fig. 2.36. Bead chain urethrocystogram, in same case as Fig. 2.35, showing decreased descent of the bladder neck and improved alignment of the proximal urethra to the postero-superior border of the symphysis, following successful colposuspension.

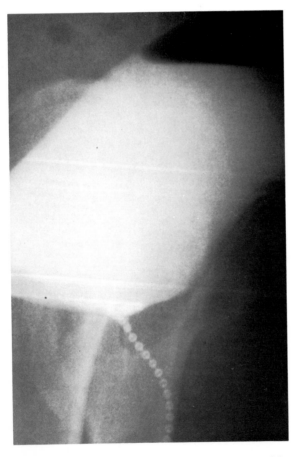

Fig. 2.35. Bead chain urethrocystogram showing descent of the bladder neck on straining, in relation to the symphysis pubis, in a patient with urethral sphincter incompetence prior to continence surgery.

The pubococcygeal portion of the pelvic floor is localised by passing the needle 1 cm lateral to the external urethral meatus and 1–3 cm deep and parallel to the urethra. The exact location of the electrode is confirmed by a good signal-to-noise ratio on an electromyograph. Additional practical information is obtained if simultaneous cystometry is performed and EMG activity recorded from the sphincter mechanism during filling, straining or coughing, voiding and voluntary interruption of the urinary stream (Blaivas 1983).

The indications for EMG investigation are:

1. Overt or suspect neuropathic bladder

2. Voiding disorders (Fig. 2.40)

3. Investigation of obscure or resistant cases of incontinence.

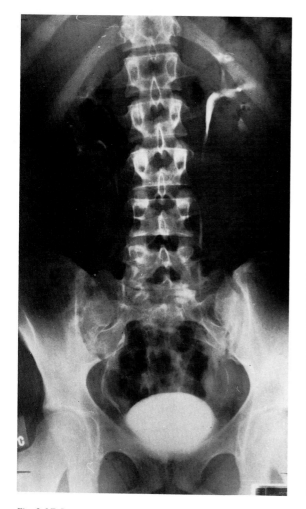

Fig. 2.37. Intravenous urogram showing right ectopic ureter.

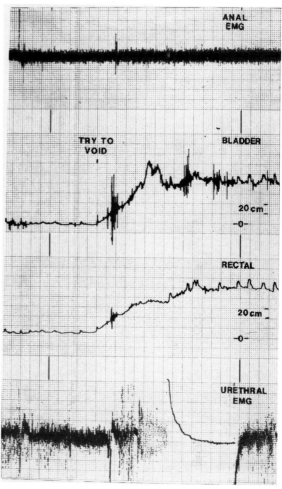

Fig. 2.38. Discrepancy between external anal and urethral sphincter EMG. Voiding is initiated by straining and accompanied by an increase in external urethral sphincter EMG activity. Coincident with the onset of a detrusor contraction, there is relaxation of the external urethral sphincter but no change in the anal sphincter EMG. Coaxial needle electrodes were used. (Courtesy of J. Blaivas and Neurourol and Urodynamics)

More elaborate electrophysiological testing may be performed by measuring:

1. *Sacral evoked responses.* These test the integrity of the sacral spinal nerve reflex. Clinically the bulbocavernosus reflex is elicited by squeezing the clitoris or pulling the bulb of a Foley catheter against the bladder neck and observing a reflex contractile response of the external anal sphincter. Care should be exercised in interpreting the results as a bulbocavernosus reflex is only present in some 70% of normal women. To measure the latency of this reflex, the clitoris is stimulated electrically with 1 mSEC rectangular pulses of a frequency duration of 0.5–1/s with a voltage increase from zero to just below the pain threshold, with simultaneous recording of EMG of the external anal sphincter.

2. *Cerebral evoked responses.* Cortical responses in the midline of the sensory cortex may be detected following urethral stimulation using a urethral ring electrode and a computer averaging technique (Gerstenberg et al. 1981). This may help in the investigation of afferent pathways from the urinary tract to the cerebral cortex.

3. *Visual evoked potentials.* These are measured by stimulation of the patient's eye using light patterns which generate electrical potentials in the retina and are transmitted to the occipital cortex. The potential produced is recorded from the scalp using a cyclical average. The visual evoked potentials are

NORMAL EMG

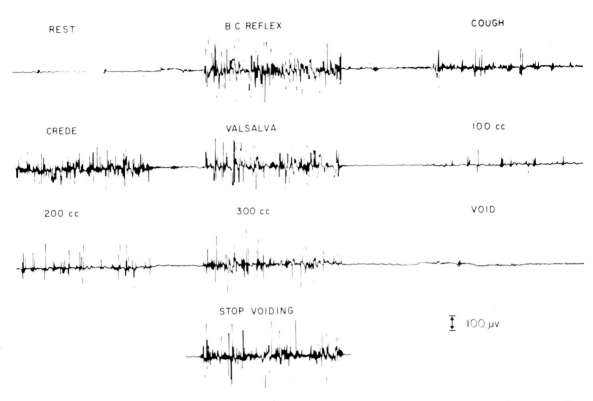

Fig. 2.39. Normal EMG of the external urethral sphincter. There is minimal activity at rest when the bladder is empty. A complete interference pattern is seen during coughing, crede and Valsalva. As the bladder fills, there is increasing EMG activity. Voluntary micturition is preceded by electrical silence. The command to stop voiding results in a complete interference pattern. (Courtesy of J. Blaivas and Neurourol and Urodynamics)

helpful in the investigation of bladder symptoms thought to be due to multiple sclerosis.

Ultrasound

Ultrasound investigation of the lower urinary tract is indicated for the following:

1. Calculation of residual urine (Poston et al. 1983). A static B scan is used to measure the greatest supero-inferior and antero-posterior measurement in the sagittal plane and the greatest transverse measurement in the transverse plane (Fig. 2.41). The product of these, when multiplied by a correction factor of 0.7 (as the bladder is not a true cuboid shape), will give the bladder volume with a minimal percentage error of 21%.

2. Assessment of change in position of bladder base and urethra on movement, e.g. straining, using either a linear array scanner with an abdominal transducer or a transrectal probe.

3. Detection of urethral and bladder diverticulae, ureterocele and periurethral cysts (Fig. 2.42).

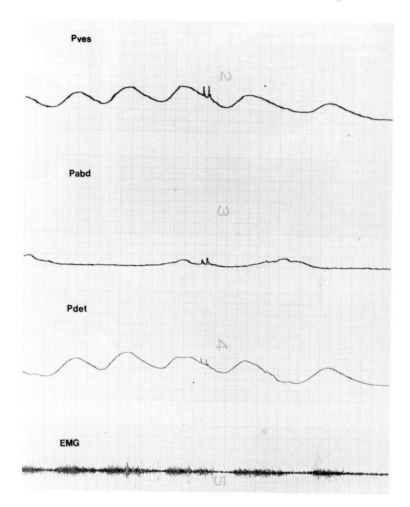

Fig. 2.40. Detrusor sphincter dyssynergia with simultaneous increase in bladder pressure (*Pdet*) and EMG activity of the external urethral sphincter. (Courtesy of J. Blaivas)

The advantages of ultrasound are:

1. It is a harmless investigation without observable side-effects.
2. It is not invasive and therefore without risk of urinary tract infection.
3. It can be used during pregnancy.

The limitations of ultrasound depend on a change of interface, and the distinction between bladder and urethra can be difficult without the presence of a urethral catheter. Ultrasound is unlikely to delineate as much detail as radiological screening; phased array will improve resolution, but this is very costly.

Perineal Pad Test

An objective test to demonstrate incontinence qualitatively and quantitatively is needed (a) to confirm the patient's claim that incontinence is present, when it thus far has not been detected either clinically or following CMG or VCU, and (b) to provide

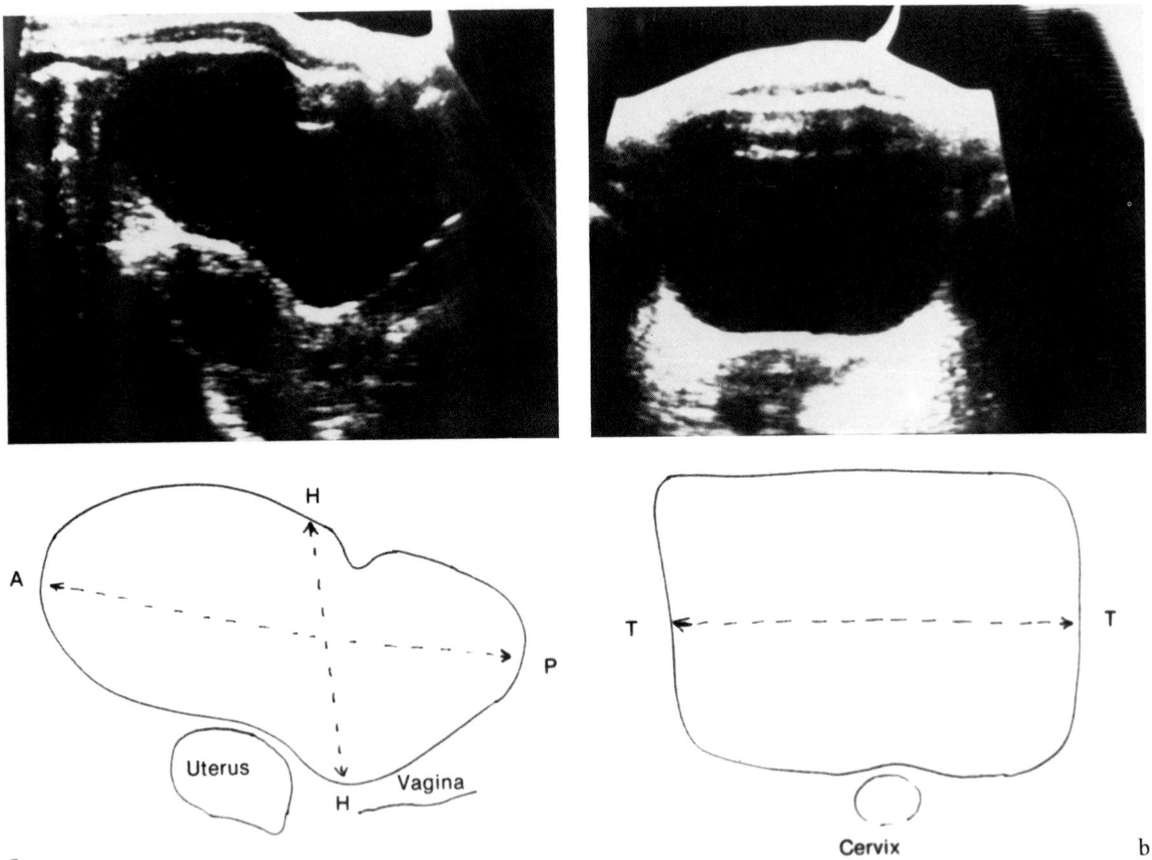

Fig. 2.41. a *Above,* longitudinal ultrasound scan at maximum height of bladder to show a full bladder. *Below,* tracing of longitudinal scan showing dimensions. *AP,* anteroposterior length; *HH,* height. **b** *Above,* transverse scan at maximum height of bladder. *Below,* tracing of transverse scan showing dimensions. TT, transverse width. (Courtesy of Dr. R. H. Patel)

objective assessment of the patient following incontinence surgery.

James et al. (1971) devised a disposable nappy (diaper) with electrodes which could detect and measure leakage, but these were not entirely reliable. Sutherst et al. (1981) weighed perineal pads following a simple exercise schedule and this has been developed into a standard 1-h test (Fig. 2.43) by the International Continence Society (1983).

The Future

A greater demand for urodynamic investigation has resulted from the increased knowledge base of the lower urinary tract, compounded by an appreciation of poor results of surgical and conservative treatment, and increasing use of technology in other fields of medicine and the unfortunate increase in the incidence of litigation.

Present investigations fall short on the ability to inform reliably about the function of the urethra and the urethral sphincter mechanism. It is likely that these investigations will continue to be invasive. Although ultrasound is an appealing technique, it is unlikely to displace radiography as a method of displaying lower urinary tract morphology. It is likely that function will be pursued at a cellular rather than at organ level, with histochemical tests becoming more prominent.

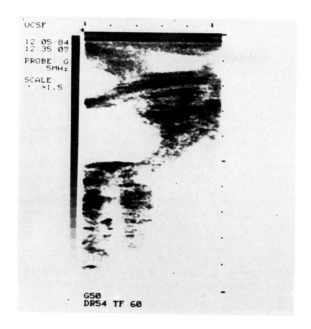

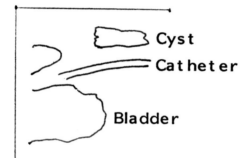

Cyst

Catheter

Bladder

Fig. 2.42. *Above,* longitudinal scan showing urethral cyst or diverticulum, catheter and bladder. *Below,* tracing of scan.

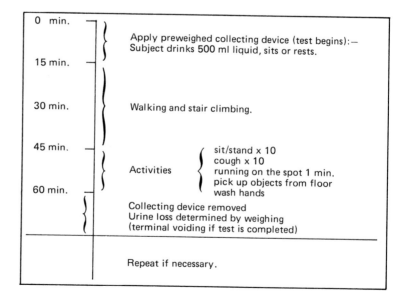

0 min.	Apply preweighed collecting device (test begins):— Subject drinks 500 ml liquid, sits or rests.
15 min.	
30 min.	Walking and stair climbing.
45 min.	Activities {sit/stand x 10, cough x 10, running on the spot 1 min., pick up objects from floor, wash hands}
60 min.	Collecting device removed. Urine loss determined by weighing (terminal voiding if test is completed)
	Repeat if necessary.

Fig. 2.43. Diagrammatic representation of extended perineal pad test.

References

Anderson R (1984) A neurogenic element to urinary genuine stress incontinence. Br J Obstet Gynaecol 91:41–45

Blaivas J (1983) Sphincter electromyography. Neurourol Urodynamics 2:269–288

Blaivas J, Labib K, Bauer S, Tetik A (1977) A new approach to electromyography of the external urethral sphincter. J Urol 117:773–777

Cardozo L, Stanton SL, Bennett AE (1978) Design of a urodynamic questionnaire. Br J Urol 50:269–274

Cardozo L, Stanton SL (1980) Genuine stress incontinence and detrusor instability—a review of 200 patients. Br J Obstet Gynaecol 87:184–190

Enhorning G, Miller E, Hinman F Jr (1964) Urethral closure studied with cine roentgenography and simultaneous bladder-urethral pressure recording. Surg Gynecol Obstet 118:507–516

Farrar D, Whiteside G, Osborn J, Turner-Warwick R (1975) Urodynamic analysis of micturition symptoms in female. Surg Gynecol Obstet 141:875–881

Gerstenberg T, Hald T, Meyhoff H (1981) Urinary cerebral evoked potentials mediated through urethral sensory nerves—a preliminary report. In: Zinner N, Sterling A (eds) Female incontinence. Alan R. Liss, New York, pp 141–143

Gillon G, Stanton SL (1984) Long term follow-up of surgery for urinary incontinence in elderly women. Br J Urol 56:478–481

Gosling J, Dixon J, Humpherson J (1983) Functional anatomy of the urinary tract. Churchill Livingstone, Edinburgh, pp 5–18

Hafner R, Stanton SL, Guy J (1977) A psychiatric study of women with urgency and urgency incontinence. Br J Urol 49:211–214

Hertogs K, Stanton SL (1983) Urethral function tests: limits to certainty. Proceedings of the 13 Annual Meeting ICS, Aachen, pp 155–157

Hodgkinson CP (1953) Relationships of female urethra and bladder in urinary stress incontinence. Am J Obstet Gynecol 65:560–573

Holmes D, Plevnik S, Stanton SL (1985) Distal urethral electric conductance test (DUEC) for the detection of urinary leakage. Proceedings of the 15th Annual Meeting of the International Continence Society, London

International Continence Society (1983) Fifth report on standardisation of terminology of lower urinary tract function. Internal report of Standardisation Committee

James ED, Flack F, Caldwell KP, Martin M (1971) Continuous measurement of urine loss and frequency in incontinent patients. Br J Urol 43:233–237

Last RJ (1977) Anatomy, regional and applied, 6th edn. Churchill, London

Macauley A, Holmes D, Stanton SL, Stern RS (1985) A clinic survey of the mental state of 211 women attending a urodynamic unit. Proceedings of the 15th Annual Meeting of the International Continence Society, London

Nordling J, Meyhoff H (1979) Dissociation of urethral and anal sphincter activity in neurogenic bladder dysfunction. J Urol 122:352–356

Plevnik S, Vrtacnik P, Janez J, Brown M (1983a) Effect of catheter stiffness on rotational variations on urethral pressure. Proceedings of 13 Annual Meeting ICS. Aachen, pp 149–151

Plevnik S, Vrtacnik P, Janez J (1983b) Detection of fluid entry into the urethra by electric impedance measurement: electric fluid bridge test. Clin Phys Physiol Meas 4:309–313

Poston G, Joseph A, Riddle P (1983) The accuracy of ultrasound and the measurement of change in bladder volume. Br J Urol 55:361–363

Snooks S, Swash M, Setchell M, Henry M (1984) Injury to innervation of pelvic floor sphincter musculature in childbirth. Lancet I:546–550

Stanton SL (1978) Diseases of the urinary system: drugs acting on the bladder and urethra. Br Med J I:1607–1608

Stanton SL, Cardozo L, Chaudhury N (1978) Spontaneous voiding after surgery for urinary incontinence. Br J Obstet Gynaecol 85:149–152

Stanton SL, Ozsoy C, Hilton P (1983) Voiding difficulty in the female: prevalence, clinical and urodynamic review. Obstet Gynecol 61:144–147

Sutherst J, Brown M (1980) Detection or urethral incompetence in women using the fluid bridge test. Br J Urol 52:138–142

Sutherst J, Brown M (1984) Comparison of single and multi channel cystometry in diagnosing detrusor instability. Br Med J 288:1720–1722

Sutherst J, Brown M, Shawer M (1981) Assessing the severity of urinary incontinence in women by weighing perineal pads. Lancet I:1128–1130

Walter S, Vejlsgaard R (1978) Diagnostic catheterisation and bacteriuria in women with urinary incontinence. Br J Urol 50:106–108

3 Congenital Causes of Incontinence

Anthony M. K. Rickwood

Introduction

Wet girls feature large in paediatric practice and come in three general categories:

1. Most numerous are those with no identifiable organic disease; the presenting complaints cover a wide spectrum from pure nocturnal enuresis to a small number with quite severe diurnal incontinence. Urodynamic abnormalities, notably detrusor instability, can often be demonstrated but their significance is debatable in the almost complete absence of urodynamic data from symptomless children. Most of these girls can be regarded as having delayed maturity of bladder control and the natural history of these complaints is, in consequence, generally one of spontaneous resolution.

2. Less numerous, but still many, are those who have organic disease in the form of recurrent urinary infections and who are variably incontinent when they are infected but are usually dry otherwise. Most have uncomplicated cystitis but a sizeable minority have some urological abnormality (most commonly vesicoureteric reflux) which may be the cause of the infections or merely an incidental feature. Even when present, such abnormalities are

not themselves the cause of the incontinence and girls in this group as a whole can be regarded as similar to those in the first category with the difference that it requires the stimulus of infection to trigger the voiding disorder. It does appear that many girls with reflux have detrusor instability (Koff 1983) and an appreciable number are enuretic even when their urine is clear.

3. There remains a very small but important residuum of girls whose incontinence results directly from congenital anomalies which are either *structural*, comprising ureteric ectopia, urogenital sinus abnormalities and exstrophic anomalies, or *neurological*, from some congenital lesion of the spinal cord. Patients in the latter category are appreciably more numerous.

There exists also a small group of girls who do not fit readily into any of these categories and who, for want of a better term, may be labelled as having "occult neuropathic bladder" (Williams et al. 1974). Some, it seems, have no organic disease but rather an extreme form of functional voiding disorder, often with detrusor–sphincter dyssynergia and sometimes secondary upper renal tract changes in consequence. Others appear to have some subtle autonomic neuropathy, as yet undefined.

Assessment of the Wet Girl

General

It is clearly crucial to identify those few girls with congenital abnormalities from the remainder. Given a purposeful history and examination, this is not usually difficult and indeed if there is some congenital anomaly, its nature is often evident from clinical assessment alone.

The general features of history, examination and investigation are covered in Chap. 2; in girls these differ only in points of emphasis.

History Taking

1. For those not dealing regularly with children the main difficulty lies in the wide spectrum of "normality" and in particular the considerable variation in age at which girls become dry, first by day and

then by night. That said, most of those with incontinence caused by congenital anomalies have, even as early as 3 years of age, a pattern of micturition which is grossly abnormal.

2. Frequency of micturition is not a major complaint of wet girls nor is it itself a cause of incontinence; parents of children with congenital anomalies may sometimes encourage frequent voiding in a usually futile attempt to achieve continence.

3. Urgency of micturition is the principal complaint of most girls with diurnal incontinence and suggests detrusor instability or, less often, sensory urgency. Except for urinary infection, instability seldom has any organic basis in girls. Patients with congenital but incomplete cord lesions may also have urgency, usually gross, and which is due to detrusor hyper-reflexia.

4. A complaint of involuntary (and allegedly unknowing) leakage of urine is common; it is usually due to detrusor instability and certainly not necessarily indicative of organic disease. Similarly "giggle incontinence", a condition as unrewarding to investigate as it is to treat.

5. Stress leakage is an uncommon symptom in girls and, if genuine, usually means some congenital anomaly.
Provoked instability, easily mistaken for stress leakage, is more common.

6. The complaint of "always being wet" is much over-used, but if really true is almost certainly caused by a congenital anomaly; sometimes it occurs only by day (e.g. with ectopic ureter).

7. Abnormal bowel habit suggests a neurological problem though it may also occur in girls with occult neuropathic bladder.

Physical Examination

1. Vulval examination should ensure the presence of separate urethral and vaginal orifices, so excluding urogenital sinus abnormalities.

2. Neurological assessment need normally comprise no more than examining leg reflexes, the feet for deformities, motor activity in the pelvic floor and sensation (particularly for temperature) in the sacral dermatomes. The ano-cutaneous reflex is important in girls with neuropathic bladder.

3. The lower spine should be palpated to exclude sacral agenesis. Most cutaneous abnormalities asso-

ciated with spina bifida occulta are obvious. Pits overlying the tip of the coccyx are without significance, in contrast to those at higher levels.

Investigations

Straight Spinal X-ray. Whether isolated laminal defects at L5 or S1 are of significance in the absence of an overlying cutaneous lesion or neurological signs continues to excite passions. It is the author's view that they are not.

Urinary Tract Ultrasound. This has partially supplanted the IVU and is invaluable in detecting renal duplication anomalies associated with ureteric ectopia. It is also a harmless means of reassuring anxious parents that their child has no major abnormality.

Contrast Radiology. IVU and cystography (a thoroughly unpleasant examination for girls) have no place in the routine work-up of childhood incontinence and should be reserved for specific indications.

Radio-isotopes. These are useful both for detecting duplication anomalies and for assessing differential function between kidneys or between the poles of one kidney.

Urethroscopy. Except in girls suspected of having urogenital sinus anomalies or single system ectopic ureters, urethroscopy is largely useless, except, possibily, as an exercise in psychotherapy.

Urodynamics. Neither in patients suspected of having functional voiding disorders nor in those with structural anomalies is urodynamic investigation routinely necessary. The facility should certainly be available for girls with neuropathic bladder and for disentangling the problems of those with occult neuropathic bladder. The investigation is best combined with simultaneous video-radiological studies.

Ureteric Ectopia

Embryology

Readers interested in the embryogenesis of these conditions may consult Williams (1982). Features relevant to clinical practice are:

1. Ureteric buds which give rise to major degrees of ectopia, causing incontinence, make unsatisfactory contact with the developing metanephros so that there is always some degree of renal dysplasia. The ureter itself has deficient musculature, is usually dilated and may exhibit poor or absent peristalsis. In duplex systems only the upper pole is affected, in single systems the entire renal unit.

2. In duplex systems with incontinence, the accessory ureteric bud fails to make contact with the urogenital sinus and breaks through into the müllerian system so that the ectopic orifice is vestibular, vaginal or, rarely, uterine.

3. In single system ectopia, because the usual separation of ureter and wolffian system has not occurred, the trigone is not formed on the affected side, while in bilateral disease the bladder neck is grossly deficient also.

4. Single ectopic ureters nearly always enter the urethra, usually just below the bladder neck; very rarely they have a vaginal termination.

Duplex System Ureteric Ectopia

Presentation

When the ectopic orifice is vestibular, vaginal or uterine, the history is classically one of continual incontinence superimposed upon an otherwise normal pattern of micturition. Because function in the upper pole is generally poor there is dampness rather than wetness. At the extreme, efflux from the ectopic system may be interpreted as vaginal discharge rather than urine.

The child may be dry overnight if urine pools in a grossly dilated system. Occasionally there is a misleading history of a previous period of complete dryness and it seems that a few girls can, for a while, exert some control from the muscles around the introitus. Although the pattern of micturition is ordinarily unremarkable, habitual frequency may result if parents encourage the child to void at ever-decreasing intervals in an attempt to become dry.

Apart from vulval dampness, physical examination is usually unremarkable; ectopic orifices can seldom be located except under anaesthetic.

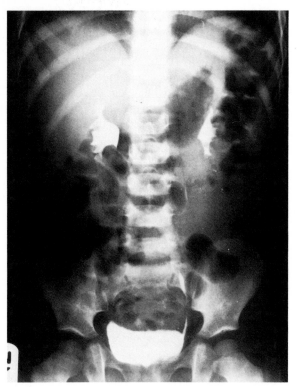

Fig. 3.1. Intravenous urogram. Left duplex kidney with non-visualised upper moiety and vaginal ectopic ureter. The lower pole is slightly rotated downwards and clearly displaced laterally by the adjacent dilated upper polar ureter. The uppermost calyx is shorter and less developed than that on the right.

Investigation

Previously the mainstays were IVU and examination under anaesthetic. Since function of the upper pole is usually too poor to allow direct visualisation by IVU (even with high dose of contrast and delayed films) its existence must be inferred from secondary changes in the lower pole and its ureter, namely (Fig. 3.1):

1. Downward and outward rotation (drooping flower kidney).
2. Lateral displacement of the renal pelvis caused by the dilated upper polar ureter lying medially.
3. The uppermost calyx being shorter than that on the opposite side.
4. A series of shallow curves in the ureter as it courses along with the dilated and tortuous upper polar ureter.

In any one case it is uncommon to find all four features, and the IVU appearances are often equivocal.

Under anaesthetic, vestibular orifices can usually be located by probing but vaginal orifices tend to defy the most prolonged and careful search. Attempts to locate ectopic orifices by intravenous injection of dye are almost always frustrated by poor function of the affected hemi-kidney. Alternatively, the bladder can be filled with dye via a catheter. A pad is placed on the vulva and if this becomes wet with *clear* fluid a diagnosis of ectopic ureter is likely.

Recently ultrasound and isotope scanning have made diagnosis more straightforward and reliable. If the upper polar element is at all dilated this is readily detectable by ultrasound (Fig. 3.2). On rare occasions when there is minimal or no dilatation, ultrasound is unhelpful, but the existence of a duplex system can be demonstrated by a ^{99m}Tc-dimercaptosuccinic acid (DMSA) scan (Fig. 3.3). A DMSA scan is routinely advisable in any case to assess the function of the upper pole.

Treatment

The function of the dysplastic upper pole is usually irrecoverably poor and the treatment in most cases is upper pole nephrectomy with excision of as much associated ureter as convenient through the one incision. The residual distal ureter seldom causes complications and it is certainly not routinely necessary to excise it through a separate suprapubic incision.

Upper pole nephrectomy is generally a straightforward procedure. The kidney is approached through a standard loin incision (rib resection is not necessary in young girls). There are often adhesions around the upper pole requiring sharp dissection to free the kidney from its bed. The vascular anatomy must be clearly displayed. This is variable, the most usual arrangement being one of two or three fine upper polar vessels arising from the main renal artery and a single vein feeding into the main renal vein. These are ligated and divided once the anatomy has been established. The two renal pelves and upper ureters are next separated from one another and the upper polar ureter divided and passed behind the main renal vessels before it is dissected to its hilum. The line of demarcation between normal lower pole and dysplastic upper pole is usually clear. If possible capsular flaps are raised from the upper pole, which is then freed from its fellow

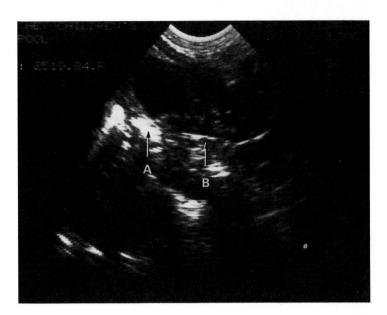

Fig. 3.2. Left duplex kidney with non-visualised upper moiety on IVU. Ultrasound clearly shows the hydronephrotic upper pole (*A*), the lower pole being normal (*B*).

by blunt dissection. After securing haemostasis with fine chromic catgut sutures, the capsular flaps are closed over the defect. If flaps cannot be raised, the upper pole is amputated and the defect closed with 2–0 or 3–0 chromic catgut mattress sutures passing through the capsule of the lower pole. Finally the upper polar ureter is traced as far distally as convenient, dissecting close to it so as not to disturb the blood supply of its fellow. The distal stump can be ligated or left open with drainage. It is advisable to fix the remaining hemi-kidney to the psoas muscle with two or three absorbable sutures.

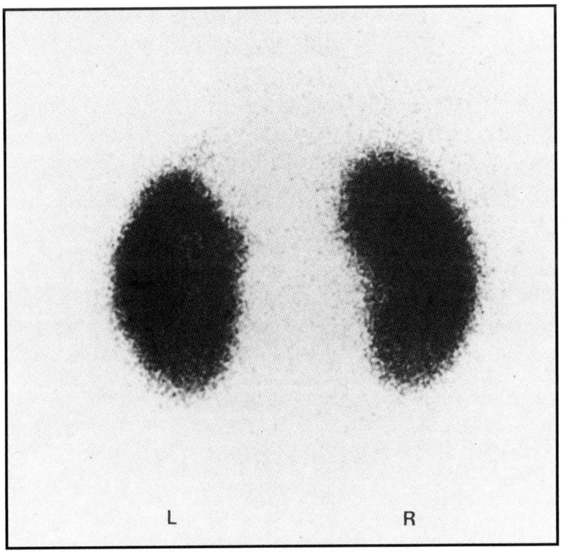

Complications of this procedure are few and rare. Very occasionally, follow-up investigation reveals no function in the remaining lower pole. This could possibly result from torsion if it had not been fixed, but a more likely cause is spasm of the main renal artery due to mobilisation and dissection. This is sometimes recognisable per-operatively and can be reversed by topical application of papaverine or lignocaine solution.

In the occasional case where DMSA scan indicates useful function in the upper pole, there exists the temptation to conserve this by performing pyelo-pyelostomy rather than heminephrectomy. Except where uptake of isotope by the upper pole is well nigh perfect, this temptation is best resisted since:

1. Even in patients with bilateral disease, excision of both upper poles still leaves a handsome reserve of renal function.

2. Pyelo-pyelostomy may be technically unsatisfactory, involving, as it does, anastomosis of a large thick walled upper renal pelvis to a small thin walled lower pelvis.

3. The upper pole is often chronically infected; pyelo-pyelostomy ensures that the lower pole becomes infected also.

Fig. 3.3. DMSA scan. Left duplex system with vaginal ectopic ureter. IVU was equivocal and ultrasound unhelpful. Compared with the right, uptake of isotope is deficient superomedially and there is a thin rim of uptake superolaterally by the dysplastic upper pole.

Single System Ureteric Ectopia

Unilateral Single Ectopic Ureter

Presentation. If the orifice lies in the upper urethra, the symptoms are principally those of infection with urgency as a secondary feature. Rarely the bladder neck mechanism is affected to an extent which allows stress leakage. Vaginal single ectopic ureters, of course, present with continuous dribbling and normal micturition otherwise.

Investigation. There is usually sufficient function for the system to be visualised by IVU although it is usually evident that the system is dilated and dysplastic (Fig. 3.4). The diagnosis can be confirmed by a combination of cystography (which shows reflux into the ectopic system during voiding) and endoscopy.

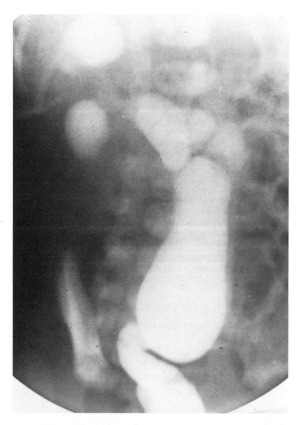

Fig. 3.4. Single ectopic ureter (in a solitary kidney) with urethral termination. Antegrade pyelogram showing a grossly dilated tortuous and dysplastic ureter. Peristalsis was minimal.

Treatment. Nephroureterectomy, with excision of the ureter as close to its ectopic termination as possible, is advisable in most cases. Reimplantation of the ureter into the bladder may be considered if the function is unusually good or if the opposite kidney is compromised in some way.

Bilateral Single Ectopic Ureters

Presentation. In this rare but major abnormality the trigone is absent and the bladder neck grossly incompetent. The bladder itself is usually small and may have deficient musculature. The kidneys are always dysplastic, sometimes severely so, while the ureters are dilated and may have poor peristalsis.

The presenting complaint is one of continual dribbling of urine, without normal micturition otherwise, and the diagnosis is suggested by a combination of normal vulval appearances and absence of neurological signs.

Investigation. In each case details of the anatomy and function must be pursued by a combination of urography, endoscopy and isotope studies. If reconstructive surgery is contemplated, urodynamic studies may be performed to assess detrusor contractility and compliance.

Treatment. The results of treatment remain generally unsatisfactory (Williams 1982). In principle it can be managed by reimplantation of the ureters into the bladder, reconstruction of the bladder neck (Chap. 10) [or placement of an artificial sphincter (Chap. 11)] and, if necessary, enhancement of capacity by bladder augmentation. Where there is marked bilateral renal dysplasia or grossly impaired ureteric peristalsis, such surgical heroics are likely to further compromise renal function. The alternative is some form of urinary diversion (Chap. 12), usually terminal ureterostomy.

Urogenital Sinus Abnormalities

Urogenital sinus abnormalities comprise several rare and somewhat disparate anomalies with the one common feature of a single vulval orifice (Williams and Bloomberg 1976). Only three forms result in urinary incontinence.

Vaginal Atresia and Wide Urethra (Fig. 3.5a)

Here the bladder neck is incompetent to a greater or lesser degree but the bladder itself is normal. The presentation is essentially that of genuine stress incontinence with a fairly normal pattern of micturition otherwise. Patients with a minor degree of bladder neck incompetence may respond to treatment with ephedrine or imipramine. Those with more severe degrees require surgery in the form of bladder neck repair (Chap. 10) or suspension (Chaps. 5,6), or placement of an artificial sphincter (Chap. 11). Vaginoplasty is also necessary.

Vaginal Confluence with Wide Bladder Neck (Fig. 3.5b)

Because there is wide confluence between bladder and vagina, urine dribbles continually. Associated anomalies of the upper renal tracts are common and include vesicoureteric reflux and renal agenesis. The bladder is often small.

If the bladder is of adequate size, it is possible to construct a sphincteric zone by the anterior detrusor tube technique (Chap. 10) with reasonably satisfactory results (Williams and Snyder 1976).

An alternative approach, pioneered by Hendren (1980), concentrates on constructing a distal neourethra from anterior vaginal mucosa and which is covered by a transposition flap from the skin of the perineum (Fig. 3.6). This has the advantages that resistance in the neourethra (particularly distally, where it is covered by the bulbocavernous and ischiocavernous muscles) may be sufficient to produce continence and that if necessary it enables intermittent catheterisation to be practised. If bladder outlet resistance remains insufficient it is still possible to perform a bladder neck repair or implant an artificial sphincter. In cases where the bladder is small and the detrusor low-compliant, this may be corrected by bladder augmentation.

Points essential to the success of this repair are:

1. The patient should be prone with the thighs abducted and the knees flexed; the pubis is supported to avoid extending the lumbar spine.

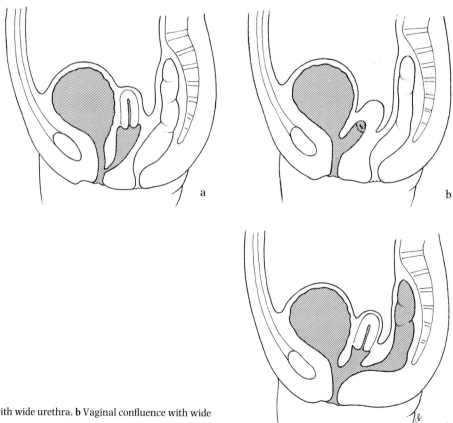

Fig. 3.5. a Vaginal atresia with wide urethra. **b** Vaginal confluence with wide bladder neck. **c** Cloaca.

2. The width of the vaginal strip should be generous and the neourethra should extend as far distally as possible, almost to the clitoris, so that it may be covered by introital muscle.

3. The base of the perineal flap should be wide.

4. A urethral catheter should be left in situ for 2 weeks.

Cloaca (Fig. 3.5c)

Only those patients with wide confluence of bladder and vagina are usually incontinent of urine. A number of girls also have a degree of sacral agenesis so that the problems of neuropathic bladder are added to those of the structural anomaly. Treatment is

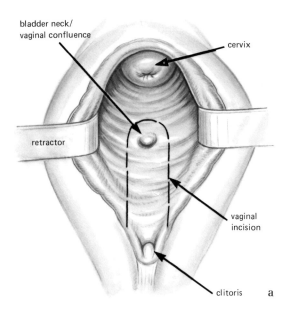

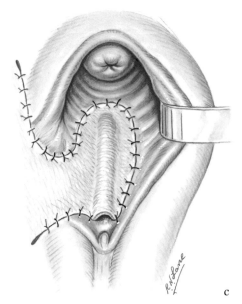

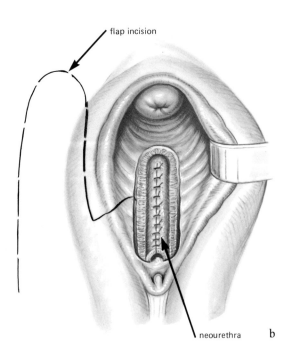

Fig. 3.6a–c. Female urethral reconstruction (Hendren 1980). a The vaginal incision encircling the urethrovaginal confluence and delineating the strip of vaginal mucosa to be tubularised. b After tubularising the vaginal mucosa to form the urethra; the perineal skin flap has been marked out. c The perineal flap inset into the vagina to cover the urethral repair. The base of the flap is divided some 3 months later.

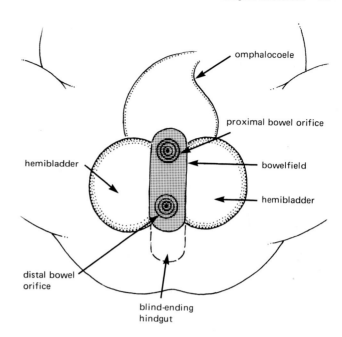

Fig. 3.7. The anatomy of cloacal exstrophy.

broadly along the lines of the previous section and the reconstructive possibilities in this major condition are admirably described by Hendren (1982).

Exstrophic Anomalies

Embryology

The aberration common to all exstrophic anomalies is failure of primitive streak mesoderm to invade the allantoic extension of the infra-umbilical membrane. As a result, this membrane disintegrates along with the cloacal membrane proper and the pelvic viscera become laid open at the surface. The unusual extent of the membrane serves to separate the developing structures of the abdominal wall, resulting in wide divergence of the recti and pubic bones. The same mechanism may also cause partial or complete duplication of the female genital tract.

Variants depend both on the extent of the membrane and on when dehiscence occurs. Classical exstrophy, the commonest anomaly, results from the breakdown of an extensive membrane after completion of the uro-rectal septum so that the primitive urogenital sinus is exteriorised. A less extensive infra-umbilical membrane leads to epispadias only. Cloacal exstrophy is due to earlier

dehiscence, before formation of the uro-rectal septum, so that there is a central bowel field (at the ileocaecal junction) separating the two bladder fields (Fig. 3.7).

Bladder Exstrophy

Presentation

Bladder exstrophy occurs in 1 in 30 000–50 000 live-born females. The size of the bladder varies from one which is almost normal (Fig. 3.8) to one where little more than the trigone is formed. At birth the mucosa is normal and the detrusor supple. Within a few days the mucosa becomes polypoid with squamous metaplasia; these changes reverse if the bladder is closed. Deterioration in the detrusor is slower but irreversible; the muscle becomes infiltrated with fibrous tissue so that the bladder contracts and can no longer be inverted. The urethra is open along its whole length, the clitoris is bifid and the labia widely separated. The anus is anteriorly displaced and the umbilicus lies immediately above the apex of the bladder.

At birth the upper renal tracts are almost always normal but the ureters angle sharply forwards to enter the bladder so that there is potential for vesicoureteric reflux.

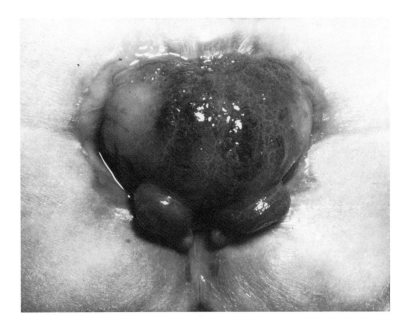

Fig. 3.8. Exstrophy in a female neonate; in this case the bladder is of good size.

Investigation

No more is required than an IVU or ultrasound examination to determine the state of the upper renal tracts.

Treatment

Although active treatment is always advisable, the results are by no means perfect and there are still divergent views as to the effort that should be expended to secure the ideal of full continence *per via naturalis*. A consensus view of basic management is:

1. Primary reconstruction should be attempted in all but the occasional case where the bladder is so small as to be unusable.
2. The results of primary closure are better if undertaken in the neonatal period and combined with closure of the bony pelvic ring.
3. This procedure is intended simply to close the bladder without attempting to prevent vesicoureteric reflux or to produce a fully competent bladder neck; procedures to deal with these problems are deferred until the child is older.
4. Urinary diversion as primary management is reserved for those few cases unsuitable for bladder

closure and as secondary management for patients in whom further attempts to achieve a continent bladder are unlikely to be rewarded.

Primary Bladder Closure. In the first 24–48h of life it is possible to approximate the pubic bones without pelvic osteotomy although the author's preference is for osteotomy even at this age. With the infant prone, the iliac bones are divided through vertical incisions just lateral to the sacro-iliac joints. The halves of the pelvis are then pressed together to stretch the ligamentous and muscular structures which still tend to hold them apart.

The bladder is closed at the same session. Sterile stockings cover the legs so that they can be manipulated when closing the pelvis. The skin incision encircles the bladder and umbilicus (Fig. 3.9a) and the latter is excised after ligating the umbilical vessels. It is usually necessary to free the detrusor from the rectus sheath on each side by sharp dissection, after which the bladder is readily mobilised extra-peritoneally around some two-thirds of its circumference. At the bladder neck, incisions are carried down on each side to isolate a urethral strip some 12–15 mm wide. These incisions can also be extended upwards for 5 mm and triangular areas of bladder muscle and mucosa excised on each side (Fig. 3.9a). This serves to elongate the urethra and further define the bladder neck. Immediately below the bladder neck bands of fibrous tissue (allegedly

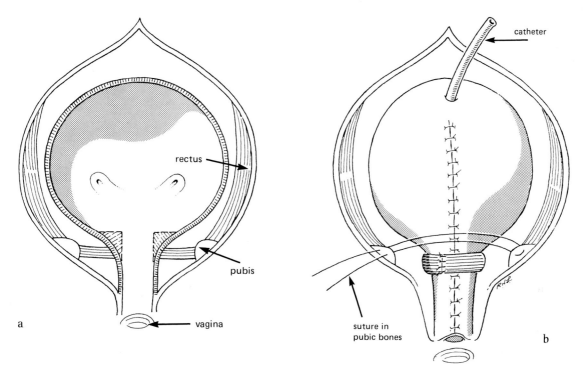

Fig. 3.9. a The incision encircles the bladder and umbilicus (which is excised) and the bladder is mobilised extra-peritoneally. A urethral strip is isolated and triangular areas (shaded) excised at the bladder neck. The tips of the pubic bones are exposed and the ligamentous bands extending from them to the urethra defined. **b** The bladder and urethra have been closed and the ligamentous bands overlapped around the bladder neck. A suture has been placed to approximate the pubic bones.

representing remnants of the urethral sphincter) extend laterally to the pubic bones. These are dissected free and detached from the bones.

A Malecot catheter (10–12F) is brought into the bladder high on its posterior wall and the bladder is then closed in two layers of chromic catgut, a running 4–0 suture for the mucosa and interrupted 3–0 for the muscularis. The urethra is closed with a single layer of 3–0 suture and the previously isolated fibrous bands sutured around the bladder neck (Fig. 3.9b).

The legs are flexed and internally rotated to approximate the two halves of the pelvis, which are then sutured together with strong (No. 1) chromic catgut passed through the bones. The bladder catheter is brought out at the "normal" umbilical site and the recti approximated with 2–0 or 3–0 polyglycolic acid (Dexon) sutures. The skin is closed vertically and the two halves of the clitoris brought together. Urethral catheter drainage is unnecessary and may even be disadvantageous (Jeffs 1983).

In neonates it is sufficient to protect the repair for 2–3 weeks with one crepe bandage around the pelvis and another holding the legs together. Infants and older children should be immobilised in gallows or Bryant's traction for 4–6 weeks. Three to four weeks postoperatively the urethral repair is examined under anaesthetic and if this is satisfactory the bladder catheter is removed.

A minor degree of breakdown of the distal urethral repair is common and of little consequence. Occasionally the entire repair disintegrates; this does not preclude a further attempt at repair later.

Secondary Procedures. Few girls become dry following primary closure as described since the bladder neck is not usually competent. Although functional capacity remains small, cystometrograms usually show a slow increase over a period of years. The timing of further surgery depends on this increase. Jeffs (1983) considers a cystometrogram capacity of 50 ml at 3 years of age sufficient to embark on bladder neck repair.

The repairs employed are those of Young–Dees (Young 1919; Dees 1949) or Leadbetter (1964) (Chap. 10), the former often modified by tubularising mucosa only and using the resulting muscle flaps to reinforce the bladder neck. The ureters are reimplanted at a higher level in the bladder to prevent reflux.

Failure of this repair may be due to:

1. Continuing incompetence of the bladder neck. A further attempt may be considered; alternatively success has been reported in a limited number of patients using the artificial sphincter (Light and Scott 1983).
2. Persistently small bladder capacity (detrusor low-compliance); in principle this can be treated by bladder augmentation although the patient may need to practise intermittent self-catheterisation afterwards.
3. Overflow incontinence resulting from a combination of a well repaired bladder neck and poor detrusor contractility; this is unusual but can be managed effectively by intermittent catheterisation.

Upper Renal Tract Complications. These may occur after primary or secondary procedures and comprise ureterovesical obstruction and pyelonephritis as a result of reflux; a recent estimate is that they occur in some 15% of cases (Turner et al. 1981).

Urinary Diversion. Inevitably a proportion of patients come to urinary diversion. Provided anal control is adequate and the upper renal tracts normal (or nearly so), ureterosigmoidostomy has been favoured although the emerging long-term risk of juxta-anastomotic colonic carcinoma is modifying this view. The best alternative is probably a non-refluxing colonic conduit (Altwein et al. 1977).

Epispadias

Presentation

Epispadias is very rare in girls. The dorsal aspect of the urethra is variably deficient and the clitoris bifid. As a rule the urethral sphincter is absent and the bladder neck wholly incompetent so that the child dribbles urine continuously. The bladder may be small and thin walled.

Investigation

An IVU or ultrasound examination is advisable to assess the upper renal tracts and a filling urodynamic study may be helpful in estimating detrusor compliance and contractility.

Treatment

The urethra may be repaired prior to bladder neck reconstruction or simultaneously, the latter usually being undertaken at 3–6 years of age. The techniques employed may be as for exstrophy (though with rather superior results because of better quality tissues) or the Tanagho repair (Chap. 10). Johnston (1977) reports that following a posterior reconstruction of the urethra, the bladder can fall forwards into the prevesical space so that the internal meatus lies high on the posterior wall of the bladder and may cause difficulty in micturition. This can be prevented by using an omental graft to fill the dead space in front of the bladder.

Cloacal Exstrophy

Presentation

In this most extreme form of exstrophy (Fig. 3.10) boys outnumber girls but because the penis is usually bifid and rudimentary, most are re-assigned as females after castration. Associated anomalies are many and common and include omphalocoele, blind-ending hindgut, short bowel proximally, spinal anomalies (hemi-vertebrae, spina bifida, sacral agenesis) and abnormalities of the upper renal tracts.

Management

As an initial procedure, the bowel field is separated from the two halves of the bladder, which are then sutured together in the midline. The bowel field can either be reconstructed, and the distal blind-ending hindgut brought as a colostomy, or separated, with the proximal end brought out as an ileostomy and the distal bowel left in situ in the hope that it may later be used for some reconstructive purpose. In principle, at least, the bladder can later be repaired

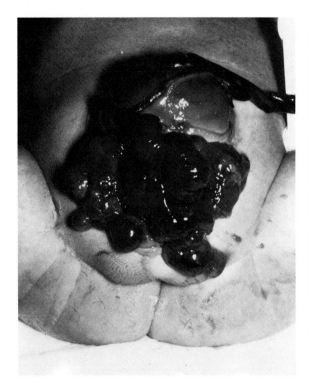

Fig. 3.10. Cloacal exstrophy in a neonate. Bowel has prolapsed between the two bladder fields. There is an associated omphalocoele.

as with exstrophy but although a few wholly successful reconstructions have been reported, the more usual final result is two abdominal stomata, the one for faeces, the other for urine.

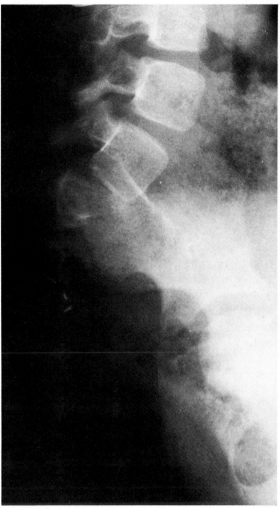

Fig. 3.11. Sacral agenesis.

Congenital Neuropathic Bladder

Several congenital lesions of the spinal cord cause neuropathic bladder, much the commonest being myelomeningocoele. Other anomalies are quite rare and include lipoma of the cauda equina (lumbosacral lipoma), diastematomyelia and intra-spinal lipomata and dermoid cysts. Sacral agenesis (Fig. 3.11) is an example of caudal regression rather than spina bifida, although the neurological impact on the bladder is similar. For many of these patients, the bladder disorder is their major handicap and their quality and expectation of life are largely dependent on how well it is managed.

As well as incontinence, neuropathic bladder may cause secondary deterioration of the upper renal tracts. This is less common in girls than boys and tends to occur in infancy rather than later in childhood. The first priority is, therefore, protection of renal function with continence a secondary objective. Dryness is ideally achieved without use of urinary appliances or diversion and in a way the patient can practice independently. Essential for appliance-free continence are:

1. *Adequate functional bladder capacity*

2. *Complete emptying of the bladder*: this both maximises effective capacity and helps maintain normality of the upper renal tracts.

3. *Voiding at will*: patients with neuropathic bladder never void normally, so some abnormal method must be used.

Clean intermittent self-catheterisation (CISC), the major advance in recent years, may be used to illustrate these principles; the process achieves both emptying and voiding at will but will only make the patient dry if the bladder has adequate functional capacity.

Presentation

Usually the diagnosis is obvious. A few myelomeningocoele patients with incomplete cord lesions achieve a form of control erroneously labelled "normal" (q.v.) and some patients with skin-covered lesions escape detection in early childhood although elementary attention to history and examination should identify these. Sacral agenesis is more easily missed since the neurological deficit is often minimal and bowel control usually normal, but the sacral deficiency is easily felt and there is frequently a characteristic flattening of the upper buttocks.

Classification and Pathophysiology

Classically, neuropathic bladder dysfunction has been considered in relation to the cord lesion:

1. Supra-sacral cord lesion (*hyperreflexic bladder*): the sacral reflex arcs are intact but isolated by a lesion higher in the cord so that the patient voids reflexly but unknowingly.

2. Sacral cord lesion (*autonomous bladder*): the bladder (and urethral sphincter) is centrally denervated, so that the patient voids by overflow or by raising intra-vesical pressure by abdominal compression or straining.

The reality is much more complex, but for present purposes this classification is retained.

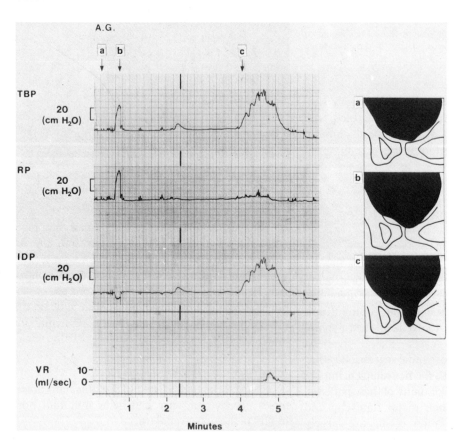

Fig. 3.12a–c. Hyperreflexic bladder in a male myelomeningocoele patient. **a** The bladder neck is closed at rest and **b** remains so during a rise in intra-abdominal pressure. **c** It opens at the onset of a hyperreflexic detrusor contraction but there is initial complete detrusor–sphincter dyssynergia lasting approximately 30 s.

Hyperreflexic Bladder

This occurs in around a third of myelomeningocoele patients and a still smaller proportion of those with other lesions. Clinically the ano-cutaneous reflex is positive and the patient voids spontaneously. As a rule no urine can be passed by abdominal straining or compression although in some suprapubic compression provokes hyperreflexic detrusor contrac-

tions, so giving the spurious impression that the bladder is "expressible".

The urodynamic features are fairly consistent. Usually the bladder neck is competent and there is no stress leakage (Fig. 3.12). Major degrees of detrusor low-compliance are uncommon. Filling ultimately provokes a hyperreflexic detrusor contraction, usually generating above normal pressure. Detrusor-sphincter dyssynergia is almost invariably present (Fig. 3.13) and is initially complete so that

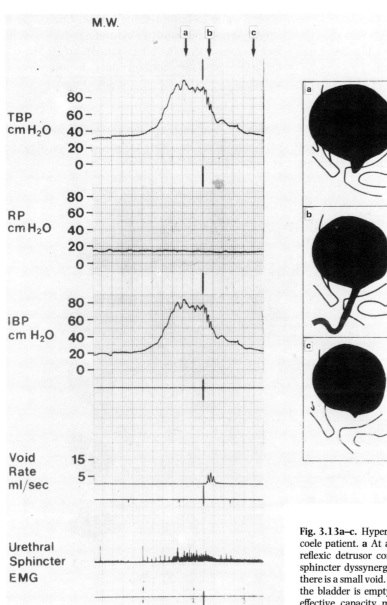

Fig. 3.13a–c. Hyperreflexic bladder in a male myelomeningocoele patient. **a** At a filling volume of 120 ml there is a hyperreflexic detrusor contraction with initially complete detrusor–sphincter dyssynergia. **b** After 1 min the sphincter relaxes and there is a small void. **c** The detrusor contraction fades away before the bladder is empty. The functional capacity is small and the effective capacity minute. [Reproduced from Rickwood AMK (1984) The neuropathic bladder in children. In: Mundy AR, Stephenson T, Wein A (eds) Urodynamics: principles and practice and application, Churchill Livingstone, Edinburgh, p 331]

no urine passes for a period of a few seconds to a minute or two. As the sphincter relaxes (often incompletely) voiding occurs but the detrusor contraction often fades away before the bladder is empty (Fig. 3.13) (non-sustained detrusor contraction).

An important subcategory exists in patients with incomplete cord lesions with retention of spinothalamic sacral sensation. Clinically they have marked urgency since they are aware of detrusor contractions yet cannot control them. If they have adequate functional and effective capacity, good mobility and prolonged complete initial detrusor–sphincter dyssynergia, they can be continent, albeit somewhat precariously. It is important that they are not labelled as having a "normal" bladder since their upper renal tracts remain at risk.

Autonomous Bladder

Clinically the ano-cutaneous reflex is usually negative. Patients tend to dribble urine but can also void

a stream by abdominal straining or compression and some void spontaneously also. The urodynamic features are variable and best considered separately.

Sphincter Weakness Incontinence (SWI). This is always present by definition; were it not it would be impossible to void by straining or compression. The degree of SWI varies widely. At one extreme it is gross, so that residual urine and functional capacity are small, and at the other it is mild, resulting in a bladder of good functional but small effective capacity due to large residual urine. Gross SWI is comparatively unusual in girls and is reflected in the fact that series of spina bifida patients treated by the artificial sphincter contain only a minority of females.

Detrusor Low-Compliance. This is common but only of importance if occurring in the physiological range of capacity (Fig. 3.14).

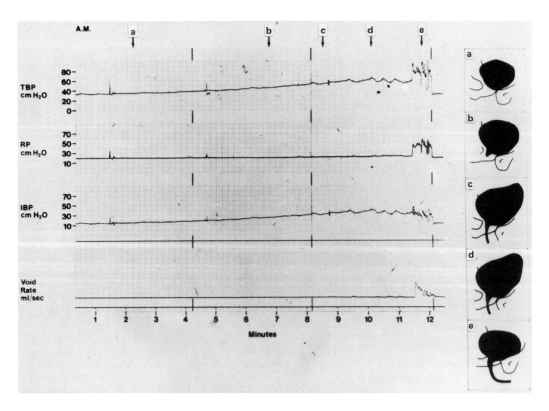

Fig. 3.14a–e. Detrusor low-compliance in a male myelomeningocoele patient. End-filling pressure of 35 cmH$_2$O at filling volume of 150 ml. **a** The bladder neck is initially closed but **b** opens as the intravesical pressure rises. **c** Later there is overflow and **d** then a series of very low pressure detrusor contractions with small voids. **e** The patient strains to void and when the bladder is empty, the baseline pressure returns to normal. [Reproduced from Rickwood AMK (1984) The neuropathic bladder in children. In: Mundy AR, Stephenson T, Wein A (eds) Urodynamics; principles and practice and application, Churchill Livingstone, Edinburgh, p 334]

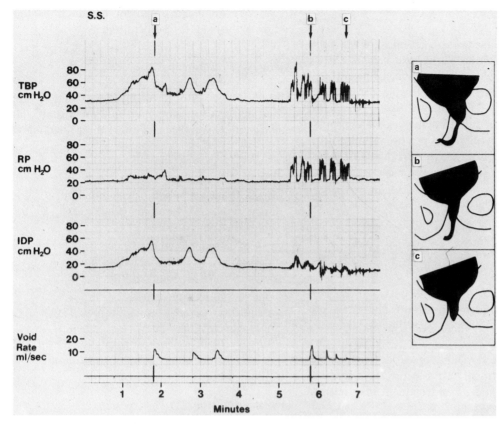

Fig. 3.15a–c. Mixed urodynamic picture in a male patient with lipoma of the cauda equina. **a** There is a series of hyperreflexic voiding contractions. **b** Later the patient voids by straining with **c** obstruction at the level of the urethral sphincter (isolated distal sphincter obstruction). [Reproduced from Rickwood AMK (1984) The neuropathic bladder in children. In: Mundy AR, Stephenson T, Wein A (eds) Urodynamics; principles and practice and application, Churchill Livingstone, Edinburgh, p 336]

Detrusor Hyperreflexia. The true autonomous bladder is quite flaccid, but in practice low pressure contractions are often observed (Figs. 3.14, 3.15); these usually contribute little to total voided volume but often serve to limit functional capacity.

Bladder Outlet Obstruction. Outlet obstruction, if present, is almost always located at the level of the urethral sphincter. If occurring in the absence of a detrusor contraction, it is not, by definition,

detrusor–sphincter dyssynergia and has been termed "isolated distal sphincter obstruction" (Rickwood et al. 1982). The cause is not always clear but this is of little practical consequence.

Factors which limit the ability of the neuropathic bladder to fill and empty are summarised in Table 3.1; it should be appreciated that in any one patient, several may be operative simultaneously.

Causes of Upper Renal Tract Deterioration

1. Bladder outlet obstruction: there is usually, but not always, residual urine; upper tract complications are uncommon if the bladder empties fully and easily.

2. Vesicoureteric reflux

3. Urinary tract infections: these are probably only of consequence if there is also vesicoureteric reflux.

4. Detrusor low-compliance.

Table 3.1. Factors affecting the performance of congenital neuropathic bladder

---

Causes of reduced functional capacity
    Detrusor hyperreflexia
    Detrusor low-compliance
    Sphincter weakness
Causes of failure to empty
    Detrusor–sphincter dyssynergia
    Isolated distal sphincter obstruction
    Non-sustained detrusor contraction

Investigation

The state of the upper renal tracts must be regularly monitored, ultrasound being most convenient for this purpose, supplemented as required by IVU and isotope studies. The nature of the bladder dysfunction can often be adequately assessed by careful clinical judgement, but urodynamic studies provide more exact information and are essential if SWI is to be treated surgically. The investigation is best combined with simultaneous video-radiological examination.

Management

Principles

1. Maintenance of renal function is always the primary concern; most important is that bladder outlet obstruction be treated.

2. Because bladder dysfunction varies considerably, so too must treatment, and because the disorder is often complex, methods of treatment may need to be used in combination.

3. Management must be realistically related to the patient's physical and intellectual abilities: girls with neuropathic bladder frequently have other disabilities, which include paralysis, deformity and, with myelomeningocoele, intellectual impairment;

these may influence treatment as much as the nature of the bladder disorder itself.

Methods of Treatment

The desirable aspects of bladder function are adequate capacity, emptying and voiding at will, and treatment is considered under these headings.

Inadequate Functional Capacity

1. Due to detrusor hyperreflexia
   Medication: oxybutynin, propantheline
   Surgery: sacral rhizotomy (Clarke et al. 1979), bladder augmentation

2. Due to detrusor low-compliance
   Medication: oxybutynin, imipramine
   Surgery: bladder augmentation

3. Due to sphincter weakness
   Medication: ephedrine, imipramine (effective only when SWI is mild)
   Surgery: bladder neck reconstruction (Chap. 10) or suspension (Chaps. 5, 6, 8), artificial sphincter (Chap. 11).

Inadequate Emptying

1. Medication
   Detrusor–sphincter dyssynergia: diazepam, baclofen, dantrolene (rarely effective)
   Isolated distal sphincter obstruction: phenoxybenzamine (inconsistently effective)

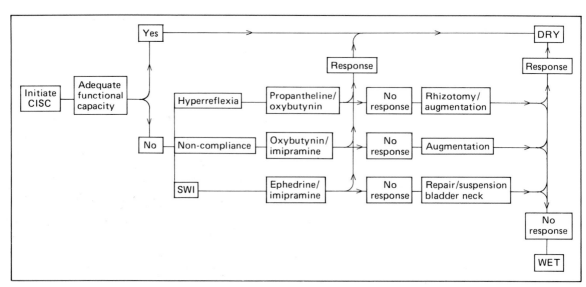

Fig. 3.16. Management of neuropathic bladder by clean intermittent self-catheterisation. This scheme assumes that there is only one factor operating to limit functional capacity; if there is more than one, methods must be used in combination (see Fig. 3.17).

2. Surgery
   Bladder flap urethroplasty (Scott et al. 1973)
   Otis urethrotomy (Chap. 13) (Rickwood 1982)
3. Catheters
   Intermittent
   Indwelling

Means of Voiding at Will

1. Abdominal compression or straining (autonomous bladders): Often this does not empty the bladder unless outlet resistance is low, in which event functional capacity is likely to be low also; the method is most effective when used in conjunction with the artificial sphincter.
2. Clean intermittent self-catheterisation: This is the only way patients with hyperreflexic bladders

can void at will and is the preferred method in patients with autonomous bladders when compression or straining leaves an appreciable residual urine.

Synthesis of Management

Individual methods of treatment must often be used in combination. As a rule, when SWI is absent or mild, CISC is the treatment of choice in conjunction with appropriate medical or surgical measures if functional capacity is lacking (Fig. 3.16). If there is gross SWI, the alternatives are use of CISC with repair or suspension of the bladder neck (Fig. 3.17) or elimination of all outlet resistance and implantation of an artificial sphincter. Patients considered

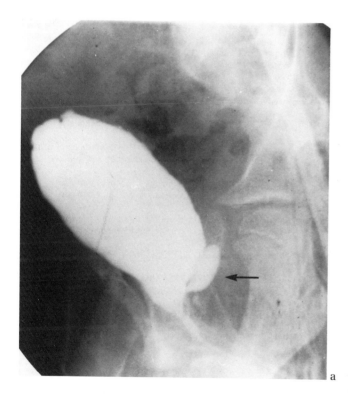

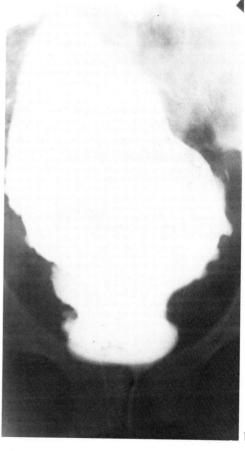

Fig. 3.17. *Left:* Myelomeningocoele patient wet on CISC. The bladder neck is grossly incompetent with reflux into the stump of a urethral ectopic ureter (*arrow*). Urodynamic study showed low compliance (end-filling pressure 35 cmH$_2$O at 150 ml filling volume) and low pressure hyperreflexic contractions. *Right:* Situation following bladder augmentation with sigmoid colon and Marshall-Marchetti-Krantz bladder neck suspension. The bladder neck is competent and contrast fills the augmentation superiorly and the bladder inferiorly. End-filling pressure is 15 cmH$_2$O at 400 ml. Voided volumes on CISC are 350 ml plus: patient dry.

Table 3.2. Criteria for implanting AMS prosthetic sphincter

The patient
  Adequate motivation
  Adequate manipulative skill
  Ability to strain (motor level below D12)
The upper renal tracts
  Good function
  No dilatation
  No reflux
The bladder
  Absent or minimal hyperreflexia (controlled by medication if necessary)
  Good compliance
  Not thick walled
  No outlet obstruction (preliminary surgery if present)

for this device should satisfy fairly stringent criteria (Table 3.2).

Appliance-free continence is not always a realistic goal, especially for more severely disabled girls. Here, the possibilities are:

1. Urinary diversion (Chap. 12): The poor long-term results of refluxing ileal or colonic conduit diversions performed in childhood are well documented (e.g. Middleton and Hendren 1976); non-refluxing colonic conduits give superior, if not ideal, results (Altwein et al. 1977).

2. Indwelling urethral catheter: The humble catheter remains a largely unregarded expedient, yet gives generally satisfactory results if handled properly (Rickwood et al. 1983).

References

Altwein JE, Jonas U, Hohenfellner R (1977) Long-term follow-up of children with colon conduit urinary diverion and ureterosigmoidostomy. J Urol 118:832–836

Clarke SJ, Forster DMC, Thomas DG (1979) Selective sacral neurectomy in the management of incontinence due to detrusor instability. Br J Urol 51:510–514

Dees JE (1949) Congenital epispadias with incontinence. J Urol 62:513–520

Hendren WH (1980) Construction of females urethra from the vaginal wall and perineal flap. J Urol 123:657–664

Hendren WH (1982) Further experience in reconstructive surgery for chloachal anomalies. J Pediatr Surg 17:695–717

Jeffs RD (1983) Complications in exstrophy surgery. Urol Clin North Am 10:509–518

Johnston JH (1977) Exstrophy of the bladder and epispadias. In: Williams DI (ed) Operative surgery: urology, 3rd edn. Butterworths, London, p 228

Koff SA (1983) Disordered vesicourethral function in the pathogenesis of urinary infection and vesicoureteric reflux. In: Johnston JH (ed) Management of vesicoureteric reflux. Williams and Wilkins, Baltimore, pp 67–81

Leadbetter GW (1964) Surgical correction of total urinary incontinence. J Urol 91:738–745

Light JK, Scott FB (1983) Treatment of epispadias–exstrophy complex with the AM 792 artificial urinary sphincter. J Urol 129:738–740

Middleton AW, Hendren WH (1976) Ileal conduits at the Massachusetts General Hospital from 1955–1970. J Urol 115:591–595

Rickwood AMK (1982) Use of internal urethrotomy to reverse upper renal tract dilatation in children with neuropathic bladder dysfunction. Br J Urol 54:292–294

Rickwood AMK, Thomas DG, Philp NH, Spicer RD (1982) Assessment of congenital neuropathic bladder by combined urodynamic and radiological studies. Br J Urol 54:512–518

Rickwood AMK, Philp NH, Thomas DG (1983) Long-term catheterisation for congenital neuropathic bladder. Arch Dis Child 58:111–116

Scott FB, Bradley WE, Timm GW (1973) Treatment of urinary incontinence by implantable prosthetic sphincter. Urol 1:252–258

Turner WR, Ransley PG, Williams DI (1981) Patterns of renal damage in the management of vesical exstrophy. J Urol 124:412–415

Williams DI (1982) Ureteric duplications and ectopia. In: Williams DI, Johnston JH (eds) Paediatric urology, 2nd ed. Butterworths, London, pp 167–187

Williams DI, Bloomberg S (1976) Urogenital sinus in the female child. J Pediatr Surg 11:51–56

Williams DI, Snyder H (1976) Anterior detrusor tube repair for urinary incontinence in children. Br J Urol 48:671–677

Williams DI, Hirst G, Doyle D (1974) The occult neuropathic bladder. J Pediatr Surg 9:35–42

Young HH (1919) An operation for the cure of incontinence of urine. Surg Gynecol Obstet 28:24–90

4 Anterior Repair

David Warrell

Introduction

Over the last decade or so there has been a swing away from vaginal to suprapubic surgery as first time treatment of women with genuine stress incontinence. This has come about because of dissatisfaction with the low cure rates obtained from vaginal repair operations. However, some surgeons, e.g. Green (1980) have achieved a satisfactory cure rate from vaginal surgery by the selection of patients for this approach using lateral cystourethrography. The philosophy of selection of patients with stress incontinence for either a vaginal or abdominal approach is one that commends itself to me, since each approach has inherent advantages and disadvantages. If all patients are treated vaginally the cure rate is likely to be lower than if all patients are treated by a suprapubic operation. On the other hand vaginal surgery is unlikely to produce other problems, as can occur after suprapubic surgery. The high position of the urethro-vesical junction achieved by suprapubic surgery causes long-term voiding difficulties for some women and may initiate urgency and urge incontinence in others. It would be ideal to be able to pick out patients who would stand a good chance of being cured by vaginal surgery and reserve a suprapubic approach for the rest. This chapter explores the basis of selection and outlines a technique of vaginal surgery.

The two major factors in genuine stress incontinence are the competence of the sphincter mechanism intrinsic to the urethra and the site of the urethrovesical junction. Traditionally bladder neck prolapse has been associated with stress incontinence, but this is not always the case, and there are many women suffering from genuine stress incontinence who have no more bladder descent and mobility than continent multipara. Measurement of the occlusive forces generated by the urethral sphincter mechanism has shown that women with stress incontinence have weaker urethral closure forces than the continent. However, there is overlap, and up to now it has not been possible to discriminate individually between the continent and the stress incontinent by measurement of urethral closure forces (Henriksson 1979). A third factor in urinary control is the extent of the forces expelling urine. Obesity is important because the intravesical pressure of obese women in the erect position is two or three times greater than in thin women. Women suffering from stress incontinence often generate cough pressures well in excess of those seen in continent women.

Urinary control can be likened to an equation. As a working hypothesis this author believes that continence is determined by the extent of the expelling forces, the strength of the occlusive forces generated by the urethral sphincter and the position of the urethrovesical junction, the latter probably determining how increases in intra-abdominal pressure affect the urethra. If there is no prolapse, increases in abdominal pressure are transmitted to the bladder as forces opening the urethra, and to the urethra as forces occluding it. The effect of urethrovesical prolapse is to maximise the opening effect and to lessen the transmission of forces occluding the urethra. Thus, if the sphincter is very weak, stress incontinence may occur with minimal prolapse. Conversely, even if there is considerable prolapse and the sphincter generates normal closure forces, the woman will be continent.

When there is genital tract prolapse other factors may contribute to continence. For example, acute rises in intra-abdominal pressure may cause a large cystocele to kink the urethra, or a large rectocele may press against the urethra and occlude it. Ideally, before deciding therapy, the forces expelling urine, the urethral closure forces and the degree of urethrovesical prolapse should all be objectively assessed, and a judgement made on the interrelationship and importance of the factors causing incontinence.

If urethrovesical prolapse is the major factor causing incontinence then restoration of the urethrovesical junction to its pre-parturition position should restore control. However, if the expelling forces are great, the sphincter is feeble and there is little descent, then a vaginal repair operation which alters the position of the bladder neck but which cannot affect the occlusive forces generated by the urethral sphincter is unlikely to restore control. Such a patient needs to be considered for suprapubic surgery.

Pre-operative Evaluation

It is self-evident that the correct diagnosis must be made and patients must indeed be suffering from genuine stress incontinence and not from any other type of incontinence. There are many ways of establishing a confident diagnosis. The investigations available for the assessment of a woman suffering from incontinence have been described in Chap. 2. In order to avoid repetition only the features which seem important to this author will be highlighted.

The History

Women suffering from genuine stress incontinence alone should not suffer from disturbance of bladder behaviour; symptoms such as nocturia and urge incontinence suggest other causes. Urine is lost only during activities which increase intra-abdominal pressure.

Examination

A number of physical signs need to be elicited. Most important, stress incontinence needs to be demonstrated and if it cannot then it is most unlikely the patient has any material degree of sphincter weakness, certainly not sufficient to warrant surgical treatment. However, care is needed during examination to be sure about the presence or absence of this physical sign. First, the patient has to have urine in the bladder. Preferably she should not have voided for at least an hour before examination. Second, the external meatus needs to be visualised for stress incontinence to be distinguished from the more prolonged jet of urine which may be seen in a cough-provoked bladder contraction. If stress incontinence can be easily demonstrated with the patient supine then it is likely the patient has a severe degree of sphincter weakness. If stress incontinence cannot be demonstrated supine the patient should be stood up, the external meatus visualised and the patient asked to cough hard. If stress if not seen then it is most unlikely that the patient has genuine stress incontinence. Next the type and degree of prolapse should be established. This necessitates the use of a Sims speculum and requires formal recognition of descent of the different parts of the genital tract, in particular the urethra, the urethrovesical junction and the trigone. Having assessed prolapse with the patient on the couch she should then be re-examined erect. The examiner who is not in the habit of doing this will be surprised by the change in the degree of descent. It is particularly important to assess urethrovesical descent in this fashion, for what has been thought to be a reasonably supported urethrovesical junction may be found to descend outside the vulva when the patient is examined erect.

The pelvic floor should be assessed for tone, bulk and episiotomy damage. Many cases of sphincter weakness have a thin, poor tone pelvic floor. It seems likely that partial denervation is an important factor in the aetiology of both stress incontinence and genital tract prolapse (Smith 1984). Clinical evidence that the pelvic floor is severely affected is an adverse sign for successful vaginal surgery. The bladder and urethra should be palpated. Tenderness of the bladder or trigone or tenderness and thickening of the urethra suggests the presence of a lesion causing a sensory abnormality of bladder function which is incompatible with the diagnosis of simple stress incontinence. Lastly, the extent of the forces expelling urine, i.e. chronic cough and obesity, should be assessed.

Investigations

The purpose of investigation is to confirm the clinical diagnosis of genuine stress incontinence and to measure the factors concerned with control. The simplest, cheapest and probably most useful investigation is to ask the patient to fill in a micturition/volume chart for a few days (Chap. 2).

Cystometry is important as it provides objective assessment of bladder function. During the filling phase it is important to note the ability of the patient to inhibit bladder contractions. At capacity, the patient should stand, move about and reproduce the activities causing incontinence without provoking a contraction of the bladder. About 10% of women with genuine stress incontinence have an impaired capacity to void and these patients may have voiding difficulties following surgery. In these women, damage to both sphincter mechanism and the autonomic nerve supply to the bladder may have occurred with parturition.

Without doubt the most important test of sphincter competence is the demonstration of stress incontinence.

The previous author of this Chapter (Green 1980) based the choice between a vaginal or suprapubic approach on a lateral X-ray of the bladder taken at rest and strain, the bladder being outlined with contrast material and the urethra with a Bead chain. His view was that if there was loss of the posterior

urethrovaginal angle alone, good results are obtained with vaginal surgery. However, if there was loss of the urethrovesical angle and an axial rotation of the bladder base, then vaginal surgery alone was unlikely to cure the patient. It seems likely that these two appearances portray differing degrees of pelvic floor damage, the latter appearance reflecting underlying severe tissue damage. In these cases a less than satisfactory result of vaginal surgery may occur, owing to the difficulty of permanently supporting the bladder neck in its pre-parturition position by a technique relying on suture of intrinsically weakened tissues.

Patient Selection

At the conclusion of assessment, the investigator should have a concept of the extent of the expelling forces, the degree of weakness of the urethral sphincter mechanism and the type and degree of prolapse. The choice of surgery is based on these factors.

It needs to be emphasised that there is no place for a second vaginal approach if the first has failed to cure the patient, as the cure rate in these circumstances will be less than 30%.

Contraindications

The following are contraindications for a vaginal approach and would be better managed by a suprapubic operation:

1. High expelling forces
2. A very weak urethral sphincter mechanism with gross stress incontinence and clinical evidence of partial denervation of the pelvic floor
3. Stress incontinence in the absence of prolapse
4. Previous unsuccessful continence surgery

It is my practice to operate vaginally on patients with bladder neck prolapse and moderate stress incontinence. These comprise about 80% of patients with primary stress incontinence.

Pre-operative Preparation

There are no special preparations and there is no routine chemotherapy cover.

Operative Technique

Anterior repair or anterior colporrhaphy are general terms describing the repair of a cystocele or a cysto-urethrocele. The term urethroplasty or bladder neck buttress should be used for the surgery of stress incontinence, with the operative site confined to the urethra, urethrovesical junction and trigone. Where appropriate it will form part of an anterior repair. What follows is a description of the urethroplasty.

The aim of surgery is to restore permanently the urethrovesical junction to its position prior to childbirth, with restoration of pressure transmission to the urethra (Weil et al. 1984). This can be achieved by plication of the pubocervical fascia beneath the bladder neck. However, the tissues beneath the urethra may be poor. Beck and McCormick (1982) have emphasised the need to take a deep bite of tissue either side of the bladder neck in order to achieve substantial elevation.

The choice of suture material is important. Fibroblasts take 3–4 months to mature. It seems rational to use suture material that will maintain the bladder neck in its new position for as long as possible. In practice this is a choice between Dexon or Vicryl and non-absorbable suture material. My own preference is for the non-absorbable suture Mersilene, the only disadvantage of this being the occasional extrusion of a suture. Beck and McCormick (1982) have achieved a 80% 2-year cure rate from vaginal surgery with Dexon.

It is helpful but not essential to inject the subepithelial tissues of the anterior vaginal wall with a 1:200 000 solution of adrenaline to minimise bleeding (Fig. 4.1).

A mid-line incision is made into the anterior vaginal wall skin from near the external meatus extending towards the cervix for say 8 cm (Figs. 4.2, 4.3). The skin edges are grasped with tissue forceps and the vaginal skin is separated from the underlying fascia with sharp dissection until the subpubic arch is reached. (Figures 4.4 and 4.5 show the plane of dissection.)

At this point the fascia lying underneath the urethra and trigone can be separated from the vaginal skin and vaginal fascia with blunt dissection (Fig. 4.6). If the correct plane has been found this manoeuvre is usually avascular. The dissection

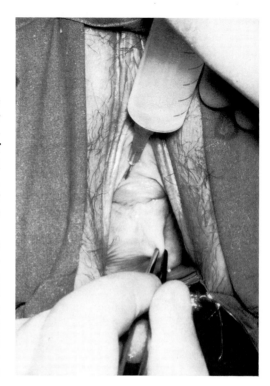

Fig. 4.1. Injection of adrenaline.

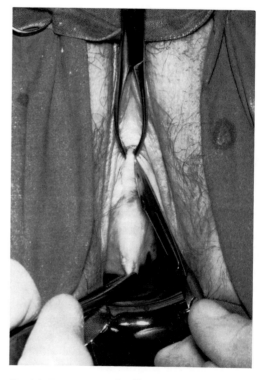

Fig. 4.2. Anterior vaginal wall incision.

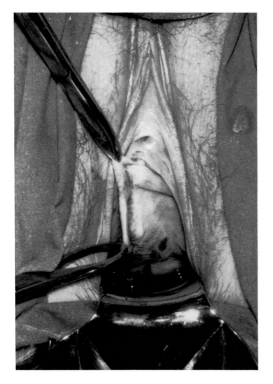

Fig. 4.3. Extent of incision.

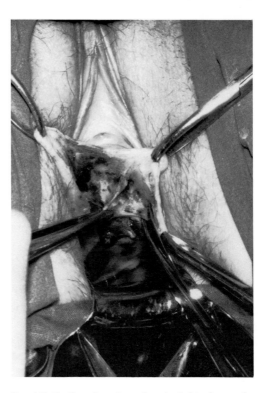

Fig. 4.5. Further dissection of vaginal skin from pubocervical fascia.

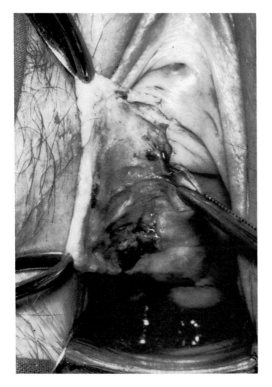

Fig. 4.4. Separation of vaginal skin from underlying pubocervical fascia.

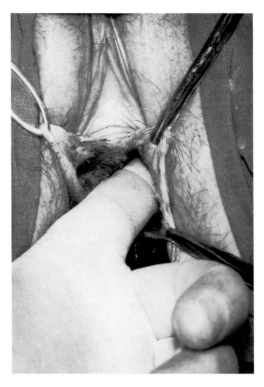

Fig. 4.6. Blunt dissection extending laterally.

must be carried out for 6–7 cm lateral to the mid-line. This distance is necessary in order to achieve satisfactory elevation of the bladder neck. (Figure 4.7 shows the completed dissection.) At this stage the urethra and trigone can usually be recognised. If not it is helpful to determine the position of the internal urethral meatus with a Foley catheter. The aim is to elevate the area of the urethrovesical junction as high as possible. The pubocervical fascia is grasped and a deep bite is taken either side of the urethra (Figs. 4.8–4.10). Three or four number 0 Mersilene sutures are placed in the fascia as high as possible on either side of the urethra, the urethrovesical junction and the proximal trigone. Since they are placed lateral to the urethra it is safe to take a generous bite of tissue. The sutures are tied so as to approximate the pubocervical fascia underneath the urethra and proximal trigone (Figs. 4.11, 4.12). They should not be tied too tight or the tissue encompassed by the suture will be devitalised and the suture material will cut out. The fascia now supports the bladder neck in a sling. Next the skin edges are trimmed and sutured with number 1 chromic catgut, tacking it to the fascia in an attempt to

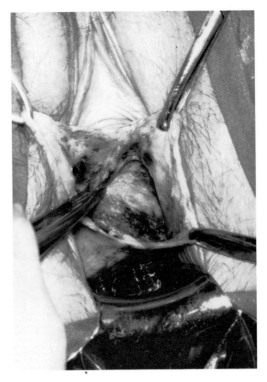

Fig. 4.8. Site of deep suture.

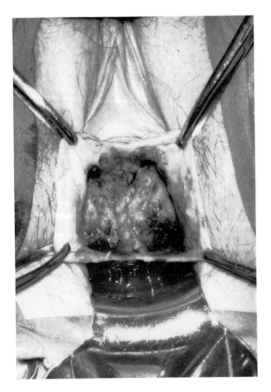

Fig. 4.7. Extent of dissection.

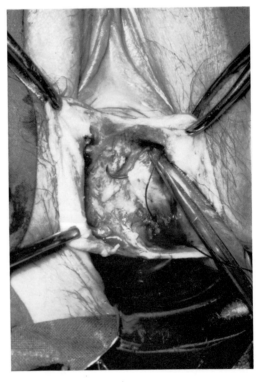

Fig. 4.9. Insertion of deep suture into pubocervical fascia, lateral to the urethra.

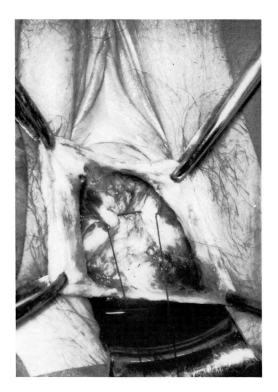

Fig. 4.10. First Mersilene suture in position.

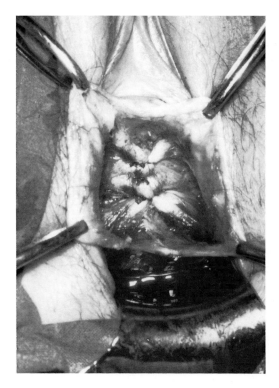

Fig. 4.12. Bladder neck support complete.

obliterate dead space (Figs. 4.13, 4.14). It is important not to excise too much vaginal skin for this will fix the anterior vaginal wall. The ideal result is a well-supported bladder neck with preservation of normal mobility (Fig. 4.15).

At the conclusion of surgery, a suprapubic catheter is inserted, for many patients take up to a week before voiding without leaving a residual urine. A vaginal pack is inserted to obliterate dead space and minimise the chance of haematoma formation.

Post-operative Management

Care

The pack is moved within 24 h. The suprapubic catheter is clamped on the 7th day and removed when the patient is voiding easily and has a residual of less than 50 ml.

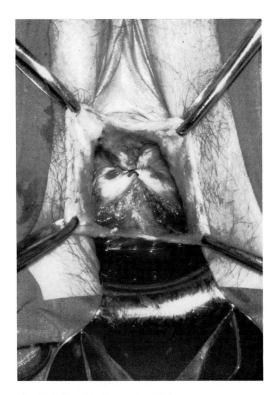

Fig. 4.11. First Mersilene suture tied.

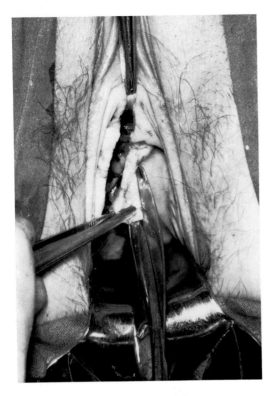

Fig. 4.13. Trimming of excess vaginal skin.

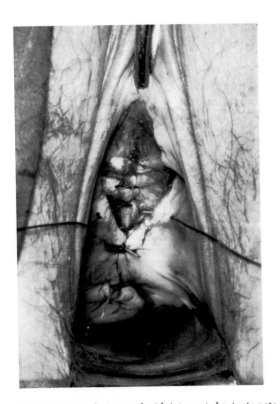

Fig. 4.14. Skin edge sutured with interrupted catgut: note the suture includes underlying fascia to obliterate dead space.

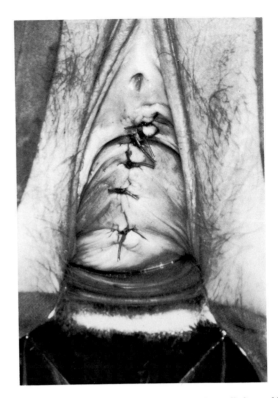

Fig. 4.15. Anterior vaginal wall closed and a well elevated bladder neck is produced.

Complications

Failure to find the right anatomical plane may result in entry into the urethra or bladder. The main postoperative complication is haematoma formation. Voiding difficulty and detrusor instability are not usually found as a result of this operation.

Follow-up Assessment

The patients are seen at 6 weeks for clinical assessment and 6 months post-operation for repeat urodynamic evaluation. They are tested for urine loss by being asked to cough forcefully with a full bladder in the standing position.

Results

Over 150 women have been operated on with this technique and the initial 6-month cure rate is between 80 and 90%. A series of 20 patients has been followed for 3 years. Continence has been assessed by giving Pyridium (phenazopyridine hydrochloride) by mouth and wearing pads for the day before assessment. The 3-year cure rate has been 80%. No patient has been found to have any adverse change in cystometric findings or been unable to empty the bladder satisfactorily.

Mechanism of Failure

Failure to restore continence usually has one of two causes. The chief cause is incorrect assessment of the patient with a severe degree of tissue damage which would have been better dealt with by a suprapubic approach. A lesser cause of failure is of haematoma formation with subsequent extrusion of suture material.

The virtue of the operation is that it is short, simple and relatively uncomplicated. Like all surgery designed to correct disorders of function, successful results will only be obtained when the operator has a clear idea of the pathology which is present and the limitation of the operation.

References

Beck PR, McCormick S (1982) Treatment of urinary stress incontinence with anterior colporrhaphy. Obstet Gynecol 59:269–274

Green TH Jr (1980) Vaginal repair. In: Stanton SL, Tanagho, EA (eds) Surgery of female incontinence, 1st edn. Springer, Berlin Heidelberg New York, pp 31–45

Henrikkson L, Anderson KE, Ulmsten U (1979) The urethral pressure profile in continent and stress incontinent women. Scand J Urol Nephrol 13:5–10

Smith ARB, Warrell DW (1984) A neurogenic aetiology of stress urinary incontinence and uterovaginal prolapse. Proceedings of the 14th Annual Meeting of the International Continence Society, Innsbruck, 485–487

Weil A, Reves H, Bischoff P, Rottenberg RD, Krauer I (1984) Modifications of the urethral resting and stress profiles after different types of surgery for urinary stress incontinence. Br J Obstet Gynaecol 91:46–55

5 The Marshall–Marchetti–Krantz Procedure*

Kermit E. Krantz

Introduction

True anatomical stress incontinence accounts for roughly 75% of all female urinary incontinence and should be relieved by a properly selected and executed surgical procedure. Approximately 25% of women who complain of uncontrollable loss of urine do not have anatomical stress incontinence, but one of several other conditions that may affect the mechanism of continence. These include urgency incontinence, bladder neuropathies, congenital or acquired urinary tract anomalies, psychogenic conditions, and detrusor dyssynergia. Careful differential evaluation of the various abnormalities leading to urinary incontinence is mandatory before instituting surgical correction.

Stress incontinence is the involuntary loss of urine through the intact urethra as a result of sudden increase in intra-abdominal pressure. In anatomical stress urinary incontinence, urine is lost in the absence of detrusor contraction without any sensation of urgency or urination. The loss of urine is in spurts, concomitant with sudden increase in intra-abdominal pressure. In the case of neuropathies, dribbling of urine occurs during and after stress; a time-factor lag is evident. Adherence to the definition that true stress incontinence is immediate loss of urine without warning upon coughing, sneezing, laughing, or other physical activity that may result in an increase in intra-abdominal pressure, will simplify the number and types of evaluation procedures.

Indications and Contraindications

Indications

Where there is primary stress incontinence and where anterior colporrhaphy or other approaches have not been successful.

If there is uterine prolapse, a vaginal hysterectomy can be performed.

If a cystocele is present, a repair from above and a Marshall–Marchetti–Krantz operation can be performed.

---

* The reference list at the end of this chapter is intended as a guide to further reading, not as a comprehensive set of references to the original literature.

Contraindications

—Where there is significant neurological lesion, e.g. multiple sclerosis. Bladder studies are required.

—Recurrent interstitial cystitis.

—A urethral length less than 2 cm. A Marshall–Marchetti–Krantz operation can be performed after lengthening of the urethra has been carried out.

—A bladder capacity of less than 200 ml.

—A large trabeculated bladder with a capacity in excess of 700 ml and where overflow incontinence is present.

Pre-operative Evaluation

Physical examination is also an important facet of pre-operative evaluation. Urethral detachment should be demonstrated during the examination, and the physician should be alert to the presence of a cystocele, urethral diverticula, vaginal scarring, or other abnormalities. Because there is a considerable overlap among the symptoms associated with common causes of urinary incontinence, objective testing is necessary as a confirmatory measure.

The standard procedure for patients with true stress incontinence who have not had previous surgery may include a cystometrogram, a check of residual urine, observation of the presence or absence of incontinence with a full bladder, and demonstrated correction of stress incontinence through elevation of the vesical neck. The latter may be achieved by placing the patient in the dorsolithotomy position and filling the bladder with 250–350 ml of water. If incontinence upon coughing and straining is observed either in the prone position or when the patient is asked to stand, the physician may insert two fingers into the vagina and with one finger on either side, elevate the vesical neck. If incontinence upon further coughing and straining ceases, indications are favourable for surgery. If no incontinence is observed when the patient stands, the test is repeated at 100 ml increments until a level of 500 ml is reached.

If the patient does not demonstrate true stress incontinence or has had previous surgery for stress incontinence, other pre-operative investigations should be considered, including cystoscopy to detect urethral abnormalities or the presence of urethral and bladder diverticula, as well as chain cysto-graphy. In addition an intravenous urogram can be of value to rule out abnormalities of the urinary tract.

Operative Technique

In 1949, Marshall, Marchetti and Krantz described a vesicourethral suspension in a 54-year-old male who had developed urinary stress incontinence following an abdomino-perineal resection. Subsequently they reported an 82% success rate for the same procedure performed on 44 women who had urinary stress incontinence.

Experience of over 30 years with the operation has allowed the author to refine the technique to offer success in approximately 95% of primary and repeat operations.

Precise suture placement and permanent fixation are the critical factors and cornerstones of long-term success in surgery for stress incontinence. Most of the author's patients are referrals who have had previous failed vaginal or suprapubic urethral suspension operations.

The patient is placed in a low dorsolithotomy position, allowing the surgeon to operate with one hand in the vagina and the other suprapubically in the space of Retzius. After preliminary cleansing of the vagina, perineal and lower abdominal regions, the patient is draped in a fashion permitting easy access to the lower abdomen and to the introitus. An 18F or 20F Foley catheter with a 5 ml balloon is inserted into the bladder through the plastic drape placed over the abdominoperineal region. Approximately 100–150 ml diluted methylene blue is instilled into the bladder.

A Pfannenstiel incision is made approximately 2 cm above the pubic symphysis. This allows good access to the space of Retzius and minimises the degree of retraction necessary. The incision is carried down through Scarpa's fascia and onto the aponeuroses of the external and internal oblique and transversus which are incised—reflected anteriorly and posteriorly and the rectus muscles separated in the mid-line. Attention is then turned to the bladder; palpation of the bladder is easily achieved because of the fluid within it. Ballottement identifies the bladder with ease. With the operator standing on the patient's left side at the operating table, the left hand of the operator is then placed into the vagina with the right hand moving into the space of Retzius by the index and second finger following along the pubic rami to the right and dropping into the space of Retzius between the bladder and the pubic bone. At this point the right hand is gently moved downward toward the vagina and held in position as its index and second finger come into contact on the right side of the patient with the index and second finger that are in the vagina. Holding the fingers in this position, an assistant then feeds an open Raytex sponge (4 × 12 cm) down between the fingers and the pubic rami. The right hand is then brought upward and placed between the pubic rami and the sponge. Gentle pressure brought to bear on the fingers of the left hand causes a stripping motion toward the mid-line and backward. The pressure is primarily against the fingers within the vagina; however, the sponge, acting against the base of the bladder, allows the bladder to be stripped backward and off the vagina. This is repeated once, twice, or frequently three times; the abdominal hand is withdrawn and a Deaver is placed to retract the bladder towards the mid-line

and hold it into place in order that the sutures can now be positioned.

If chromic catgut sutures (2–0) are to be employed, two or three sutures are inserted. The first suture is placed halfway down the urethra and a double bite is taken starting from the mid-line, looping over to the opposite side, and coming back through the mid-line. It is placed against the finger in the vagina; using the same technique, the second suture is placed approximately 0.5 cm above it and the third suture is placed opposite the vesicourethral junction.

If a non-absorbable suture material is used (2–0 braided Mersilene) it is placed at the vesicourethral junction, at right angles to the urethra and parallel to the vesical neck. A double bite is taken similar to that described previously, beginning on the inside looping toward the urethra, the loop being brought over and down through the vaginal musculature and back up again (Fig. 5.1). This gives a pulley effect. A double bite ensures that the suture will not pull through and secondly gives a 4:1 lift whereas one would only have a 2:1 lift in a single bite.

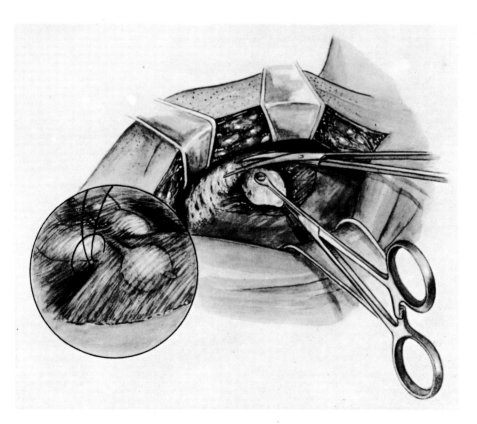

Fig. 5.1. Marshall–Marchetti–Krantz procedure. First stage. Mild traction of the catheter keeps the balloon at the vesical neck. *Inset:* Tips of the index and middle fingers of assistant elevating the anterior vaginal wall on each side of the proximal urethra. A double bite of the vaginal wall is taken on each side of the urethra at the region of the vesical neck (urethrovesical junction).

The procedure as described is then carried out on the opposite side; the dissection is performed with the left hand in the vagina, the two fingers being brought over onto the vaginal side of the urethra affording a position for lift. In order that one can be sure of placing the sutures into the muscularis of the vagina and avoid going through the mucosa, the surgeon's hand is placed in the vagina. Following the placement of the sutures, the point of fixation of the urethra to the pubic symphysis can be determined. This is achieved by placing the index finger on one side of the urethra and the second finger on the opposite side, with the Foley bulb brought into the vesical neck. The two fingers are then lifted up and the point where the vesical neck comes in contact with the pubic symphysis is the position in which the sutures will be placed into the pubic periosteum (Fig. 5.2). The suture is then placed with ease by placing the needle from the inside alongside the urethra against the periosteum and turning it with a simple wrist action to place the suture in position. It may involve the cartilage itself in the mid-line depending upon the width, the

thickness, and the availability of the periosteum. Each side is placed accordingly. The sutures are anchored to the periosteum on the posterior surface of the symphysis pubis, elevating the urethrovesical junction with the index and third fingers, and tying the suture to immobilise it. If there is venous bleeding it is controlled by pressure with a sponge stick. After satisfactory haemostasis, the rectus abdominis muscles are approximated with a horizontal mattress suture of 2–0 chromic catgut.

The rectus sheath is closed with an interlocking suture of 2–0 absorbable suture material. The subcutaneous tissue is closed with 3–0 chromic catgut placed in Scarpa's fascia, and the skin is closed with a subcuticular stitch of 4–0 absorbable suture material or 5–0 Nylon. These sutures are removed in 6 days.

At this time, pressure upon the bladder will demonstrate incontinence. As the suture is tied on either side, the incontinence will diminish. This is proof that the operation will be successful. Following this the methylene blue solution in the bladder is drained. No sutures are placed in the vesical neck

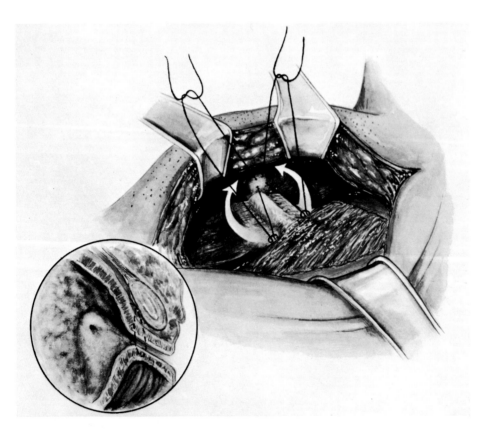

Fig. 5.2. Marshall–Marchetti–Krantz procedure. Suture placement. *Inset:* The proximal urethra and urethrovesical junction are elevated under the symphysis pubis.

for it has been the author's experience that they are of little value and in fact may overtly fix the urethra. A cystopexy is not carried out because this fixes the bladder to the abdominal wall and sets the stage for involuntary incontinence during sexual activity.

If a patient has a urethra that measures less than 2.5 cm, lengthening of the urethra must be carried out. Prior to the placement of any sutures, the length of the urethra should be checked. A position approximately 0.5 cm below the vesical neck is marked with a 4–0 chromic suture and a diamond-shaped wedge of muscularis of the vesical neck and bladder is removed by sharp dissection (Fig. 5.3). This diamond shape is approximately 2.5 cm in length and approximately 1.5 cm in width. Following the removal of the tissue, the transitional epithelium of the bladder is closed with interrupted or continuous sutures in a locked fashion retro to the mucosa—so that no suture material is present within the urethra or bladder (Fig. 5.4). Interrupted sutures are then placed in the muscularis of the bladder employing 4–0 chromic catgut. When this has been completed, the lengthened urethra is sus-

pended in the same manner as previously discussed using either chromic catgut or non-absorbable sutures. The urethra is measured following surgery. The additional length of the urethra will be approximately 1.5–20 cm. This can be critical in the control of incontinence.

If the uterus is acting as an additional traction force on the vesical neck and the patient has no desire for further childbearing, then an abdominal hysterectomy with or without bilateral salpingo-oophorectomy is carried out according to the age and the desires of the patient and the surgeon's assessment. The peritoneum is closed and then the suprapubic urethral suspension is carried out. This is done to minimise the chances of cross-contamination.

Drainage of the retropubic space is only carried out when there is an indication such as venous bleeding (this is not easily controlled as a result of involvement of the large extensive venous plexus around the bladder). This is carried out through a stab wound outside the incision. A Penrose drain is placed through Hesselbach's triangle and down

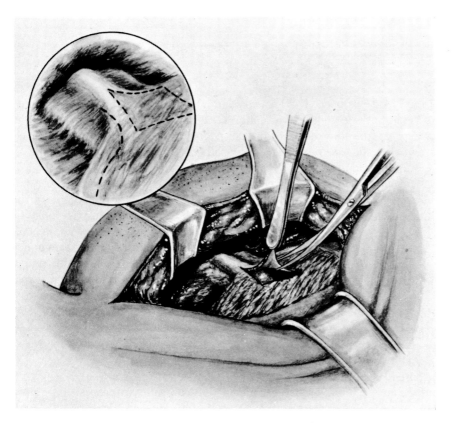

Fig. 5.3. Urethral lengthening. *Dotted line:* new urethral position. *Inset:* The area shown is resected to lengthen the urethra anatomically. The incision is made by cutting or resecting the diamond-shaped piece of urethrovesical wall.

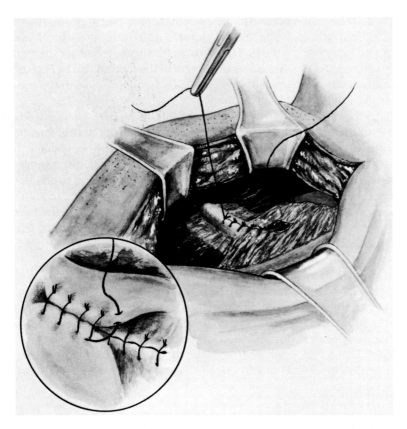

Fig. 5.4. Urethral lengthening. Suture placement. *Inset:* The mucosa is closed with continuous or interrupted 4–0 chromic catgut sutures. A second layer of interrupted sutures is placed in the muscularis.

into the space of Retzius. If the bladder is opened on entrance into the space of Retzius, it is left open during the operative procedure to be sure that the sutures are properly placed and that they do not involve the bladder itself. The author has found little cause to open the bladder in repeat surgical procedures unless there is a compelling reason. An indwelling Foley urethral catheter is inserted.

Post-operative Management

Following surgery, the vagina is packed with gauze to help reduce haematomas and disruption of the operation due to post-anaesthetic coughing. The packing is removed when the patient is fully awake.

If the bladder has been entered and repaired, the catheter is left in place until the urine is microscopically clear of blood. It may otherwise be removed on the day following surgery.

The patient is advised about straining, coughing, and lifting. When indicated, antibiotics and chemotherapeutics are employed prior to surgery prophylactically or to control infection, primarily if bacteriuria was present before surgery. In 3 or 4 weeks the patient may resume normal activity, but is cautioned to refrain from lifting heavy objects. The degree of relief of stress incontinence must be measured by the patient and her physician in comparison with her pre-operative state. Pregnancy may be anticipated without difficulty and vaginal delivery, while not preferred, is not contraindicated.

Complications

The following complications can occur.

—Osteitis pubis—caused by using a cutting rather than a round-bodied needle. Treatment is antibiotics and incision and drainage if abscess formation occurs.

—Failure to secure elevation and fixation of the bladder neck owing to incorrect placement of sutures.

—Injury to bladder during dissection. The bladder should be closed in two layers using absorbable suture material and drained by the urethral catheter for 14 days.

—Haematoma formation in the retropubic space.

Follow-up Assessment

Routine follow-up assessment is through clinical history and examination. If concern is felt about an effective cure, objective assessment using urethral pressure measurements and cystometry is performed.

Results

To date, 3861 patients have been personally treated by the Marshall–Marchetti–Krantz procedure. Follow-up has continued for up to 31 years in some cases. A cure rate of 96% has been obtained.

Summary

The place of the Marshall–Marchetti–Krantz operation in modern gynaecological surgery is well accepted. It should not be relegated to cases of failure of other procedures, either vaginal or abdominal, but should be considered as a primary approach to stress incontinence when a predictably high rate of success is desired.

References

Green TH (1975) Urinary stress incontinence: Differential diagnosis, pathophysiology, and management. Am J Obstet Gynecol 22:368–398

Hodgkinson CP (1970) Stress urinary incontinence. Am J Obstet Gynecol 108:1141–1168

Krantz KE (1950) Anatomy of the urethra and anterior vaginal wall. Am Assoc Obstet Gynecol Abdom Surg 61:31–59

Krantz KE (1951) Anatomy of the urethra and anterior vaginal wall. Am J Obstet Gynecol 62:374–386

Krantz KE (1970) The anatomy and physiology of the vulva and vagina and the anatomy of the urethra and bladder. In: Philipp EE, Barnes J, Newton M (eds) Scientific foundations of obstetrics and gynecology. Heinemann, London, pp 47–64

Marshall VT, Marchetti AA, Krantz KE (1949) The correction of stress incontinence by simple vesico-urethral suspension. Surg Gynecol Obstet 88:509–518

Shingleton HM, Davis RO (1977) Stress incontinence in perspective. Obstet Gynecol Digest 19:15–25

6 Colposuspension

Stuart L. Stanton

Introduction

Stress incontinence due to urethral sphincter incompetence (GSI) is defined as involuntary loss of urine through the intact urethra, when the intravesical pressure exceeds the intra-urethral pressure due to elevation of the intra-abdominal pressure and in the absence of a detrusor contraction (International Continence Society 1976). The patient complains of stress incontinence on physical effort, e.g. coughing, jogging or standing up, and this is accompanied by demonstrable stress incontinence and sometimes anterior vaginal wall prolapse. Continence surgery will correct the former and the same procedure may correct prolapse as well.

The original operative description is due to Burch (1961, 1968). Many variations have since been described. All have the common purpose of bladder neck elevation and achieve this by suturing the paravaginal tissue of the lateral vaginal fornix to the ipsilateral pelvic wall tissue—usually the ileopectineal ligament. This allows equal transmission of the intra-abdominal pressure to the proximal urethra (Enhorning 1961) and places the proximal urethra in an advantageous position to the postero-superior border of the symphysis, where it may be compressed by intra-abdominal forces during effort (Hertogs and Stanton, 1985). At the same time, Burch (1961) pointed out that anterior vaginal wall descent can also be corrected.

Terminology

Burch first used the term urethrovaginal fixation (1961) and then later urethrovesical suspension (1968). Colposuspension (from the Greek κολποσ) was first used by Turner Warwick and Whiteside (1970). Since then, numerous clinicians have modified this concept and used different terminology, e.g. colpocystourethropexy (Tanagho 1976), retropubic urethropexy (Hodgkinson 1980) and, more recently, the vaginal obturator shelf procedure (Turner Warwick 1984, unpublished work).

Indications and Contraindications

Prior to any continence surgery, the patient should be mentally aware of the need to be continent and physically fit enough to undergo surgery. The main indication is objective demonstration of stress incontinence due to urethral sphincter incompetence, with or without anterior vaginal wall prolapse.

Coexistent detrusor instability is a relative contra-indication and ideally it should be detected by urodynamic assessment and treated beforehand by conservative means: if stress incontinence persists and is a substantial complaint, a colposuspension may be proceeded to, provided the patient is informed that the chances of curing stress incontinence are decreased in the presence of detrusor instability and that any accompanying urgency and frequency may be made worse.

Voiding difficulty is a relative contraindication, depending on its severity as gauged by residual urine, uroflowmetry and maximal voiding pressure (Stanton et al. 1978a; Walter et al. 1982). Anecdotal experience suggests that pre-operative voiding difficulty due to distal urethral stenosis may be ameliorated by a prior urethrotomy.

Detrusor sphincter dyssynergia is more difficult to treat and often coexists with detrusor instability. Treatment of the latter using anxiolytics may sometimes be effective.

Other contraindications include the presence of a foreshortened, scarred and immobile vagina, when elevation of the lateral fornices may be unlikely. The presence of an elevated bladder neck, satisfactorily aligned to the symphysis pubis, is a contraindication as a further colposuspension is unlikely to achieve anything more.

As with any continence procedure, the patient should have completed her family beforehand as pregnancy or a vaginal delivery may weaken the bladder neck supports and lead to recurrence of incontinence. This may be mitigated by a prophylactic lower segment caesarian section, and where appropriate the argument for this course of action must be discussed prior to the colposuspension.

Because of post-operative pain associated with any lower abdominal incision, a patient with chronic obstructive airways disease should have the operation deferred until she is as fit as possible and the winter months should be avoided.

Pre-operative Evaluation

History and Physical Examination

These are detailed in Chap. 2. Of particular importance are questions to detect voiding disorder and a past history of pelvic surgery which may compromise the technique of colposuspension. This will include vaginal and abdominal hysterectomy, which if performed incompetently can lead to significant vaginal scarring and stenosis. Although obesity and lung disease (such as asthma and chronic coughing) are not contraindications to surgery, the patient should be made aware that these factors may jeopardise the results of surgery.

Gynaecological examination should include an appraisal of the capacity and mobility of the vagina and in particular the ease with which the lateral fornix can be elevated retropubically. Genital prolapse and the presence of residual urine needs to be noted. The procedure should not be performed unless stress incontinence can be demonstrated either clinically or by investigation. If prolapse or menorrhagia is present, an abdominal hysterectomy should be performed beforehand. No advantage has been found in removing an otherwise asymptomatic uterus at the same time (Stanton and Cardozo 1979). Coexistent enterocele or rectocele is managed by closure of the pouch of Douglas (Moschowitz procedure) or a posterior repair, respectively.

Investigations

Investigations are important (a) to confirm the patient's history that stress incontinence is present, especially when it cannot be detected on clinical examination, and (b) to detect detrusor instability and voiding difficulty. Therefore uroflowmetry and cystometry or videocystourethrography are relevant investigations. Urethral pressure measurements are useful to detect urethral relaxation but otherwise make little contribution to the diagnosis or the choice of a colposuspension procedure. Metallic bead chain urethrocystograms are helpful to determine the elevation and alignment of the bladder neck in relation to the postero-superior border of the symphysis pubis, especially when there has been previous failed surgery (Chap. 2).

Pre-operative Preparation

No special preparation is necessary apart from an abdominal and perineal shave. For prevention of deep vein thrombosis, 5000 international units of subcutaneous heparin are given with the premed and this is repeated twice daily until the patient is fully mobile (about the 6th day). Either general or epidural anaesthesia may be employed. If a posterior repair is to be performed, a 1-g rectal suppository of metronidazole is given with premedication.

After induction of anaesthesia, the patient is placed in the horizontal lithotomy position with the legs in Flotron or other antithrombotic boots, slightly abducted and supported in Lloyd-Davies or similar stirrups (Fig. 6.1). The abdomen, vaginal and perineal regions are prepared and draped in a sterile manner. A transurethral resection drape is used for the perineum, allowing access to the vagina during the operation by means of a sterile condom. A 14 French Foley urethral catheter is inserted and left to drain freely: this delineates the bladder neck and allows filling of the bladder after operation prior to insertion of the suprapubic catheter.

Operative Technique

A low Pfannenstiel incision is made approximately 1 finger breadth above the symphysis pubis. It is purposely low, to obtain the maximum access to the bladder neck region. If there has been previous abdominal surgery, access is made easier with less risk of opening the peritoneal cavity, by using a Cherney incision as well, which incises the recti muscles at their insertion on the symphysis. Should an abdominal hysterectomy or Moschowitz procedure be required, it is performed before the colposuspension and without the need of a Cherney incision.

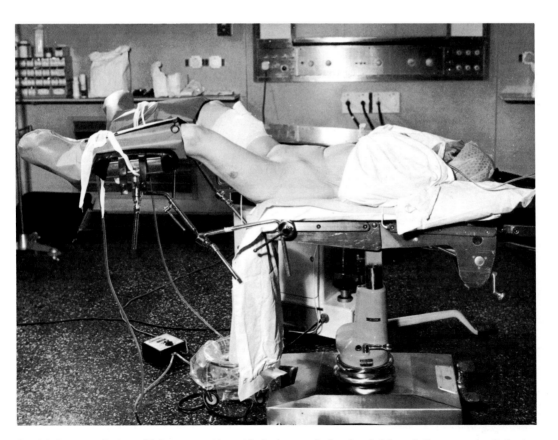

Fig. 6.1. Patient in horizontal lithotomy position with the legs gently flexed and abducted. Flotron pneumatic boots are worn to diminish the risk of deep vein thrombosis.

A Denis Browne four-bladed self-retaining ring retractor (Fig. 6.2) is used; the bladder is carefully dissected from the symphysis and the space of Retzius is exposed by blunt finger dissection (Fig. 6.3). When a previous suprapubic procedure has been performed, separation of the bladder and urethra from the symphysis is difficult and best carried out using a scalpel.

With the space of Retzius exposed, the operator places his forefinger in the vagina and elevates one or other lateral vaginal fornix (Fig. 6.4). From above, the upward pressure cone is easily identified visually and by palpation. The abdominal hand, using either a swab on a holder or a Lahey ("Peanut") mounted on a curved artery forceps (Roberts), dissects the bladder base medially off the paravaginal fascia, care being taken to start the dissection sufficiently lateral to the bladder (Fig. 6.5). Where there has been previous surgery, scissor dissection may be required. Some large perivesical veins may be encountered: these should either be moved to one side, diathermied or ligated. The paravaginal fascia is recognised as white tissue: when visible from the bladder neck to the uppermost (cephalad) extent of the vaginal cone, three sutures of number 1 polyglycolic acid suture (Vicryl or Dexon) or of unabsorbable polybutylate-coated polyester (Ethibond) suture are inserted into the fascia and then to the nearest point on the ipsilateral ileopectineal ligament. The most distal (caudad) suture is inserted opposite the bladder neck and not lower. The next two sutures are inserted more proximally (cephalad) alongside the bladder base. All are spaced approximately 1 cm apart (Fig. 6.6). It is likely that upon tying, the first pair will elevate the bladder neck and produce continence and the last two pairs will correct the cystocele and may enhance the holding power of the first sutures. As each suture is inserted into the paravaginal fascia, it is tied to provide haemostasis and to avoid the suture moving in the fascia when it is tied again to the ligament. The lateral vaginal fornix should be elevated each time by the operator's finger towards the ileopectineal ligament as the corresponding suture is being placed through the ligament, so as to position it accurately. This will ensure close approximation of paravaginal fascia to ileopectineal ligament and minimise the "bow string" effect.

Once all six sutures are in position and haemostasis is complete, the sutures can be tied, approximating paravaginal fascia to the ileopectineal ligaments (Fig. 6.7). The operator holds taut that limb of the suture passing through the ileopectineal ligament (which will elevate the lateral fornix and paravaginal fascia) and then ties the remaining limb around this in a knot. When polyester is used,

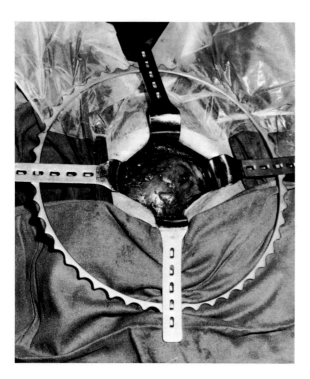

Fig. 6.2. Pfannenstiel incision with Denis Browne four-bladed self-retaining ring retractor in place.

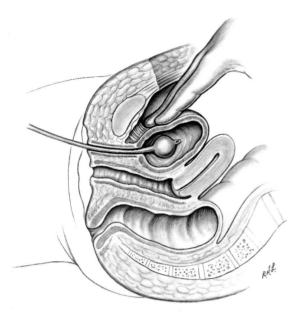

Fig. 6.3. Sagittal section showing blunt finger dissection in the space of Retzius, between the symphysis pubis and the anterior surface of the bladder and urethra.

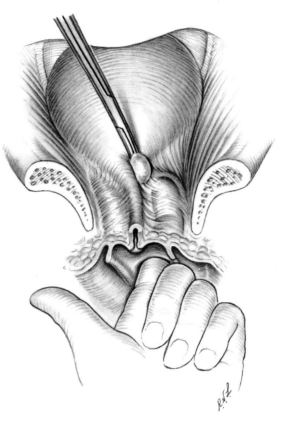

Fig. 6.5. With the operator's finger still in the vagina and elevating the lateral vaginal fornix, the bladder base is dissected medially off the paravaginal fascia.

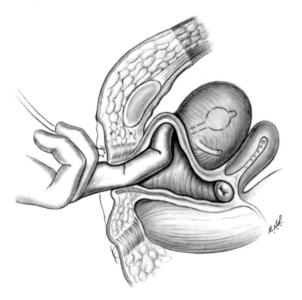

Fig. 6.4. Sagittal section demonstrating upward pressure in a lateral vaginal fornix, to aid in the abdominal dissection.

throws must be placed in opposite directions to avoid the knot slipping. The most caudal suture is tied first and then the remaining sutures are tied, moving alternately from side to side, thus ensuring even elevation (Fig. 6.8). Although it may look surgically inept, it does not matter if some "bow stringing" of the more caudal sutures occurs when

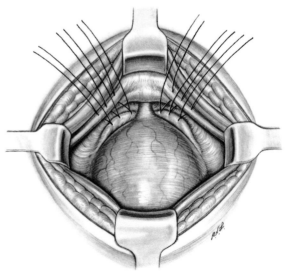

Fig. 6.6. The three pairs of sutures are in place but not tied.

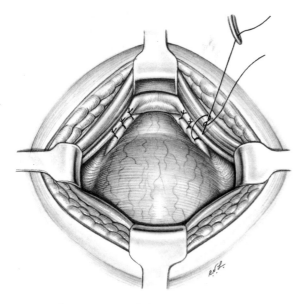

Fig. 6.7. The sutures are tied, showing approximation of paravaginal tissue to the ileopectineal ligaments. Elevation is produced by holding taut the suture which passes through the ileopectineal ligament and tying the other limb of the suture around this. The operator gauges the amount of tension required. This method obviates the need for an assistant to elevate the vagina at this stage.

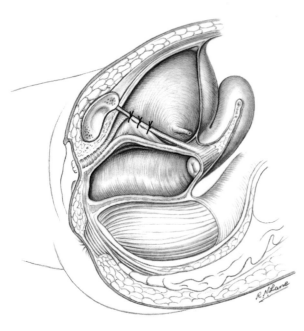

Fig. 6.8. Sagittal section showing elevation of the bladder neck and bladder base on a shelf of paravaginal fascia, sutured to an ileopectineal ligament.

the fascia fails to approximate to the ileopectineal ligament. However, successful cure of urethral sphincter incompetence is less likely if there is no meeting point at all between fascia and ligament. This is usually due to relative immobility and decreased capacity of the vagina and is a reflection on poor clinical selection of the case for colposuspension.

If there is doubt about the integrity of the bladder, either methylene blue or sterile milk can be instilled via the urethral catheter, so that a leak would be obvious. Milk has the advantage of not staining the tissues and thus allowing further instillation after the bladder has been sutured.

A suction drain is left in the space of Retzius which will also drain the rectus sheath. If the rectus insertions have been cut, they are repaired together with the rectus sheath in one layer using a number 1 loop nylon. Otherwise the sheath is closed with number 1 nylon or number 1 polyglycolic acid suture.

If a vaginal examination is performed now, the anterior vaginal wall would be found to be well elevated, with the external urethral meatus drawn upwards underneath the symphysis. A crescentic web of rectovaginal fascia may be felt on the posterior vaginal wall. If required at this stage, a posterior repair is performed.

The bladder is filled by the Foley catheter with 500 ml of sterile normal saline or water and the suprapubic catheter introduced, about 2 cm cephalad to the Pfannenstiel incision, and the Foley catheter removed.

Intra-operative complications include injury to the urethra and bladder, venous haemorrhage from paravesical veins and ureteric ligation. Injury to the urethra and bladder is repaired in a one or two layer closure using 3.0 polyglycolic acid suture and the bladder drained for 8–10 days with a 14–16 French gauge urethral catheter as well as the suprapubic catheter. When the urethra is injured, I rely only on a wide bore suprapubic catheter with an irrigation channel, such as a 16 gauge Argyle Ingram catheter (Chap. 19). The patient is placed on a suitable chemotherapeutic agent (e.g. cephradine). Venous haemorrhage is managed by diathermy, oversewing or the use of Sterispon. Any remaining venous bleeding usually ceases as soon as elevation of the paravaginal fascia has been completed. Ureteric ligation is fortunately rare, and avoided by always ensuring that sutures are placed only into the white paravaginal fascia.

Post-operative Management

The author places his patients on cephradine 500 mg q.d. for 48 h starting at operation. Regular catheter specimens of urine are sent for culture and sensitivity. The patient is on an accurate input and output chart and is encouraged to drink between 2 and 2.5 litres per day.

The post-operative care is usually straightforward. Gradual mobilisation is commenced on day 1 and suction drainage is removed within 24–36 h of operation. On the morning of day 2, the catheter is clamped for the first time for 8–10 h and the patient is allowed to void spontaneously. At the end of this time, the patient is encouraged to void once more and then the catheter is unclamped and any urine which drains off over a 30-min period is termed the residual urine. If the patient cannot void and has pain, the catheter is unclamped earlier and the residual is measured. Once she voids amounts greater than 200 ml and the residual urine is less than 100 ml, the catheter is clamped overnight. She is woken by the nursing staff on one or two occasions to void and the morning residual urine is measured in the same fashion. Provided the patient voids amounts in excess of 200 ml and neither develops retention nor has been incontinent, it is safe to remove the catheter. The residual urine is usually less than 300 ml. The final catheter specimen of urine is sent for culture and sensitivity and

the trimethoprim is stopped. The benefits of early clamping of the catheter are illustrated by Fig. 6.9, where it is seen that 28 out of a total of 43 patients (65%) voided by the third post-operative day and 17 patients (39%) had their suprapubic catheter removed by the fifth post-operative day (Montz and Stanton 1985).

If the post-operative progress is satisfactory, the patient may be discharged home on the 6th or 7th post-operative day. She is asked to avoid sexual intercourse for 2 months because dyspareunia may occur due to a ridge of rectovaginal fascia in the posterior vaginal wall. Strenuous lifting should be avoided for 2 months and preferably for ever if convenient. This is because effective long-term elevation of the bladder neck (which is the principal effect of this operation) will only be as good as the patient's tissues, despite the unabsorbable sutures.

Complications

Post-operative complications are infrequent. Provided injury to urethra or bladder is recognised at the time of operation and dealt with properly, urinary fistula is unlikely to occur. Ureteric injury needs recognition by endoscopy, IVU and retrograde catheterisation. Treatment is outlined in Chap. 15.

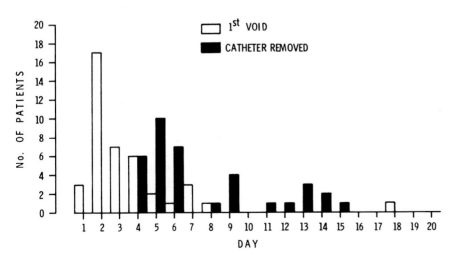

Fig. 6.9. The day of first spontaneous void and the day when the catheter was removed following colposuspension, in a series of 43 patients.

Urinary tract infection is not common, especially when using a suprapubic catheter. However, a persistent residual urine will exacerbate this and lead to recurrent infection.

Voiding difficulties are well documented following colposuspension. Stanton et al. (1978a) described voiding difficulties secondary to a pre-operative low peak flow rate and noted that cure of stress incontinence is usually accompanied by decreased peak flow rate and a raised maximum voiding pressure (Stanton and Cardozo 1979). Walter et al. (1982) found voiding difficulties occurred with correction of an anterior rather than a posterior bladder suspension defect. Dundas et al. (1982) analysed the aetiology of voiding difficulties following colposuspension and found them to be due to reduced mobility and "super elevation" of the bladder neck. A follow-up of patients who underwent colposuspension 2–5 years previously, indicated that 17% had some objective evidence of impaired flow (Dwyer and Stanton, to be published). No relationship was found between post-operative voiding difficulty and subjective operative finding of bladder neck elevation or approximation of paravaginal tissue to the ileopectineal ligament. There was no relationship between the time taken to void spontaneously following colposuspension and subsequent voiding difficulty or between the cure of stress incontinence and presence of voiding difficulties. Post-colposuspension detrusor instability was more common in the voiding difficulty group ($P<0.05$). Most patients with voiding difficulties may be successfully managed by prolonged catheter drainage and adjunct drugs (Chap. 19). Some may benefit from urethrotomy. Resistant cases may require intermittent self-catheterisation. However, the most important lesson to be learnt is prevention, by detecting the likely cases prior to surgery and by use of a suprapubic rather than a urethral catheter for post-operative bladder drainage.

Detrusor instability was first reported following colposuspension by Cardozo et al. (1979). Five per cent of patients undergoing colposuspension for urethral sphincter incompetence were found to have incurred systolic detrusor instability. This has also been found following sling procedures and insertion of an artificial urinary sphincter, and appears to be more common in patients who have undergone previous bladder neck surgery. Steel et al. (to be published) reviewed patients for up to 5 years with detrusor instability following colposuspension and found that 60% appeared to be

symptomatic, although 16% were improved by drug therapy. A statistical trend was found only for previous bladder neck surgery as a causative factor.

Follow-up Assessment

Clinical review and urodynamic assessment are carried out 3–4 months after surgery: thereafter the patient is followed annually by clinical review, uroflowmetry and a urilos/perineal pad test for 5 years. If, during that time, incontinence recurs, invasive urodynamic studies are only performed if the patient complains of her incontinence and wants it treated.

Results

Comparable results are difficult to evaluate because most follow-up series in the literature are clinical and not objective. Burch's original study (1961) indicated that all 45 cases were cured at 17 months follow-up. A later study (Burch 1968) showed that 133 out of 143 patients (93%) were subjectively cured, over a follow-up period of 2–60 months. Stanton and Cardozo (1979) reported on a series of 88 patients followed for 1 year with objective outcome measures. Incontinence was cured in 88%. Walter et al. (1982) described an 84% cure or improvement rate in a series of 38 patients with a median follow-up of 14 months. In a larger series, Stanton et al. (1982) reported on the results of 42 patients followed for 5 years. There was an overall objective cure rate of 80%, with a 91% cure rate for patients who had not had previous bladder neck surgery. With previous surgery, the cure rate fell to 67%. At 5 years the overall success rate was 78%, with a cure rate of 86% for patients without previous bladder neck surgery, again decreasing to 67% for patients with previous surgery. Four patients developed an enterocele, of whom one required corrective surgery. Cystocele and cystourethrocele were encountered pre-operatively in 16 patients, and at 5 years only two recurrences were detected. In the elderly, Gillon and Stanton (1984) found an 89% objective cure rate in a series of 35 patients followed for between 3 and 5 years.

The incidence of frequency and urge incontinence before and after colposuspension is shown in Table 6.1 (Stanton and Cardozo 1979), and this shows

Table 6.1. Incidence of frequency, urgency and urge incontinence before and after colposuspension (Stanton and Cardozo 1979)

Symptom (%)	Pre-operative (n = 146)	1 year (n = 88)	2 years (n = 43)
Diurnal frequency	62	40	39
Nocturnal frequency	39	25	30
Urgency	66	43	44
Urge incontinence	53	20	26

that despite recurrence of detrusor instability as previously reported, there was an overall decrease in the post-operative incidence of frequency, urgency and urge incontinence.

Causes of Failure

The reasons for failure are (a) inability to adequately elevate the bladder neck, (b) occurrence of post-operative detrusor instability and (c) para-urethral and urethral fibrosis affecting bladder neck and proximal urethra.

Urgency and frequency without instability are still adverse pre-operative factors. Post-operative weight gain does not adversely affect the cure rate. Increasing age and a past history of bladder neck surgery are deleterious factors (Stanton et al. 1978b). Occasionally, a patient reports a tearing feeling following exertional straining, associated with return of incontinence. Concern about the integrity of absorbable sutures after 1 month and the subsequent gradual deterioration of the objective cure rate within 5 years has led me to use a permanent suture (polyester—Ethibond) instead of polyglycolic acid suture; over the 4 years of its use I have not had any reason to regret this, despite the suture something being passed through the total thickness of the vaginal wall. There has been no instance of infection due to the use of a braided suture.

References

Burch J (1961) Urethrovaginal fixation to Cooper's ligament for correction of stress incontinence, cystocele and prolapse. Am J Obstet Cynecol 81:281–290

Burch J (1968) Cooper's ligament urethrovesical suspension for stress incontinence. Am J Obstet Gynecol 100:764–772

Cardozo L, Stanton SL, Williams J (1979) Detrusor instability following surgery for genuine stress incontinence. Br J Urol 51:204–207

Dundas D, Hilton P, Williams J, Stanton SL (1982) Aetiology of voiding difficulties post-colposuspension. Proceedings of 12th Annual Meeting of the International Continence Society, Leiden, p 132

Dwyer P, Stanton SL (to be published) Voiding difficulty following Burch colposuspension

Enhorning G (1961) Simultaneous recording of intravesical and intraurethral pressure. Acta Chir Scand [Suppl] 276:1–68

Gillon G, Stanton SL (1984) Long term follow-up of surgery for urinary incontinence in elderly women. Br J Urol 56:478–481

Hertogs K, Stanton SL (1985) Mechanism of urinary continence after colposuspension: barrier studies. Br J Obstet Gynaecol 92:1184–1188

Hodgkinson CP (1980) Retropubic urethropexy or colposuspension. In: Stanton SL, Tanagho E (eds) Surgery of female incontinence, 1st edn. Springer, Heidelberg Berlin New York, pp 55–68

International Continence Society (1976) Standardization of terminology of lower urinary tract function. Br J Urol 48:39–42

Montz F, Stanton SL (1985) Suprapubic bladder catheterization: Use and management in the gynecologic patient. Contemp Obstet Gynecol 25:31–46

Stanton SL, Cardozo L (1979) Results of colposuspension for incontinence and prolapse. Br J Obstet Gynaecol 86:693–697

Stanton SL, Cardozo L, Chaudhury N (1978a) Spontaneous voiding following incontinence surgery. Br J Obstet Gynaecol 85:149–152

Stanton SL, Cardozo L, Williams J, Ritchie D, Allan V (1978b) Clinical and urodynamic factors of failed incontinence surgery in the female. Obstet Gynecol 51:515–520

Stanton SL, Hertogs H, Cox C, Hilton P, Cardozo L (1982) Colposuspension operation for genuine stress incontinence: a 5 year study. Proceedings of the 12th Annual Meeting of the International Continence Society, Leiden, pp 94–96

Steel S, Cox C, Stanton SL (to be published) Long term follow-up of detrusor instability following colposuspension. Br J Urol

Tanagho E (1976) Colpocystourethropexy: the way we do it. J Urol 116:751–753

Turner Warwick R, Whiteside G (1970) Investigations and management of bladder neck dysfunction. In: Riches E (ed) Modern trends in urology, 3rd edn. Butterworths, London, pp 295–311

Walter S, Olesen K, Hald T, Jensen H, Pedersen P (1982) Urodynamic evaluation after vaginal repair and colposuspension. Br J Urol 54:377–380

7 Sling Procedures

Rudolf Hohenfellner and Eckhard Petri

Introduction

Suburethral sling operations have won favour throughout the world for cases of recurrent stress incontinence associated with pelvic floor weakness, especially after repeated incontinence surgery. Whilst living muscle tissue has been employed previously, strips made of fascia, synthetic material, or lyophilised dura are currently coming into use, simplifying the procedure considerably. The chances of curing incontinence are excellent; primary success in over 90% has been reported. After the pioneer work by von Giordano (1907, quoted by Ullery 1953) and Stoeckel (1917), sling procedures fell into discredit during the pre-antibiotic era as a result of abscess formation in the paravaginal space. More recently, however, they have experienced a renaissance through reports published by Bracht (1956), Anselmino (1952), Zoedler (1961) (alloplastic strips) and Narik and Palmrich (1962) (fascial slings) (Table 7.1).

Table 7.1. History of sling procedures (dates refer to first clinical use)

1907	Von Giordano	Sling formation using gracilis muscle
1910	Goebell	Pyramidalis muscle
1911	Squier	Levator ani and transversus perinei profundus
1914	Frangenheim	Pyramidalis muscle and strip of rectus fascia
1917	Stoeckel	Pyramidalis muscle and strip of rectus fascia
1919	Solms	Suburethral sling using the round ligament
1923	Thompson	Prepubic sling using rectus fascia
1925	Hans	Strips of the rectus fascia
1931	Baumm	Simple sling of rectus fascia
1942	Aldridge	Rectus fascia
1947	Meigs	Duplicating strips of rectus muscle
1947	Millin and Read	Strips of rectus muscle and fascia
1951	Bracht	Nylon sling
1952	Anselmino	Perlon sling
1960	Zoedler	Nylon sling
1962	Narik and Palmrich	Strips of external oblique muscle fascia
1972	Havlíček	Lyophilised dural sling

Indications

The primary indication for a sling operation is severe, recurrent incontinence following one or more operations, and urodynamic proof of pure stress incontinence. The procedure should not be performed until gynaecological precautions such as hysterectomy or correction of a cystocele are taken, as a prolapsed uterus causes a relative pressure increase in a caudal direction. Under these conditions, a sling implanted in the presence of the uterus may cause steady traction on the urethra. These operations may be performed prior to, or simultaneously with, a sling procedure.

In selected cases with neuropathic bladder dysfunction, considerable improvement of the psychosocial status of the patient is made possible. Residual urine and an increase in uninhibited detrusor contractions, however, are the calculated risks involved.

Classification

—Fascial sling as fascia lata (Beck and Lai 1982; Parker et al. 1979) or inguinovaginal sling (Narik and Palmrich 1982)

—Dural sling (Havliček 1972)

—Alloplastic sling (Anselmino 1952; Zoedler 1961; Kersey 1983; Sexton 1983; Stanton et al. 1985).

Whilst the fascial sling procedure uses autogenic material, the dural sling implantation involves an allogenic transplantation, and the nylon sling employs alloplastic material. The dural sling is a strip of dura mater cerebri cleansed of its antigenic properties and obtainable in lengths of 2×25 cm or 2×30 cm. Alloplastic slings are available in different materials, some still in a developmental stage.

Pre-operative Evaluation

Urine is sent for culture and sensitivity, and intravenous urography, a resting and a straining lateral cystourethrogram and voiding cystourethrogram recorded on videotape, are carried out. In addition, simultaneous recording of intravesical and intrarectal pressures, measurement of urinary flow and volume, and pelvic floor electromyography are performed. Simultaneous urethral and bladder pressures are recorded with either a four-channel polyvinyl chloride membrane catheter or a Gaeltec catheter tip pressure transducer, withdrawn mechanically at a constant speed of 3 mm/s.

Operative Technique

In most of the techniques described, the construction of a fascial, muscular or alloplastic sling and insertion around the vesical neck and the base of the urethra by a suprapubic approach has been combined with a vaginal approach through which the pubocervical fascia is plicated beneath the urethra and the bladder neck. A notable exception to this is the technique described by Millin and Read (1948), in which the repair is carried out entirely through a suprapubic approach. While it was thought that the use of muscular tissue for the sling would replace the "missing sphincter", slings made of fascia, dura and synthetic material achieve suspension and fixation of the critical bladder neck region; the fibrous tissue to the os pubis is additionally supported by the sling. The inguino-vaginal fascial sling procedure is described in detail below; the other operations are discussed in their divergent stages.

The patient is placed on the operating table in a lithotomy position. The legs should be movable as necessary without disturbance of sterile conditions. Both abdominal and vaginal operative fields should be cleansed and draped before the onset of the operation.

Inguinovaginal Fascial Sling

Skin incision starts at the pubic tubercle and is directed toward a point medial to the superior iliac spine (Fig. 7.1). If hysterectomy is planned in the same surgical procedure, a Pfannenstiel incision is performed.

The dissection of the fascial strip from the aponeurosis of the external oblique muscle is best performed using two short, parallel preliminary incisions starting close to the pubic tubercle and about 2 cm apart. These initial incisions are then continued to the iliac spine for a distance of about 12 cm, up to the point where the fibres of the external oblique muscle continue into the fascia

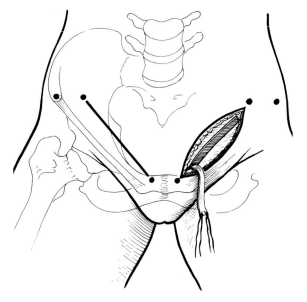

Fig. 7.1. Skin incision; preparation of fascial strip.

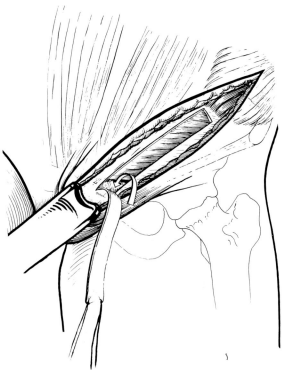

Fig. 7.2. Preparation of fascial strip; site of perforation (*arrow*).

(Fig. 7.2). The proximal end of the strip is then clamped and cut, marking each angle with a suture of a different colour (e.g. black and white silk) to avoid connection of contorted strips later on. The strip is then mobilised, preserving a broad attachment of the fascial strip to the pubic tubercle.

The triangular space above the tubercle, which is confined by the rectal sheath on the medial side and by the lower part of the internal oblique muscle on the lateral side ("suprapubic trigone"), is then perforated (transverse fascia), leading straight into the paravesical space (space of Retzius) (Fig. 7.2). The index finger in introduced and carefully pushed downward as far as the inferior pubic artery. Instrumental manipulations within the retropubic tunnel should be avoided, as they carry the danger of injury to the bladder or branches of the pudendal, obturator or epigastric vessels. It is of great importance always to use the posterior face of the os pubis as a guideline.

Having prepared both fascial strips and the retropubic tunnels, the vaginal stage of the operation is started. (One assistant remains in attendance at the abdominal operative field.) An anterior colpotomy is performed, exposing the urethrovesical junction and the paraurethral and paravesical spaces.

After perforation of the pelvic fascia (Fig. 7.3) the operator introduces the index finger into the paravesical space while the assistant at the abdomi-

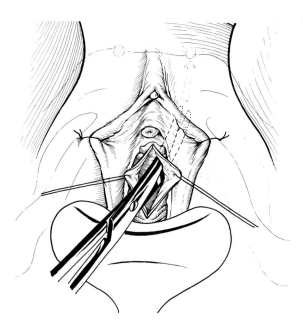

Fig. 7.3. Perforation of pelvic fascia.

nal field passes the index finger through the retropubic tunnel (Fig. 7.4). Their aim should be to bring their fingers into contact by blunt dissection.

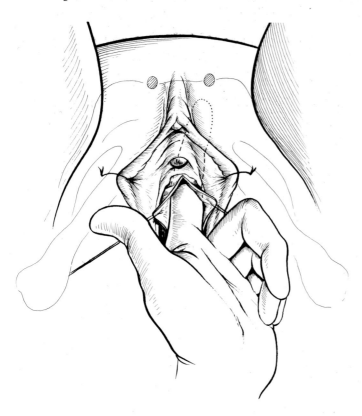

Fig. 7.4. Insertion of index finger into the retropubic tunnel.

A long curved clamp is introduced through the vaginal incision. [Narik and Palmrich (1962) have developed a special instrument which they call an "elephant's tooth".] Having attached the fascial strip, the instrument is pulled downward. A rather lateral course of direction should be taken when inserting the clamp in order to bypass the urethra and bladder. Having pulled out the instrument to its full length, the fascial strip is freed and clamped. The same procedure is then performed on the contralateral side (Fig. 7.5).

The fascial strips are approximated and united at a level close to the bladder neck. Suture is accomplished by means of fine silk and small round needles. At least three sutures should be placed to secure a firm union of the strips (Figs. 7.6, 7.7).

Different ways of determining suspension effectiveness have been described: the bladder may be filled with 200 ml of saline and the loss of fluid through the urethra checked following pressure upon the suprapubic region. Although this test seems of reduced value because of relaxation of the pelvic floor during general anaesthesia, it gives some hint as to urethral closure pressure. We insert the tip of the little finger into the triangle between the urethra and the connected fascial strips and place additional sutures when more than the tip can be inserted. Overlapping parts of the strips are then everted and sewn to the pubovesical fascia. Following resection of the vaginal edges and reconstruction of the pelvic floor (see Chap. 4), the colpotomy incision is closed. A suprapubic catheter is inserted in the bladder.

Prior to closing the inguinal incisions, the vaginal team should change gloves. Abdominal incisions are closed by interrupted sutures after having placed haemovac drains through the subcutaneous tissue, into the paravesical space.

Dural and Alloplastic Sling

Operations using dural sling or alloplastic material start with the vaginal stage of the procedure. Anterior colpotomy and preparation of the retropubic tunnel are performed using the technique described above.

A second assistant makes a transverse suprapubic incision of 8–10 cm. The sling is prepared by fixing chromic catgut or Dexon sutures to its ends, which

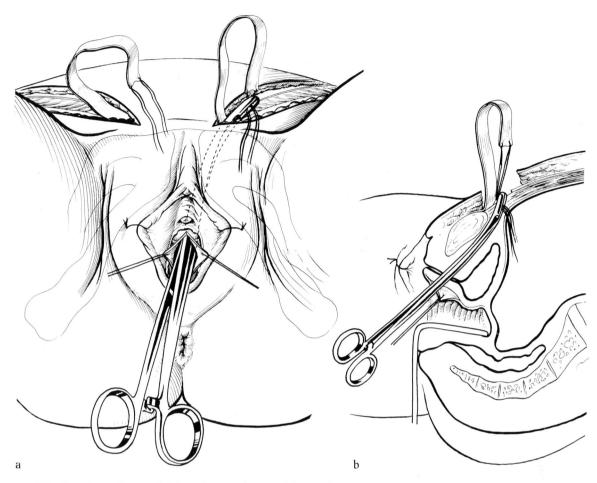

Fig. 7.5. a Fascial strips being pulled through retropubic tunnel. **b** Lateral view.

are then gripped by a long, slightly curved clamp and inserted into the retropubic tunnel from the anterior colpotomy. The abdominal fascia is incised at the point where the clamp is palpable. The sutures are then drawn through the incision and fixed to the rectus sheath or the abdominal fascia.

The main difference between the fascial sling and alloplastic band procedures is the tension of the band on the urethra. Too little tension of the organic sling causes failure, while too much may lead to dysuria or urinary retention. The growth of fibrous tissue through the holes of the nylon net is thought to hold the bladder neck in position with a minimum of tension.

It is of great importance, regardless of the type of sling used, that surgery be restricted to reconstitution of the physiological state, i.e. support and elevation of the bladder neck. If compression of the urethra is induced by the operation, an obstruction might result, leading to residual urine and urine retention.

It must be pointed out that it is not necessary to terminate the operation if an intra-operative bladder injury occurs during blunt retrosymphysial dissection, as happens following previous suprapubic surgery (e.g. a Marshall–Marchetti–Krantz procedure). The lesion is usually located retrosymphysially, and rarely requires further operative treatment.

Post-operative Management

During the post-operative period, patients are given prophylactic antibiotics to prevent any infection which might endanger the sling. The suprapubic

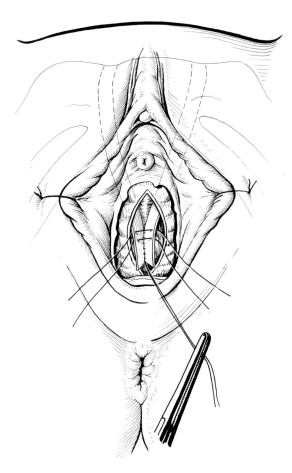

Fig. 7.6. Suture of fascial strips.

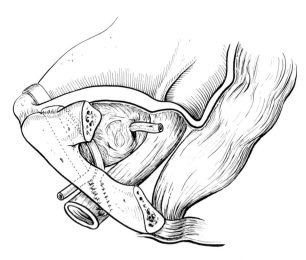

Fig. 7.7. Correct position of fascial strip under bladder neck.

catheter is removed after 10 days, if repeated measurements of residual urine are less than 100 ml. Patients not voiding satisfactorily are discharged with the catheter in place and reviewed after 10–14 days.

Complications

Post-operative complications (7.2%), with the exception of one case, occurred only in the years before 1973. Apart from one instance of pulmonary embolism (which was not fatal), two women (who were very obese) developed local abdominal wall infection and hernia in the area of the inguinal fascial scar. Injury to the lower urinary tract, as is occasionally seen with alloplastic slings, was not observed at all. Incompatibility reactions, infections or fistula formation were not observed. Table 7.2 shows complications which may accompany sling procedures as well as their cause and suggestions for treatment.

Follow-up Assessment

Culture and sensitivity, and measurements of residual urine are repeated at frequent intervals. Symptoms of dysuria or strangury persisting for more than 6 months or positive urine culture or recurrence of pre-operative symptoms indicate further urodynamic evaluation. Women who are dry and asymptomatic with sterile urine and without residual urine are followed up by the family physician or the referring specialist.

Results

Depending on patient selection and indication, cure rates for incontinence of up to 90% have been reported for sling operations (Table 7.3), although late results of several techniques have not yet been published. In contrast to the technically simpler and less involved implantation of one of the many modified alloplastic slings, the fascial sling operation is a relatively complex procedure. The not inconsiderable number of complications resulting from alloplastic slings referred to our clinic for correction, however, has raised some doubt as to the use of alloplastic material.

Table 7.2. Complications of sling procedures

Complications	Cause	Therapy
A. Intra-operative		
Bladder perforation	Inadequate preparation	Careful dissection Closure of perforation
Severe haemorrhage (paravesical veins)	Inadequate preparation	Tamponade with gauze pack for several minutes Release the catheter to look for haematuria indicating bladder trauma
B. Post-operative		
Residual urine/ retention	Sling too tight Op-indication correct?	Transurethral bouginage Vaginal severance of the band
Dysuria	Band too tight Incorrect position	Conservative Severance if necessary
Parametritis	Incomplete separation of the vaginal and abdominal op-fields	Conservative
Urethrovaginal fistula	Urethral lesion unrecognised	Fistula closure
C. Late complications		
Fistula (alloplastic slings)	Infection (Diabetic?)	Conservative Removal if necessary
Ulceration of bladder or urethra (alloplastic)	Placement incorrect or too tight	Transurethral severance of the sling or single fibres Removal
Direct hernia (fascial sling)	Incorrect fascial suture	Herniotomy
Pain in the scar region	(Multiple pre-operations)	Scar revision

Since 1968, we have performed more than 100 inguinovaginal sling operations in our Department. The average age of patients was 53 years; the oldest patient was 76 years. There were no intra- or post-operative deaths. Sixty per cent of the women had had up to ten previous incontinence operations. In the last few years, hysterectomy was performed at the same time by a gynaecologist (if not performed previously). In 12 patients with vaginal descent, an anterior and posterior repair were performed. In three patients, urethrovaginal fistulae resulting from previous incontinence operations were closed during the sling procedure.

Non-neuropathic

Continence was achieved in 84.4% of patients with urodynamic proof of pure stress incontinence in a follow-up period of up to 12 years. The success rate was similar for primary and recurrent incontinence. However, with increasing duration of follow-up, there was a marked increase of recurrences (Table 7.4).

Neuropathic

Continence was successfully achieved in 14 of 21 (66.7%) specially selected patients with neuropathic bladder disturbance, some of whom had serious psychosocial conditions before the operation. As could be expected, dysuria and urgency (19%) and residual urine (28.6%) occurred more frequently than in women with pure stress incontinence. This,

Table 7.3. Results of sling operations for incontinence

Sling operation	Author	No. of patients	Continent/ improved (%)	Continent (%)	Improved (%)
Zoedler sling	Wienhöwer et al. (1976)	136	90	—	—
	Zoedler (1970)	250	98	—	—
Silicone tendon	Sexton (1983, unpublished work)	127	—	35.4	50.4
Polyglactin mesh	Fianu and Soderberg (1972)	21	95.2	—	—
Gauze hammock	Kersey (1983)	105	—	60.2	25.2
Dural sling	Heidenreich et al. (1976)	48	94	—	—
	Gaudenz (1976)	28	61	—	—
	Hägele et al. (1983)	127	86.3	—	—
Fascial sling	Parker et al. (1979)	50	—	84	10
	Beck and Lai (1972)	88	—	88.6	6.8
	Altmann et al. (1976)	193	84.4	—	—
	Petri et al. (1983)	106	—	86	9

Table 7.4. Long-term results of sling operations for incontinence (Petri et al. 1983)

Result	Post-operative (%)	< 2 yrs (%)	> 2 yrs (%)	> 5 yrs (%)
Continent	50	86	64	52
Improved	1	9	14	19
Primary retention	45	—	4	—
Failure	2	—	15	26
Urge incontinence	2	5	3	3
	$n=106$	$n=21$	$n=73$	$n=63$

however, was a calculated risk, and had been discussed with the patients pre-operatively.

Failure

Analysis of 18 operative failures and 5 recurrences demonstrated a non-functional urethra during pre-operative urodynamic investigation in eight women; a further seven had congenital or acquired neurological disease, and another three had severe diabetes mellitus or had undergone radical gynaecological surgery with radiation therapy. There was no explanation for failure in five women, so that the possibility of operative error has been considered. Ten women complained of dysuria, probably due to excessive sling tension, which could be treated by bouginage or anticholinergic drugs (e.g. indomethacin or flavoxate hydrochloride).

Summary

Sling procedures have found a permanent place among the operative procedures to correct incontinence in women, especially in instances of recurrent incontinence.

In addition to achieving continence, it is necessary to consider such side-effects as dysuria, urgency, increased amounts of residual urine and, in particular, secondary injuries to the lower urinary tract when judging the success of the operation.

Operative results can be improved by:

—Pre-operative exclusion of neuropathic bladder dysfunction by a sophisticated urodynamic evaluation.

—Carrying out simultaneous gynaecological operations (e.g. hysterectomy, or correction of a cystocele).

—Avoiding operative errors by careful preparation and correct positioning of the sling.

The ideal sling operation should be technically as simple as the alloplastic procedures, whilst healing should be as good, and with as little risk of later lesions of the lower urinary tract as with the fascial sling operation. Long-term observations of the dural band—with its shorter duration of surgery and less complex procedure than the fascial sling—are necessary to determine whether this method provides a viable alternative.

References

Altmann P, Georgiades E, Rudelstorfer B (1976) Zur Technik der inguinovaginalen Schlingenoperation (Modifikation nach Narik–Palmrich) und ihre Spätergebnisse. In: Verh Ber Dtsch Ges Urol 27. Tagung, Springer, Berlin Heidelberg New York, pp 213–215

Anselmino KJ (1952) Eine neue Schlingenoperation zur Behandlung der hochgradigen Urininkontinenz des Weibes. Geburtshilfe Fraunheilkd 12:277

Beck RP, Lai AR (1982) Results in treating 88 cases of recurrent urinary stress incontinence with the Oxford fascia lata sling procedure. Am J Obstet Gynecol 142:649–651

Bracht E (1956) Eine besondere Form der Zügelplastik. Geburtshilfe Fraunheilkd 16:782–790

Fianu S, Söderberg G (1983) Absorbable Polyglactin mesh for retropubic sling operations in female urinary stress incontinence. Gynecol Obstet Invest 16:45–50

Gaudenz R (1976) Die Bedeutung einer Zusatzoperation bei der primären operativen Behandlung einer Urethralinsuffizienz. Geburtshilfe Fraunheilkd 39:393–401

Hägele D, Frühwirth O, Kriesche H, Nol C, Berg D (1983) Ergebnisse nach Schlingenoperation mit Tutoplast-Dura. Geburtshilfe Fraunheilkd 43:762–765

Havlíček S (1972) Schlingenoperationen mit Lyoduraband bei rezidivierender Harninkontinenz der Frau. Geburtshilfe Frauenheilkd 32:757

Heidenreich J, Faber P, Beck L (1976) Suspension mit Lyoduraband. In: Verh Ber Dtsch Ges Urol 27. Tagung, Springer, Berlin Heidelberg New York, pp 221–222

Kersey J (1983) The gauze hammock sling operation in the treatment of stress incontinence. Br J Obstet Gynaecol 90:945–949

Millin T, Read C (1948) Stress incontinence of urine in the female. Postgrad Med J 24:3–10, 51–56

Narik G, Palmrich AH (1962) A simplified sling operation suitable for routine use. Am J Obstet Gynecol 84:400–405

Narik G, Palmrich AH (1965) Inguinovaginale Schlingenoperation zur Behandlung hochgradiger Harninkontinenz. Urologe [Ausg A] 4:205–207

Parker RT, Addison WA, Wilson CJ (1979) Fascia lata urethrovesical suspension for recurrent stress urinary incontinence. Am J Obstet Gynecol 135:843–852

Petri E, Frohneberg D, Thüroff JW (1981) Problems of loop grafts. Akt Urol 12:31–33

Petri E, Beckhaus I, Frohneberg D, Thüroff JW (1983) Inguinovaginal fascial sling according to Narik and Palmrich— indication, problems, long-term results. Akt Urol 14:286–290

Sexton GL (1983) The risks and complications of the epiurethral suprapubic vaginal suspension for the correction of recurrent postoperative-stress incontinence. Gynec Urol Soc New Orleans Nov 2–5 1983

Stanton SL, Brindley G, Holmes D (1985) Silastic sling for urethral sphincter incompetence in the female. Br J Obstet Gynaecol 92:747–750

Stoeckel W (1917) Über die Verwendung der Musculi pyramidales bei der operativen Behandlung der Incontinentia urinae. Zentralbl Gynakol 41:11–19

Ullery JC (1953) Stress incontinence in the female. Grune & Stratton, New York

Wienhöwer R, Merten M, Zoedler D (1976) Ergebnisse urologischer Rezidiv-Inkontinenz-Operationen. In: Verh Ber Dtsch Ges Urol 27. Tagung, Springer, Berlin Heidelberg New York, pp 222–224

Zoedler D (1961) Zur operativen Behandlung der weiblichen Stressinkontinenz. Z Urol Nephrol 54:355–358

Zoedler D (1970) Die operative Behandlung der weiblichen Harninkontinenz mit dem Kunststoff-Netzband. Akt Urol 1:28–34

8 Endoscopic Suspension of the Vesical Neck

Thomas A. Stamey

Introduction

The cure of stress urinary incontinence (SUI) in the female is dependent upon moving the internal vesical neck to a position forward and upward behind the symphysis pubis (Fig. 8.1), where sudden increases in intra-abdominal pressure presumably become additive to the resting urethral pressure and thereby prevent intravesical pressure from exceeding intraurethral pressure (Enhorning 1961).

We described an operation in 1973 which has the following advantages (Stamey 1973):

—It accurately identifies the internal vesical neck at the time of surgery.
—It strongly supports the internal vesical neck by bolstering the pubocervical and endopelvic fascia with permanent number 2 nylon suture passed through a 1-cm tube of knitted Dacron.

—It does not require open pelvic surgery, thereby decreasing operative morbidity.
—It allows physiological measurements during surgery which assure the surgeon that the incontinence has been corrected.

Indications and Contraindications

This is the ideal operation for the surgically difficult pelvis, i.e. severe fractures, radiation incontinence, multiple operative failures, obesity, etc. Because of these advantages, endoscopic suspension of the vesical neck is applicable to all females with surgically curable urinary incontinence (urethral sphincter incompetence); there are no contraindications to the use of this operation.

Spinal cord injury patients with reflex neuropathic bladders and massive urethral dilatation associated with urinary leakage around their

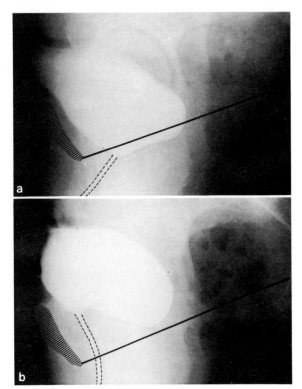

Fig. 8.1. a Pre-operative, direct, lateral view cystogram made during straining. The catheter was filled with 90% Hypaque and the bladder with 25% Hypaque. A reference line is drawn from the distal end of the fifth sacral vertebral body to the lower border of the symphysis pubis. **b** Post-operative film of the same patient following endoscopic suspension of the vesical neck. Note the substantial elevation of the internal vesical neck to a position several centimetres high behind the symphysis pubis.

Foley urethral catheters can be cured of the incontinence by combining suprapubic catheter drainage with endoscopic suspension of the vesical neck (Fowler 1978). Women with acontractile, neuropathic bladders, and large residual volume—when accompanied by demonstrable stress urinary incontinence—can also be cured of their incontinence by endoscopic suspension, but they must accept a permanent programme of intermittent self-catheterisation.

Pre-operative Evaluation

History

When patients with urinary incontinence are first seen in consultations, a detailed history is taken with a serious attempt to quantify the degree and circumstances of urinary incontinence. The following few questions are the important ones.

1. Do you lose urine only with severe stress such as coughing, sneezing, laughing (Grade I incontinence)? Do you lose urine with minimal increases in abdominal pressure such as changing from the sitting to the standing position, walking, running, etc. (Grade II incontinence)? Do you lose urine continuously without accumulation of urine in the bladder during the day (total urinary incontinence, or Grade III)?

2. Do you lose urine by small spurts (related to physical activity)? By continuous dribbling (unrelated to activity)? Do you lose urine in large amounts (a cupful or more), feeling your bladder has suddenly contracted and emptied without your control?

3. How many, and what size, perineal pads do you use per day to keep the clothing dry? Are the pads saturated or damp?

4. How often do you urinate during the day? How often at night? Is the volume of urine you usually pass large, average, small or very small?

5. Are you dry at night in bed? It should be noted here that while the answer is "yes" in Grade I incontinence, it is frequently "no" in Grade II and always "no" in Grade III incontinence.

An attempt is made to quantify the degree of urge incontinence which is present in one-third of our patients with surgically curable urinary incontinence. The question is asked as follows: When you have a desire to urinate, do you lose urine before you can get to the toilet? If so, does this urinary leakage represent a small amount, a moderate amount, or most of the total urine you lose throughout the 24 h? Urge incontinence is not uncommon with SUI and usually disappears immediately or a few months after surgical correction of SUI (Stamey et al. 1975); those patients with severe urge incontinence (with demonstrable SUI) are usually forewarned that several months may be required before they can fully control their urge incontinence. Although urge incontinence is common in our patients with demonstrable stress urinary incontinence, if the complaint is only urgency leakage and the amount of stress urinary incontinence is very minimal when examined in the standing position, it is a major error to operate upon such a patient.

Previous surgical attempts to correct the urinary incontinence and the duration of success or failure of that surgery, as well as any complications (pelvic abscess, etc.), should be carefully explored in the history. Neurological diseases (including cerebrovascular accidents) and neurosurgical or orthopaedic procedures on the spinal column should be documented, along with any residual neuromuscular defects.

The above questions are the really useful ones in evaluating urinary incontinence. Many other questions are found in some questionnaires, especially queries relating to childhood history, sensations of losing urine, sight or sound of running water causing urinary leakage, etc., but we have not found any of these questions to be useful.

Physical Examination

Stress urinary incontinence, or surgically curable incontinence, is not a syndrome. It is a *physically demonstrable* event that is curable by elevating the internal vesical neck to a position forward and upward behind the symphysis pubis. For this reason, its occurrence must be demonstrated on physical examination by the responsible surgeon. If urinary incontinence cannot be demonstrated to occur *exactly coincident* with a rise in abdominal pressure, the patient should not be operated upon, no matter how suggestive the history. Remember, the patient's history is subjective; the demonstration of SUI is an objective finding.

The procedure is simple. While taking the history, the patient is given water to drink. When the bladder is very full she is asked to void in private. The voided volume is recorded (to estimate the functional size or capacity of the bladder), and she is immediately catheterised (14F gauge) for a residual urine estimation. The catheterisation should occur quickly after voiding because the patient is hydrated: the residual urine should be 10% or less of the voided urine volume and certainly never greater than 20%. The catheter is left in the bladder so that the surgeon can fill the bladder slowly by gravity (at about 15–20 cmH$_2$O) with an open syringe or funnel in the end of the catheter.

The bladder should be filled until the patient is comfortably full but not to the point of urgency to void. The catheter is withdrawn, the patient is allowed to relax, the labia separated with one hand, and the patient asked to cough while a light is directed at the urethral meatus. Loss of urine from the urethral meatus *must occur simultaneously with the rise in abdominal pressure and immediately cease with the fall in abdominal pressure.* This is my definition of surgically curable urinary incontinence in the female. It is a specific entity, it is not complicated, it certainly is not a syndrome, and it is curable by endoscopic suspension of the vesical neck.

About 20% of patients with SUI will not demonstrate urinary loss on coughing in the lithotomy position. When this occurs, the table is tilted 45° from the horizontal, which adds additional pressure on the bladder from the weight of the intestinal contents; another 15% of patients will show SUI in this position. The remaining 5% will demonstrate SUI only in the standing position on coughing; the legs are straight and spread about 30° apart in order to hold a kidney basin between the legs about 15 cm above the knee.

The surgeon must be very careful when operating on these patients who require examination in the standing position because it is here that many unstable neuropathic bladders will also be demonstrated. It is essential to make certain that the loss of urine is exactly coincident with the cough. In such instances, the initial loss or spurt of urine occurs with the cough, but because the labia create a "dam-like" effect in the standing position, the immediate cessation of urine flow at the urethral meatus is followed by some post-cough dribbling from the labia and pubic hair. This prolonged leakage, however, should be minimal.

On the other hand, patients with unstable neuropathic bladders will often lose urine in the standing position, but urine loss never starts exactly with the cough because the detrusor contraction is relatively slow in comparison with the "mechanical" fluid loss of SUI. In my experience, urine loss from these hyperreflexic bladders is always delayed by at least 5–10 s and usually develops into a sizeable stream: the patient has great difficulty in contracting her levators and stopping the flow of urine. Hodgkinson et al. (1963) called this condition detrusor dyssynergia and later provided an excellent visual description of urinary loss from these unstable bladders (Hodgkinson 1970).

The physical examination is completed (in the lithotomy position) by (a) testing the mobility of the tissues lateral to the internal vesical neck, because it is these tissues that must hold the vesical neck in position behind the symphysis pubis, and (b) checking the degree of anterior (cystocele) and posterior (rectocele) relaxation of the vaginal wall during straining in the lithotomy position or in the standing position. If a large rectocele is present, it should be repaired at the time of endoscopic suspension because cystoceles are so elevated and corrected by the support acquired from suspending the vesical neck that rectoceles can then protrude from the introitus post-operatively, once the counterpressure from the cystocele is removed by surgery. While the speculum is helpful in deciding whether to repair a rectocele at the same time, we find a tongue blade or a single blade from the vaginal speculum much more useful in lifting up the anterior bladder wall while the patient strains to lower the rectocele.

The Bonney or Marshall–Marchetti–Krantz test is always positive in true SUI, but as it cannot be performed in the condition of unstable neuropathic bladder (as leakage does not occur simultaneously with coughing) it is not a discriminating test.

Lateral Chain Cystogram

Lateral chain cystograms are helpful in that *every* operative cure of SUI is accompanied by movement of the urethrovesical junction from a position backward and downward to a new position forward and upward behind the symphysis pubis (Fig. 8.1). A lateral chain cystogram is the only way to measure surgical movement of the urethrovesical junction accurately, so if the operation fails and the surgeon wants to know whether or not the procedure accomplished what it was supposed to do, it is necessary to obtain a pre-operative lateral chain cystogram to compare movement with a post-operative lateral chain cystogram.

We have performed over 150 pre- and post-operative lateral chain cystograms on our 450 patients operated upon by endoscopic suspension of the vesical neck; we published an analysis of 44 consecutive patients early in our series (Stamey et al. 1975). We now perform a lateral chain cystogram only on those patients with severe pelvic problems (irradiation, pelvic fractures, multiple retropubic failure, etc.) in whom we expect a difficult operation. If the operation is unsuccessful, we can immediately answer the major question: "Did we move the internal vesical neck forward and upward behind the symphysis pubis in relation to its pre-operative position?" If the answer is "no", the operation is a technical failure and no improvement can be expected in the urinary incontinence.

Although we have ceased getting lateral chain cystograms in uncomplicated cases, we have learned several lessons from the large consecutive series in which every patient had pre- and post-operative chain cystograms. Figure 8.2 shows the movement of the internal vesical neck at a point 1 cm behind the urethrovesical junction in 44 consecutive cases reported previously (Stamey et al. 1975). Note that the average movement upward of the urethrovesical junction in those successfully treated patients who had undergone previous surgery was 47 mm, almost as good as the 54 mm movement achieved in those patients who had not had previous pelvic surgery. Since the 22 patients with previous surgery (Fig. 8.2) had undergone 44 operations for SUI (including 14 Marshall–Marchetti–Krantz operations), it is clear from these radiological data that it is the failure of the pubocervical and endopelvic fascia to hold the internal vesical neck upward and forward that accounts for

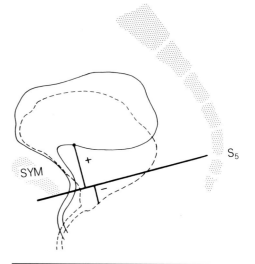

	PRE-OP	POST-OP
	mm	mm
Cures without previous surgery (N=15)	−19 (−40, −5)	+35 (+10, +45)
Cures with previous surgery (N=19)	−8 (−35, +20)	+39 (+10, +60)
Failures with previous surgery (N=3)	+3 (−22, +10)	+40 (+15, +50)

Fig. 8.2. The pre-operative (*broken line*) and post-operative (*solid line*) position of the posterior base-plate of the bladder 1 cm from the posterior urethrovesical junction during straining. The mean of the three patient groups, together with the minimal and maximal value observed, is presented for each category. + indicates those positions above the symphyseal (SYM)-fifth sacral vertebral (S$_5$) line; − indicates those positions below the line (Stamey et al. 1975).

operative failures. These data show that the surgeon achieves about the same movement of the vesical neck in patients who are previous surgical failures as in patients who have not had previous surgery, at least when endoscopic suspension is the method of elevating the vesical neck.

Whilst funnelling of the vesical neck with loss of the posterior urethrovesical angle is found in patients who have not had previous retropubic surgery for SUI (Jeffcoate and Roberts 1952), we have a dozen or more patients with SUI who have had unsuccessful retropubic surgery, whose lateral chain cystograms show a flat base-plate without funnelling (Fig. 8.3a) and who were cured by moving their urethrovesical junction further forward behind the symphysis pubis (Fig. 8.3b), perhaps to a position free of scar tissue where intra-abdominal pressure can apply additional force to the urethra on coughing.

Cystometry

Although urethral pressure profiles, both dynamic (Constantinou et al. 1981) and resting (see Results) may serve to identify a stress incontinent urethra, cystometry is not helpful in the diagnosis of surgically curable stress urinary incontinence. Constantinou and I (Shortliffe and Stamey, 1985) recently studied 151 consecutive unselected women with incontinence, 84 (56%) of whom had demonstrable stress urinary incontinence on physical examination and 67 (44%) of whom had no evidence of stress urinary incontinence even in the standing position. Of the 84 women with stress urinary incontinence, 62% showed stable bladders, whilst 38% were unstable (involuntary, unsuppressible detrusor contractions during bladder filling that led to loss of urine.) Of the 67 women without demonstrable stress urinary incontinence to explain their incontinence, 51% were stable and 49% unstable. Therefore, if one-third of patients with surgically curable stress urinary incontinence display instability on cystometry examination, and 50% of women without demonstrable stress urinary incontinence appear stable, it is clear that cystometry (at least with currently available techniques) cannot help the surgeon in his decision as to whether or not to operate.

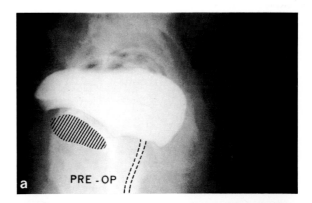

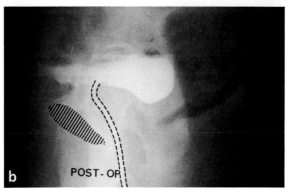

Fig. 8.3. Pre-operative **a** and post-operative **b** lateral cystograms in a patient with three previous retropubic failures for SUI, now cured of her incontinence by endoscopic suspension of the vesical neck (9 years of follow-up).

Endoscopy

Although urethroscopy will often show an open, lax urethra and a vesical neck that is not angled high behind the symphysis pubis, urethroscopy actually plays no role in the diagnosis of SUI. The diagnosis is made simply by demonstrating SUI on physical examination. Indeed, urethroscopy is not only cost-ineffective in an already overburdened health system, but is misleading to the unwary, since common diagnoses such as "trigonitis" do not even exist (Cifuentes 1947).

Operative Technique

The operation is still performed exactly as originally described (Stamey 1973). Gentamicin 80 mg is given the evening before surgery (to sterilise any unsuspected urinary infection by the next morning) and is also given in the operating room (for pelvic tissue prophylaxis against vaginal contamination). Briefly, the patient is placed in a modified lithotomy position with the lower abdomen flat and the legs extended laterally with the knees slightly bent (the same position as for cystectomy and urethrectomy). Careful attention is paid to draping the patient, especially if the cystocopy table is used, where it is important to avoid contamination of the drapes by the underlying drainage drawer. A layer of sterile plastic is used to separate the drainage drawer from the overlying drape. The rectum is separated from the vagina by a plastic half-towel which is sutured to the perineum and to the medial edge of the buttocks. The labia minora are sutured laterally to the skin to expose the vaginal introitus. A 16F Foley balloon catheter is inserted.

Abdominal Incision

Two suprapubic incisions, 3–5 cm long, are made to the left and right of the mid-line, exactly at the upper border of the symphysis pubis, and carried down to the rectus fascia by separating the fat and subcutaneous fascia with a curved Mayo clamp. The strength of the anterior rectus fascia is estimated, in case later buttressing of this fascia appears indicated at the end of the operation when the suspending nylon sutures are tied over the anterior rectus fascia.

Vaginal Incision

The urethral length is measured with the Foley catheter prior to incising the anterior vaginal wall. If the urethra is short (2.5 cm or less), the transverse incision is begun just below the urethral meatus (Fig. 8.4a). If the urethra is longer, the incision can be made closer to the internal vesical neck. In practice, especially in those patients with previous anterior vaginal surgery, a convenient fold of tissue at least 2 cm from the internal vesical neck is chosen for the transverse incision in such a way that the remaining tissue toward the vesical neck is flat rather than folded. After the transverse incision is made, Metzenbaum scissors are used to free the anterior vaginal wall from the proximal urethra and distal trigone (Fig. 8.4b). During this manoeuvre, the tip of the scissors must be directed posteriorly toward the floor at all times; in this way, the bladder will not be entered. Any freeing of the anterior vaginal wall in the region of the vesical neck should be done carefully to avoid weakening the pubocervical fascia, i.e. dissection should be on the anterior vaginal wall and not on the tissues that immediately surround it. In most instances, adequate exposure to accept a 1-cm tube of 5 mm Dacron on either side of the internal vesical neck is easily achieved by spreading the Metzenbaum scissors laterally in a posterior direction and then incising this anterior flap in the mid-line (Fig. 8.4c). The Foley balloon should be easily palpable within the incision, thereby determining exactly the internal vesical neck on the distal side of the balloon.

Stamey Needles

A series of three special but simple needles have been developed—a straight needle, a 15° angled needle and a 30° angled needle (Fig. 8.5).[1]

I always begin with the straight needle on the medial side of either the right or left suprapubic incision. The angled needles are especially useful in those patients who have had previous retropubic surgery in which the anterior bladder wall remains adherent to the symphysis pubis. Both hands are used to introduce the needle through the anterior

---

1. Pilling Company, Fort Washington, Pennsylvania, USA

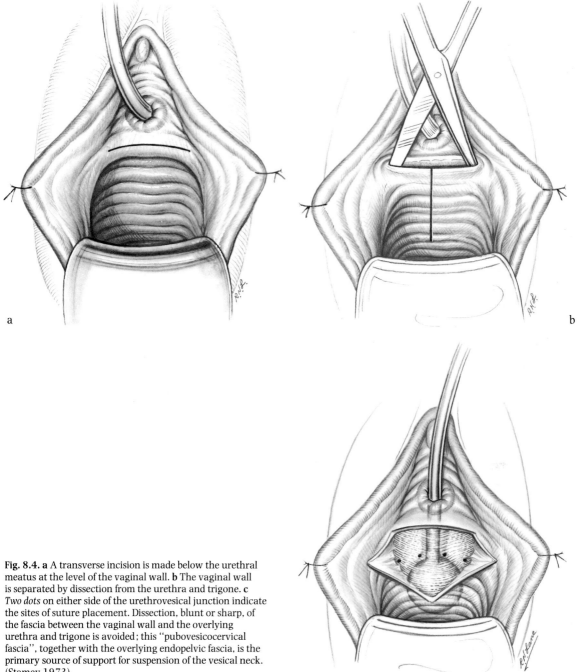

a

b

c

Fig. 8.4. a A transverse incision is made below the urethral
meatus at the level of the vaginal wall. **b** The vaginal wall
is separated by dissection from the urethra and trigone. **c**
Two dots on either side of the urethrovesical junction indicate
the sites of suture placement. Dissection, blunt or sharp, of
the fascia between the vaginal wall and the overlying
urethra and trigone is avoided; this "pubovesicocervical
fascia", together with the overlying endopelvic fascia, is the
primary source of support for suspension of the vesical neck.
(Stamey 1973)

rectus fascia just at the superior border of the symphysis pubis. After penetrating the anterior rectus
fascia, the needle is laid almost flat on the abdomen
in order to probe for the superior edge of the symphysis pubis. Once the superior edge is located, the
point of the needle is guided 1 cm behind and parallel to the undersurface of the symphysis pubis. The

needle is then returned to an almost vertical position. With one hand on the suprapubic needle, the
Foley catheter is now placed across the open palm
of the other hand, gently grasped by closing the
fingers, and the index finger is placed into the
vaginal incision at the point of the internal vesical
neck. By lifting up the pubocervical fascia with the

Use of Endoscopy

The 90° (or 70°) angle cystoscope is introduced into the bladder after first removing the Foley catheter (Fig. 8.7). By directing the cystoscope at the 1–2 o'clock or 10–11 o'clock position, the surgeon first makes sure that the needle has not entered the bladder and that it has not been placed submucosally or intramuscularly. Once the needle is known not to have entered the bladder wall, the cystoscope is withdrawn to the internal vesical neck and turned to either the 3 or 9 o'clock position. By vertically moving the needle up and down, the surgeon can readily tell whether the needle is exactly positioned beside the internal vesical neck. If the needle is distal to the neck (down the urethra), the tissues at the neck will show little movement. If the needle is proximal to the neck and to the side of the trigone, it is easily identified as such. This manoeuvre with the 70° or 90° angle cystoscope, in which it is determined that the needle is placed exactly outside the internal vesical neck, is the most important part of this operation; it is why the operation is called "endoscopic suspension of the vesical neck". Moreover, in addition to being placed exactly at the internal vesical neck, the needle should be freely movable and not fixed by scar tissue.

If the tissue feels too rigid, the needle should be passed again in an effort to find more pliable tissues. Lastly, if the bladder is filled with 200 or 300 ml of irrigating fluid, indentation of the needle outside the bladder wall between the vesical neck and air bubble should not be too great. (See film entitled *Visits in Urology. Urinary Incontinence in Women*, Norwich Eaton Film Library, 1983, Stamey.)

Once the needle is determined to be exactly at the internal vesical neck, the cystoscope is withdrawn, a weighted (Auvard) vaginal speculum is introduced, and a number 2 monofilament nylon suture is threaded through the eye of the needle. One end of the nylon suture is securely clamped in the vaginal incision and the needle withdrawn suprapubically; the suprapubic end of the nylon is also clamped (Fig. 8.8).

The Foley catheter is reintroduced, the vaginal retractor withdrawn, and the special needle introduced 1 cm lateral to the nylon suture that exits from the medial edge of the suprapubic incision. The needle is introduced and passed exactly as described above. The only difference this time is that, in addition to feeling the Foley balloon to identify the internal vesical neck, the surgeon must also feel the

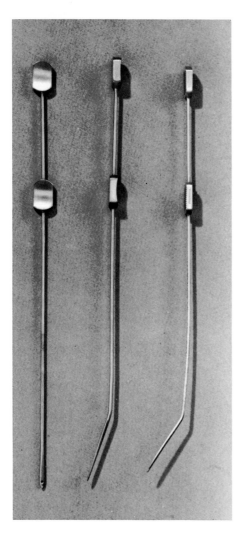

Fig. 8.5. Straight, 15° and 30° angled needles used for endoscopic suspension of the vesical neck.

index finger (Fig. 8.6a), the blunt point of the special needle, as it rests just below the rectus fascia and behind the symphysis pubis, is readily palpated. Occasionally, a vertical bouncing motion of the needle (without advancing it) is helpful in locating the point of the needle. Once the point is located on the index finger, the needle is guided downward exactly at the side of the internal vesical neck (indicated by the Foley balloon) and into the vaginal incision (Fig. 8.6b). It is important to emphasise that the initial 1 cm advancement of the needle at the upper border of the symphysis pubis, while both hands are on the needle in the suprapubic position, represents the *only* part of the operation in which needle advancement is "blind"; the rest of the needle passage is under bimanual control.

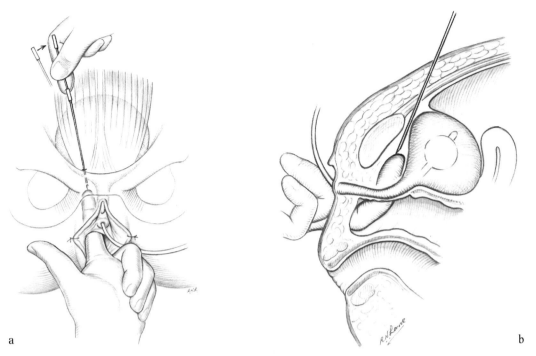

a   b

Fig. 8.6. a Sagittal view, showing a 15° angled needle passed through the right anterior rectus fascia and turned towards the under-surface of the symphysis pubis to avoid perforating small intestine that may be adherent to the top of the bladder and then guided alongside the urethrovesical junction (*inset*) (Stamey 1973). **b** Coronal view showing location of the needle point on the tip of the index finger.

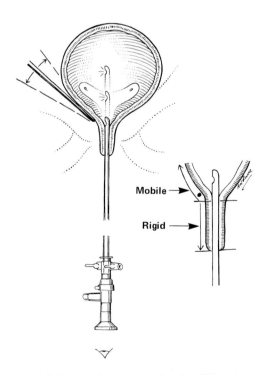

Fig. 8.7. Foley catheter removed and a 90° angle cystoscope introduced (Stamey 1973). The needle is moved vertically up and down so that it can be positioned exactly beside the internal vesical neck. *Inset*, a magnified position.

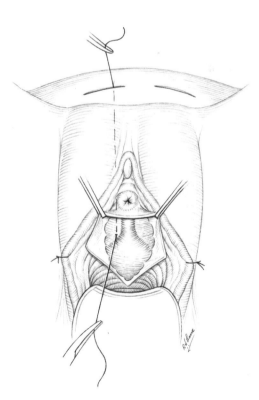

Fig. 8.8. Both ends of the nylon suture clamped following the first passage of the needle.

position of the first nylon suture against his index finger so that he can stay 1 cm lateral to it throughout this second passage of the needle. I usually place two or three Mayo clamps on the vaginal end of the nylon suture, in order to give added weight to the nylon suture before passing the needle the second time. The second passage of the needle should be 1 cm lateral to the first, exactly at the internal vesical neck, and not down the urethra distal to the first suture. In this way, the internal vesical neck—not the urethra—is suspended in position behind the symphysis pubis.

After establishing that the second needle is 1 cm lateral to the nylon suture and that it is endoscopically exactly at the internal vesical neck (as well as free from the bladder wall), the vaginal end of the existing nylon suture is first threaded through the hole of a 1 cm tube of 5 mm Dacron before engaging the eye of the needle (Fig. 8.9). The needle is then withdrawn suprapubically, pulling the nylon suture with it, thereby establishing the suspended loop with the Dacron buttress vaginally reinforcing the pubocervical and endopelvic fascia. I usually hold the Dacron tube with an Allis clamp placed on the side of it as the second needle is withdrawn suprapubically. Then, after adjusting the two exiting ends of the nylon suture in the suprapubic incision so that they are even, I observe the Dacron tube as it settles into the vaginal space to the side of the internal vesical neck.

The identical procedure is then repeated for the incision on the opposite side of the mid-line so that two separate suspending sutures, each with its vaginal Dacron buttress, are located on either side of the internal vesical neck (but not passing across beneath the neck) (Figs. 8.10).

Once both suspending loops are established on the right and left side of the mid-line, the panendoscope is introduced for the first time and is used to observe the point of urethral closure when each suspending loop is individually pulled up suprapubically (Fig. 8.11a,b). With the panendoscope in the distal urethra, the surgeon can observe: that closure occurs exactly at the internal vesical neck; that the left and right suspending loops are symmetrically placed; and the approximate amount of suprapubic tension required to close the internal vesical neck, which then serves as a guide as to how tightly to tie the nylon sutures suprapubically. These observations are best made with the bladder nearly empty: a full bladder limits movement of an otherwise mobile vesical neck.

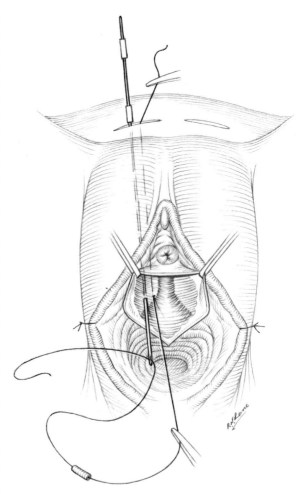

Fig. 8.9. Second passage of the needle 1 cm lateral to the first passage, with the Dacron sleeve threaded on the nylon.

Physiological observations should now be made after the urethra has been examined through the panendoscope. Before withdrawing the panendoscope, it is depressed posteriorly to relieve any suspending tension from the Dacron buttresses. As the instrument is removed, a large stream of irrigating fluid will gush from the urethra. On gently pulling up on either suspending suture, leakage of irrigating fluid should sharply cease with the slightest amount of tension. The cessation of fluid leakage with this manoeuvre is so abrupt and so complete that it allows the surgeon to predict the success of the operation with confidence. Obviously, failure to observe cessation of leakage indicates improper placement of the suspending sutures (which would also have been observed from panendoscopic examination of the urethra) and the operation should be redone. However, if the bladder

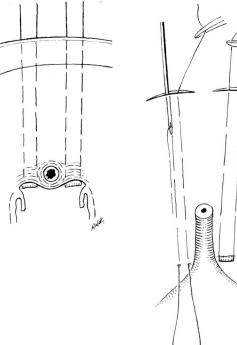

Fig. 8.10. *Right:* Diagrammatic representation showing the level of the two supporting nylon loops and their respective Dacron tubes, alongside the internal vesical neck. The loops support a shelf of pubovesicocervical fascia on either side of the internal vesical neck. *Left:* Pubovesicocervical fascia on either side of the internal vesical neck suspended by two nylon loops.

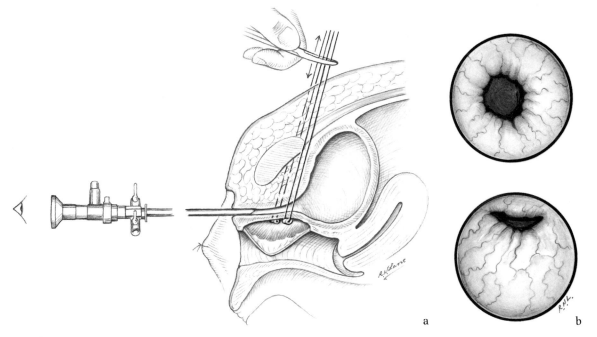

Fig. 8.11. a Position of the panendoscope prior to elevating the suspending nylon sutures to check closure of the vesical neck. **b** *Above:* the patulous appearance of the vesical neck in the open position. *Below:* exactly at the internal vesical neck when the surgeon pulls vertically on either nylon loop.

is over-filled during these physiological assessments of bladder neck closure, considerable suprapubic tension will be required to prevent urinary leakage and may incorrectly indicate inadequate placement of the suspending sutures.

The vaginal incision is closed first with continuous 2–0 or 3–0 chromic catgut before tying the suprapubic nylon sutures. Copious irrigation of the vaginal wound and vaginal Dacron buttresses with gentamicin solution is performed before closing the vaginal incision. A vaginal pack is placed for 24 h.

The nylon sutures are now tied suprapubically with minimal tension. It is important to make sure that the bladder is empty of all irrigating fluid before tying them. If the rectus fascia appears weak, each suture is passed through a 1 × 2 cm oval of flat silicone rubber and tied over the silicone which rests directly on the weakened fascia. We irrigate the suprapubic wound with gentamicin solution (80 mg/100 ml) before tying the nylon sutures. The subcutaneous tissue is closed with 4–0 chromic catgut and the skin with 3–0 nylon.

The bladder is filled to capacity through a Foley catheter (or it can be filled during the time of panendoscopic examination of the urethra) and a percutaneous 14F gauge Stamey suprapubic tube is placed in the bladder 3 cm above the symphysis pubis (Fig. 8.12).[2]

The Foley catheter is removed (the post-operative urethral length can be measured if desired—it is invariably longer) and the patient returned to the recovery room.

The New Pereyra–Lebherz Suspension

The basic principle of this procedure is the bilateral separation of the lateral attachments of the periurethral tissues and endopelvic fascia from the pubic ramus by blunt and sharp dissection through a vaginal incision similar to that shown in Fig. 8.4 (Pereyra and Lebherz 1978). This exposes the retropubic space to the vagina. The lateral edge of these periurethral tissues is grasped with a clamp and pulled into the incision in order to place a helical suture of number 0 polypropylene monofilament suture for approximately half an inch distal to the urethrovesical junction. Two helical sutures are placed on either side of the urethra.

A 1-in. skin incision is made just above the pubic symphysis to expose the rectus fascia and a special Pereyra Ligature Carrier Instrument used to puncture the rectus fascia 1 in. right of the mid-line, whilst the index finger of the opposite hand guides the needle into the retropubic space and through the vaginal incision. Both ends of the helical suture on the right side of the urethra are threaded into the needle and the instrument pulled through the suprapubic incision. This means that both suture ends exit through the same suprapubic hole; because of this, one of the ends is passed under the fascia parallel to the mid-line for about half an inch, thereby creating a fascial bridge over which the suspending suture can be tied. The procedure is then repeated on the other side of the urethra to bring the suture ends into the suprapubic incision. The vaginal incision is closed and the two suspending sutures are tied at a tension which appears to flatten and elevate the bladder neck. The suprapubic incision is then closed.

The advantage of this procedure is that the surgeon does not have to worry about entering the bladder with needles, because the entire retropubic space is open and palpable from the vaginal incision to the inferior surface of the rectus muscle. The disadvantage, however, is that the paraurethral suspending tissues and endopelvic fascia (which are left intact in the Stamey procedure) are removed from the pubic rami. Pelvic infections and retropubic haemorrhage may prove a problem in some cases since the entire retropubic space is exposed from the vaginal incision. Lastly, it is unlikely that the suspension of the Pereyra–Lebherz operation is as accurately limited to the urethrovesical junction as occurs with the endoscopic suspension operation. Nevertheless, for those surgeons unfamiliar with the cystoscope (which is the essential instrument for endoscopic suspension) the Pereyra–Lebherz procedure avoids placing suspending sutures too close to the bladder.

Post-operative Management

Care

Antimicrobial Management

Two additional doses of gentamicin are given at 8-h intervals and then discontinued. No further anti-

2. Cook Urological Inc., 1100 West Morgan Street, P.O. Box 227, Spencer, Indiana, 47460, USA

microbial therapy is used until the suprapubic tube is removed. If the tube is removed within 3 or 4 days while the patient is in the hospital and still on closed catheter drainage, the bladder urine is invariably sterile and antimicrobial therapy is unnecessary. On the other hand, if the patient is discharged with the tube in place, the great majority become infected with a variety of different bacteria and sometimes yeast. Because of the occasional occurrence of *Pseudomonas*, I give the patients 5 days of oral tetracycline at the time the tube is removed. Whatever regimen is used, including the ideal one of culturing immediately before removing the tube and treating the specific bacteria present, it is the surgeon's responsibility to make certain that the patient ultimately has a sterile bladder urine while off all antimicrobial agents. The surgeon who allows a *Proteus mirabilis* infection to go undetected in his patient commits her to infection and stone formation in the kidneys.

Removal of the Suprapubic Tube (Catheter)

On the third post-operative day, the patient is told to empty her urinary collection bag, clamp the suprapubic tube and await a strong desire to void as an indication her bladder is full. It is very important that the patient waits for a full bladder with the characteristic sensations of a detrusor contraction before attempting to urinate. She then attempts to void (the amount is measured), opens her suprapubic tube to empty the residual urine completely from the bladder into the drainage bag, and measures the amount in the drainage bag 5 min later. The suprapubic tube is removed when she voids 75% of her bladder volume on several consecutive voidings; it should not be removed when the residual is equal to the amount voided (50/50). An alternative to suprapubic catheterisation is to instruct the patient in intermittent self-catheterisation. This is especially helpful in those patients prone to bladder "spasms" from an indwelling catheter.

In 203 consecutive patients operated upon between 1973 and 1979 (Stamey 1980) the median time of suprapubic drainage was 7 days (range 1–120), with 14 patients requiring periods of more than 30 days.

Although only half of our patients have their suprapubic tube removed by the eighth day, the other half rarely mind the longer periods of suprapubic drainage because of one fact: they are no longer wet and know they will be dry once the tube is removed or intermittent catheterisation stopped.

Ambulation

All patients are mobilised the day after surgery. They are encouraged to "walk-out" any localising discomfort in the area of the suprapubic incision. Most patients can actually be discharged on the first or second post-operative day, if this is considered to be financially or environmentally necessary.

Complications

Operative

There have been no operative deaths. Blood transfusion is not required and we do not cross-match for it. In one elderly patient whose anterior pelvic peritoneum extended over the upper two-thirds of the proximal urethra, one suture passed through the mesentery of a loop of small bowel; intestinal obstruction required the removal of this suspending suture.

Post-operative

Early. One severely hypertensive patient died of either a massive coronary or pulmonary embolus on the fourth post-operative day (autopsy not performed).

One severe diabetic (fasting blood sugar 27.7 mmol/litre) developed *Staphylococcus aureus* infections of both suprapubic and vaginal wounds, necessitating removal of the nylon suture and the Dacron tubes. She remains incontinent of urine.

Urge incontinence, although not uncommon, has not been a serious problem. It was carefully analysed in our 1975 report (Stamey et al. 1975) and the data are reproduced here (Table 8.1).

Late. Out of 450 patients, 15 have had to have one suprapubic suture removed under local anaesthesia because of pain, infection, or both. Most of these complications, but not all, occurred in the earlier

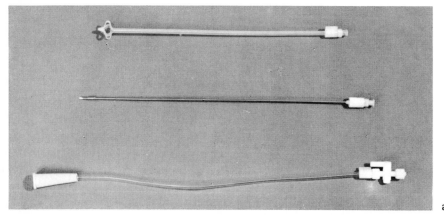

a

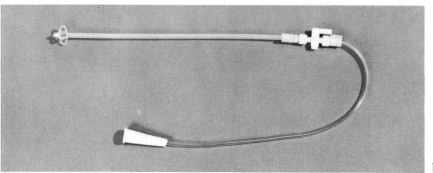

b

Fig. 8.12. a The author's percutaneous suprapubic tube. The hollow obturator needle (*centre*) Luer-locks inside the 14F suprapubic tube, thereby straightening the Malecot wings flat against the obturator and protruding as a sharp needle 3 mm through the tip end of the catheter. On puncturing the bladder, urine flows through the hollow obturator needle, thereby indicating proper placement before withdrawing the obturator and allowing the Malecot wings to re-expand. **b** After the obturator needle is withdrawn and discarded, the drainage tube connector with a stop-cock valve and Luer-lock is connected to the suprapubic tube. The suprapubic tube is taped to the abdomen and a drainage bag connected to the white, polyvinyl flared connector.

series when silk or braided nylon was the suspending suture. All patients remained continent with their single suspending suture.

In two patients the Dacron tube eroded into the vagina where it was cut free from the nylon suture. They, too, remain continent with the single remaining nylon suspension.

Follow-up Assessment

The patients are seen at appropriate intervals after surgery and assessed clinically. A mid-stream urine sample is taken for culture and sensitivity and a residual urine measured. They then reattend at 3–6 monthly intervals for a year and are seen thereafter at yearly intervals.

The mean duration of follow-up for the 44 patients in the 1975 report was 18 months (range

Table 8.1. Comparison of pre-operative and post-operative urge incontinence (Stamey et al. 1975)

Patients	Degree of urge incontience		
	None	Minimal	marked
Pre-operative			
Cures, $n=41$	17	19	5
Failures, $n=3$	0	3	0
Post-operative			
Cures, $n=41$	25	15	1
Failures, $n=3$	1	0	2

10–29 months). In the 1980 series, 47 patients were followed over 4 years, and 156 patients from 6 to 48 months.

Results

Cure Rate

We reported our operative technique in 1973 when we had treated 16 patients (Stamey 1973); there were five failures for a cure rate of 69%, but we were developing the technique and two of the five failures were clearly neuropathic bladders which should not have been operated upon. The 11 cures included one 15-year-old patient whose pelvis was fractured in a road accident and who had a frozen, stove-type urethra in which the entire urethra was fixed in an open position at the time of endoscopic suspension. She has remained totally dry since her surgery in 1969, and was delivered of a healthy infant by caesarian section in early 1979.

In 1975, we reported the next consecutive 44 patients with three failures for an operative cure rate of 93% (Stamey et al. 1975), and in 1980 we analysed an additional 203 consecutive patients (mean age 56 years, range 15–87) who had 19 failures for a cure rate of 91% (Stamey 1980). Cure is defined as complete absence of SUI, and we have included as a failure any patient who has the slightest SUI. While urgency incontinence does occur post-operatively for up to 6 months in some patients (69 of 203), it is usually minimal (Table 8.1) and if substantial and persistent, has been considered an operative failure in this series. Seven of the 203 patients in the 1980 series required a second endoscopic suspension for cure for their SUI.

A variety of surgical procedures will cure Grade I SUI because minimal movement of the internal vesical neck (less than 1 cm), such as that achieved by anterior colporrhaphy, will often suffice (Low 1967). It is, therefore, appropriate to indicate the complexity of any series undergoing surgery for SUI by analysing the severity of stress incontinence presented by the patient, as well as the number of surgical failures prior to presentation.

Severity of Urinary Incontinence

In the 1975 series of 44 patients (Stamey et al. 1975), 15 had Grade I, 20 had Grade II and 9 had total urinary incontinence (Grade III). In the 1980 series of 203 patients, 43 had Grade I, 119 had Grade II and 41 were totally incontinent (Grade III) (Stamey 1980).

It is clear that both series represent a substantially severe group in terms of severity of incontinence. Indeed, 20% of both series were totally incontinent. In fact, two of the three failures from endoscopic suspension in the 1975 report and 9 of the 19 failures in the 1980 series occurred in those patients who had total urinary incontinence. Despite this particular group accounting for most of the failures, 32 of the 41 patients with total urinary incontinence were cured by endoscopic suspension of the vesical neck. These data surely indicate that before complicated mechanical prostheses or major reconstructive operations (including urinary diversion) are undertaken for total urinary incontinence, all patients deserve the opportunity of having their internal vesical neck restored to a position of continence by endoscopic suspension.

Analysis of Previous Surgery for Stress Urinary Incontinence

In the 1973 report of 16 patients, there were 29 previous operations for SUI (Stamey 1973); in the 1975 report of 44 patients there were 48 previous operations (including 14 Marshall–Marchetti–Krantz procedures), and in the 1980 series of 203 patients there were 188 previous operations (including 74 Marshall–Marchetti–Krantz procedures).

Prior Hysterectomy

Of the 203 patients, 138 had undergone hysterectomy prior to presentation; 74 were done vaginally and 64 abdominally. There were 65 patients who had not had a hysterectomy prior to endoscopic suspension.

The 19 failures were equally distributed among the hysterectomised and non-hysterectomised patients. It is clear that the practice of routinely performing a hysterectomy in order to improve the chances of curing SUI is unwarranted and unnecessary; it simply points out the inadequacy of that operative procedure in restoring the vesical neck to a position of urinary continence and maintaining it in that position.

Urethral Observations

The anatomical urethral length at the time of surgery increased from a mean length of 2.6 cm (164 patient measurements) to 4.0 cm (130 patients) following endoscopic suspension in the 1980 series. Corresponding figures for the 1975 report were a mean of 2.5 cm (range 1.6–3.9 cm) pre-operatively to 4.0 cm (range 3.0–5.4 cm) post-operatively. Despite this increase in urethral length that occurs invariably with restoration of the internal vesical neck behind the symphysis pubis, we do not believe that urethral length is aetiologically related to SUI. For example, we commonly see incontinent patients with a 3.0–4.0 cm long urethra before surgery, whereas we have seen young women with recurrent cytitis with a 2.0 cm long urethra who are totally continent.

Urethral pressure profiles were measured on eight patients before and after endoscopic suspension of the vesical neck, all of whose bladder base-plates were radiologically raised from 2.2 cm to 4.5 cm (Stamey 1980). The maximal urethral pressure was unchanged (Table 8.2). These studies, confirmed by the report from Sweden (Henriksson and Ulmsten 1978), indicate that the defect in SUI may be unrelated to urethral pressure per se, as predicted by Enhorning (1961). It is clear that surgical operations designed to narrow or wedge the urethra itself are ill-designed and surely represent an incorrect approach. Recent observations at Stanford by Constantinou (Shortliffe and Stamey, 1985), using an 11 French gauge catheter with two microtip transducers at 180° to each other to measure resting urethral pressure profiles before and after endoscopic suspension of the vesical neck, have shown a characteristic reduction with post-operative restoration of the posterior urethral closure pressure (Table 8.3). The posterior pressure is elevated post-operatively, whilst the anterior pressure is unchanged. These diagnostic changes were undoubtedly masked by techniques measuring only mean urethral pressure profiles (Table 8.2). Hilton and Stanton (1983) were the first to recognise that rotational variations in urethral pressure as measured by a microtip transducer catheter might not be an artefact in patients with stress urinary incontinence.

Bladder Capacity and Residual Urine

Bladder capacity before surgery (either the maximal amount voided or the amount instilled during physical examination) in the 1980 series was as follows: less than 250 ml, 21 patients; 250–300 ml, 55 patients; more than 300 ml, 163 patients; no data, 24 patients. Hence, a small bladder pre-operatively has not been a contraindication to endoscopic suspension, although these patients run the risk of some increased frequency of urination; many of their bladders expand nicely with return of continence, and this even includes irradiated bladders.

Table 8.2. Urethral pressure profiles before and after endoscopic suspension of the vesical neck (Stamey 1979)

Patient	Age (years)	Previous surgery for incontinence		Maximum urethral pressure (cmH$_2$O)			Post-operative change in lateral cystogram		
		Vaginal	Retropubic	Before	After	Net change	PUV[a] (degrees)	Urethral angle (degrees)	Base-plate (cm)
1	56	1	1	70	42	− 28	30	− 20	+2.5
2	47	1		65	45	− 20	71	−105	+4.5
3	69	1		145	118	− 27	70	− 30	+4.2
4	68	1	1	52	58	+ 6	90	− 40	+4.5
5	68	0	0	100	94	− 6	85	− 88	+3.7
6	52		1	49	55	+ 6	52	− 25	+2.2
7	59	1		60	63	+ 3	35	− 60	+2.2
8	56	2		114	83	− 31	155	− 92	+2.3
			Mean	82	70	− 12			

[a] PUV, posterior urethrovesical angle (difference in degrees between pre-operative and post-operative measurements)

Table 8.3. Anterior and posterior maximum urethral closure pressures in incontinent women with and without SUI, in comparison with volunteer controls (Shortliffe and Stamey 1985)

	Volunteer controls		Women with SUI				Women without SUI	
	Stable	Unstable	Stable bladders		Unstable bladders		Stable bladders	Unstable bladders
			Pre-op	Post-op	Pre-op	Post-op		
Number of subjects	17	4	52	47	25	18	34	29
Age (years)	24 ± 4	27 ± 6	56 ± 13	55 ± 15	60 ± 11	63 ± 10	50 ± 16	43 ± 18
Maximum anterior closure pressure (cmH$_2$O) (SD)	119 ± 25	116 ± 27	60 ± 33	45 ± 43	47 ± 38*	45 ± 43	51 ± 29	82 ± 29*
Maximum posterior closure pressure (cmH$_2$) (SD)	113 ± 17	107 ± 23	44 ± 25**	58 ± 42	33 ± 20***	51 ± 34	60 ± 42**	82 ± 42***

-, **-** $= P < 0.01$
*** $= P < 0.001$

All patients without residual urine before surgery remained so at the 3-month follow-up visit following removal of their suprapubic tube or discontinuation of their intermittent catheterisation. Several patients with large residual urines and flaccid bladders pre-operatively have been unable to void post-operatively and require intermittent self-catheterisation, but such catheterisation was a planned part of their continence programme.

Summary

I have presented our operation for urinary incontinence in the female. The cure rate is 90% but 20% of the patients had total urinary incontinence before referral and almost three times as many of the remaining 80% had Grade II incontinence as had simple SUI (Grade I) (Stamey 1980). Over one-third of all referrals were failures after the Marshall–Marchetti–Krantz operation, and most of the remaining two-thirds had undergone a variety of vaginal procedures in an attempt to correct their incontinence.

The operation has been presented in detail. The advantages over retropubic urethrovesical suspension are as follows:

1. The pubocervical and endopelvic fascia that must be used to suspend the internal vesical neck is more strongly supported because of the vaginally placed Dacron buttress and the use of permanent monofilament heavy nylon (no. 2).

2. Post-operative morbidity is less because open pelvic surgery is avoided. There is less pain, minimal blood loss (no blood is cross-matched), and the patients can be discharged with their suprapubic tube on the first or second post-operative day if necessary.

3. The internal vesical neck—the absolute key to surgical cure of urinary incontinence—is accurately identified by endoscopy for suture placement.

4. Functional closure of the internal vesical neck is tested during surgery by observing complete cessation of urinary leakage before permanently tying the suspending sutures.

5. Anatomical closure of the internal vesical neck, and not the urethra, is confirmed by endoscopy of the urethra before the operation is completed.

6. It is the ideal operation for the surgically difficult pelvis, e.g. radiation incontinence, severe fractures, multiple operative failures, obesity. For example, regardless of the degree of obesity, the distance from the symphysis pubis to the anterior vaginal wall is no greater than in a thin patient.

7. In those patients who have a rectocele the surgical area is fully draped and only a few additional minutes are required for surgical repair.

8. So strong is the suspension of the pubocervical fascia by the Dacron buttress placed at the internal vesical neck that small and moderate cystoceles are automatically corrected by endoscopic suspension. Extensive cystoceles which protrude below the introitus pre-operatively are readily repaired by an extension of the anterior vaginal wall incision to the vaginal vault or cervix.

References

Cifuentes L (1947) Epithelium of vaginal type in the female trigone: The clinical problem of trigonitis. J Urol 57:1028–1037

Constantinou CE, Faysal MH, Rother L, Govan D (1981) The impact of bladder neck suspension on the mode of distribution of abdominal pressure along the female urethra. In: Zinner NR, Sterling AM (eds) Female incontinence. Alan Liss, New York, pp 121–132

Enhorning G (1961) Simultaneous recording of intravesical and intra-urethral pressure. Acta Chir Scand [Suppl] 276:1–68

Fowler JE Jr (1978) Endoscopic suspension of the vesical neck in massive urethral dilatation. J Urol 119:573–574

Henriksson L, Ulmsten U (1978) A urodynamic evaluation of abdominal urethrocystopexy and vaginal sling urethroplasty in women with stress incontinence. Am J Obstet Gynecol 131:77–82

Hilton P, Stanton SL (1983) Urethral pressure measurements by microtransducer: the results in symptom free women and in those with genuine stress incontinence. Br J Obstet Gynaecol 90:919–933

Hodgkinson CP (1970) Stress urinary incontinence. Am J Obstet Gynecol 108:1141–1168

Hodgkinson CP, Ayers, MA, Drukker BH (1963) Dyssynergic detrusor dysfunction in the apparently normal female. Am J Obstet Gynecol 87:717–730

Jeffcoate TNA, Roberts J (1952) Stress incontinence of urine. J Obstet Gynaecol Br Commonw 59:685–697

Low JA (1967) Management of anatomic urinary incontinence by vaginal repair. Am J Obstet Gynecol 97:308–315

Pereyra AJ, Lebherz TB (1978) The revised Pereyra procedure. In Buchsbaum HJ, Schmidt JD (eds) Gynecologic and obstetric urology. Saunders, Philadelphia, pp 208–222

Shortliffe LMD, Stamey TA (1985) Urinary incontinence in the female. In: Walsh PC, Gittes RF, Perlmutter AD, Stamey TA (eds) Campbells' urology, 5th edn. Saunders, Philadelphia, pp 2680–2711

Stamey TA (1973) Endoscopic suspension of the vesical neck for urinary incontinence. Surg Gynecol Obstet 136:547–554

Stamey TA (1980) Endoscopic suspension of the vesical neck for urinary incontinence in females: Report on 203 consecutive cases. Ann Surg 192:465–471

Stamey TA, Schaeffer AJ, Condy M (1975) Clinical and roentgenographic evaluation of endoscopic suspension of the vesical neck for urinary incontinence. Surg Gynecol Obstet 140:355–360

Addendum

There are two sources of further operative details.

1. Stamey TA (1981) Endoscopic suspension of the vesical neck for surgically curable urinary incontinence in the female. Monographs in Urology 2:65–98. Custom Publishing Services Inc, Princeton.

2. Film—Stamey TA (1983) Visits in Urology. Urinary Incontinence in Women. Obtainable from Norwich Eaton Pharmaceuticals Inc, Norwich, N.Y. 13815.

The article and the film complement each other and contain much practical guidance for the surgeon.

9 Abdominoperineal Urethral Suspension: The Zacharin Procedure

Robert F. Zacharin

Introduction

Stress urinary incontinence is a mechanical problem resulting from an imbalance between intra-abdominal pressure on the one hand, and the upper urethral supports on the other. The integrity of the sphincteric mechanism of the bladder in resisting sudden rises of intra-abdominal pressure lies in the suspensory mechanism of the urethra, especially the paraurethral attachment of the posterior pubourethral ligaments to the junction of the upper urethral third and the lower two-thirds (Zacharin 1963, 1968, 1977b) (Figs. 9.1, 9.2). It seems that the sphincteric mechanism functions efficiently provided there is a limitation to upper urethral descent following a sudden rise in intra-abdominal pressure, and it is the paraurethral attachment of the two posterior pubourethral ligaments, together with their levator connections, which is the anatomy responsible for this check to descent. This is the key site of continence control in the female.

Factors increasing intra-abdominal pressure are obesity, chronic cough due particularly to cigarette smoking, and poorly functioning abdominal and perineal musculature. Deterioration of the suspensory mechanism is due predominantly to pregnancy, but may also follow certain hypotensive agents and the contraceptive pill. Mechanical problems involving the pelvic floor are rare in certain racial groups—Chinese, Eskimo, American Indian, and in particular stress incontinence is most uncommon in the non-westernised Chinese.

Detailed pelvic dissection has demonstrated clear differences in the upper urethral supporting anatomy of the oriental and occidental female (Zacharin 1977a), but even though there is a superior anatomical mechanism operating in the oriental female, the functional impact of this anatomy is still exerted at the junction of the upper urethral third with the distal two-thirds (Figs. 9.3, 9.4). The reasons for such anatomical differences are race, lack of obesity, harder work and squatting for rest, childbirth and defaecation. However, deterioration will gradually occur, and mechanical pelvic floor problems begin to appear after several generations have adopted the habits of the Western world and moved away from their ethnic life-style.

Although commonly associated with genital prolapse, prolapse and stress incontinence are separate

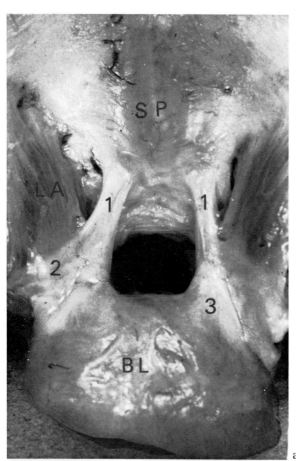

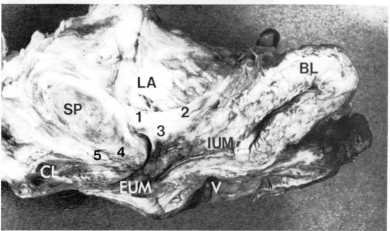

Fig. 9.1. a Pelvic surface of the symphysis pubis, viewed from above. The entire posterior pubourethral ligament (1) is shown on either side from the apical bony attachment to the broad paraurethral attachment (3). The intimate relationship to the levator muscle is shown. The potential space outlined by the subpubic arch, posterior ligaments and upper urethra may be seen clearly. SP, symphysis pubis; BL, bladder; LA, levator ani. 2, Expansion from the ligament crossing and fusing with the levator ani fascia. b Sagittal midline section through the pubic symphysis. The paraurethral attachment of the right posterior pubourethral ligament to the junction of the upper urethral third with the distal two-thirds is shown clearly. The expansion from the posterior ligament crossing and fusing with the levator fascia is seen. SP, symphysis pubis; EUM, external urethral meatus; BL, bladder; IUM internal urethral meatus; LA, levator ani. 1, posterior pubourethral ligament; 2, expansion; 3, broad paraurethral attachment; 4, intermediate ligament; 5, anterior pubourethral ligament; V, vagina; CL, clitoris. c The entire suspensory mechanism viewed from above after splitting the symphysis pubis. A metal catheter lies in the urethra and bladder.

problems, so correction of the prolapse is not necessarily followed by cure of the stress incontinence (Turner Warwick and Brown 1979; Cardozo and Stanton 1980). It is wise to point out this disparity to patients prior to vaginal reparative surgery. It is unusual for stress incontinence to be a solitary urinary symptom; usually it is associated with urge incontinence which only rarely is produced mechanically, and is accordingly very unlikely to respond to reparative surgery. It is essential that these two symptoms are separated and that the urge incontinence is treated before any consideration is given to correction of the stress incontinence.

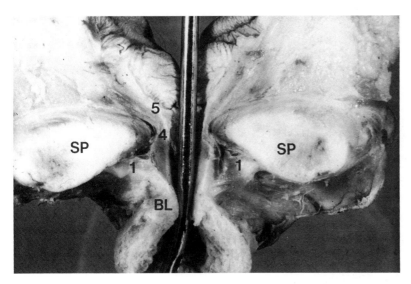

Fig. 9.1c

Indications and Contraindications

Abdominoperineal urethral suspension is indicated for recurrent stress incontinence, and may be applied regardless of the type and number of surgical corrections which have been previously attempted. The surgical technique is not difficult; the major problem lies in correct selection. Providing the diagnosis is correct and the upper urethral anatomy defective, the procedure may be applied, but there is never any urgency for the operation. Contraindications include urge incontinence, obesity, cigarette smoking and poor abdominal and perineal muscles.

Pre-operative Investigations and Preparation

Surgical intervention for recurrent stress incontinence is justified only after stringent application of conservative measures has failed. Differentiation from urge incontinence is best and most faithfully achieved by a thorough history, physical examination and cystoscopy without anaesthesia. Stress incontinence may be defined as "a sudden and involuntary loss of a small volume of urine following a sudden sharp rise in intra-abdominal pressure, and after the pressure falls, continence control is regained". This is an anti-gravity symptom predominantly and contrasts markedly with the definition of urge incontinence: "a sudden need to void unrelated to gravity and with the onset of micturi-

tion, continence cannot be reimposed until the urge diminishes". Common features in the history of stress incontinence are the onset in pregnancy, followed by remission after parturition with eventual recurrence and persistence without remission. Once persistent, the symptom will not change except temporarily with the Bonney test or long-term after surgery which changes upper urethral mechanics. The symptom is worsened by the oral contraceptive pill and before menstruation, when softening in the suspensory mechanism is accentuated. Spontaneous remission, enuresis and dribbling are not mechanical problems. Stress incontinence has only one cause and that is mechanical change in upper urethral supports, but urge incontinence has a multiplicity of causes, the least common being mechanical alteration in these supports. Neurological problems, in the absence of gross neurological disorders producing urinary symptoms, are characterised by retention with overflow presenting as dribbling incontinence and readily distinguished by a careful history. Neurological examination with equivocal urinary symptoms is quite unrewarding in terms of diagnosis and management. The fact that a urinary symptom has been relieved completely (even for a short time) by surgery is excellent evidence of an underlying mechanical problem, and must always be sought in the history. Similarly, the failure to change a symptom means imperfect surgery or a wrong initial diagnosis. Recurrent stress incontinence occurs usually without genital prolapse and in four distinct clinical groups:

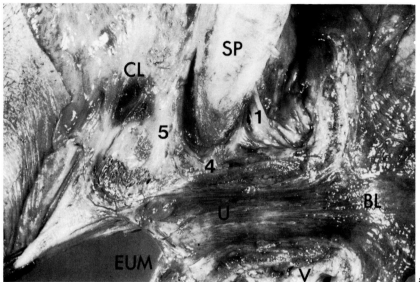

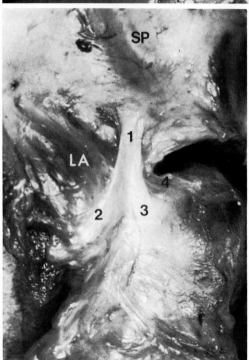

Fig. 9.2. a Close-up of the urethral suspensory mechanism with the urethra put on the stretch. b Close-up of the left posterior pubourethral ligament showing its attachments. *SP*, symphysis pubis; *EUM*, external urethal meatus; *V*, vagina; *U*, urethra; *LA*, levator ani; *BL*, bladder; *CL*, clitoris. *1*, posterior pubourethral ligament; *2*, expansion of posterior pubourethral ligament; *3*, paraurethral attachment of the posterior pubourethral ligament; *4*, intermediate ligament; *5*, anterior pubourethral ligament.

1. The common group are those in whom stress incontinence has been cured by prolapse surgery, only to recur.

2. Prolapse cured without change in the stress incontinence—it is important to repeat that prolapse and stress incontinence are separate problems and no matter how well the prolapse is corrected recurrent stress incontinence will occur in 10%–15% of patients. The other reason, of course, is that the original diagnosis of stress incontinence was incorrect.

3. The prolapse has been cured, but stress incontinence has appeared for the first time. A large prolapse may lead to reverse urethral kinking at the site of posterior pubourethral ligament support and "cure" the stress incontinence, which recurs when

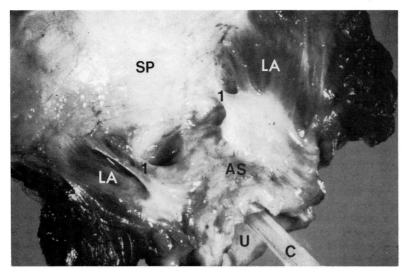

Fig. 9.3. Pelvic surface of the symphysis pubis in a young Chinese female viewed from above. The well developed levator ani muscles are shown with relatively deficient posterior pubourethral ligaments compared to the occidental female, but an exceedingly dense aponeurotic sheet extends between the levators and supports the urethra. *SP*, symphysis pubis; *LA*, levator ani; *1*, posterior pubourethral ligament; *AS*, the aponeurotic sheet; *U*, urethra; *C*, catheter.

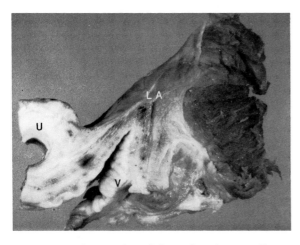

Fig. 9.4. Coronal section through the urethra of a young Chinese female at the junction of the upper third with the distal two-thirds. The method of urethral suspension by musculo-aponeurotic sling is demonstrated. *U*, urethra; *V*, vagina; *LA*, levator ani.

the vaginal inversion is reduced.

4. The so-called stress incontinence occurring in females who have never been pregnant nor suffered prolapse is most often urge incontinence, although rarely stress incontinence may be the correct diagnosis so very careful assessment is required.

Clinical examination excludes prolapse, confirms stress incontinence, and a positive Bonney test performed unilaterally with a uterine sound will limit paraurethral descent and produce temporary continence control. Cystoscopy without anaesthesia measures conscious bladder capacity: urge incontinence patients show characteristic departures from normal—slow filling rates because of suprapubic discomfort, small accommodated volumes well below normal, and moderate to marked bladder trabeculation. There is no unequivocal radiological or urodynamic picture which will give the absolute diagnosis of stress incontinence, and an equivocal X-ray or graph is of less use than an equivocal clinical picture in formulating a decision whether or not surgical intervention is reasonable. In fact, the use of this information has provided little improvement in short-term results (Cardozo and Stanton 1980; Hodgkinson and Stanton 1980; Bhatia and Ostergard 1982).

Many overweight patients on oral contraceptives who smoke and also have poor abdominal and perineal muscles will respond so well to conservative measures that surgery is no longer necessary. The level of continence control in the female is seldom perfect and conservative treatment may well return the level of control to an acceptable one. Until weight loss to a reasonable level, muscle improvement by supervised physiotherapy (Table 9.1) and absolute cessation of smoking have been achieved, surgery should be deferred—should surgery proceed in the face of such handicaps, the recurrence rate will be unacceptably high.

Table 9.1. Specific abdominal and perineal exercises (courtesy of Barbara Parker)

FIRST EXERCISE: The patient lies supine on the floor with the knees bent and the buttocks squeezed together. The perineal area is drawn up and the abdominal wall pulled in as though endeavouring to prevent micturition and this position is held for a count of 6 and repeated six times. The same exercise is done with the knees straight. The patient is told to practise the exercise frequently during the day whilst standing or sitting. She endeavours also to maintain a slight contraction of these muscles while vacuuming or sweeping.

SECOND EXERCISE: Commences as in Exercise I with the chin pulled onto the sternum with the head and shoulders lifted forward, bringing both hands first to the left knee and then repeating to the right.

THIRD EXERCISE: The patient lies supine with the knees bent and the perineal and abdominal muscles tightened as in the first exercise and the buttocks are lifted from the floor. This movement is assisted initially by pushing with the elbows but later experienced exercisers fold the arms across the chest.

FOURTH EXERCISE: Commences as in Exercise I and then with the chin on the sternum, the head, shoulders and chest are lifted to the sitting position. The movement is helped initially by holding the legs until the patient's strength improves.

Leg raising exercises are not used because they have little effect on the abdominal muscles and commonly produce a strained back in this group of women.

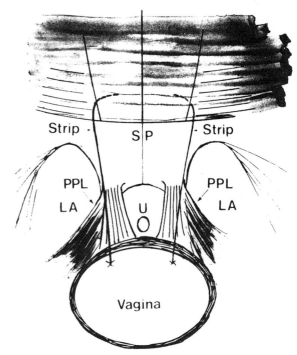

Fig. 9.5. Coronal view showing the aponeurotic bands derived from the anterior abdominal wall aponeurosis, passed through the paraurethral attachment of both posterior pubourethral ligaments and then fixed in the vagina. *SP*, symphysis pubis; *U*, urethra; *PPL*, posterior pubourethral ligament; *LA*, levator ani.

Operative Technique

The principle of the procedure is to pass two bands of aponeurosis from the abdominal wall through the paraurethral attachment of the posterior pubourethral ligament on either side, to terminate in the vagina (Figs. 9.5, 9.6). The bands are elevated by abdominal muscular wall contraction consequent upon a rise in intra-abdominal pressure, and it is believed that this mechanical restraint effectively limits urethral descent at the key site of continence control. The efficiency of the sphincter mechanism depends upon such mechanical restraint to the posterior urethra and its effect on limiting urethral descent. The principal steps in the procedure are as follows: The patient is placed in a lithotomy–Trendelenburg position, and the suspensory mechanism approached by two surgeons using a synchronous combined abdominoperineal technique. Through a Pfannenstiel incision, the abdominal surgeon commences by

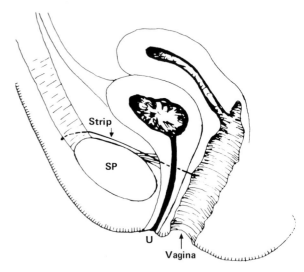

Fig. 9.6. Sagittal view showing the course taken by the strip as it passes through the retropubic space and on into the vagina. *U*, urethra; *SP*, symphysis pubis.

preparing two 10-cm strips of abdominal wall aponeurosis which include both the internal and external oblique fascia. The retropubic space is opened down to the urethrovesical region and each strip is passed from the lateral to the medial side of the corresponding rectus muscle and into the retropubic space. Later, when the strips are fixed in the paraurethral area, the rectus muscles ensure their separation and transmission of abdominal wall tension in a vertically efficient direction. In order to minimise blood loss, the perineal surgeon delays the vaginal procedure until this juncture, for his approach takes only minutes to achieve. His task is to locate accurately the paraurethral attachment of each posterior pubourethral ligament in order to be sure that the strips are passed through the correct site. Placing a metal catheter in the urethra, an inverted Y-shaped supraurethral incision is made below the crura of the clitoris and the anterior pubourethral ligament divided. A passage is developed beneath the subpubic arch by finger and blunt dissection using sharp pointed scissors curved on the flat until the retropubic space is reached. The two sharp free medial borders of the posterior ligaments are recognised with ease and certainty (Fig. 9.7). With the index finger in the supraurethral space, the thumb in the vagina and the metal catheter in the urethra, the paraurethral attachment of the posterior ligament can be palpated with confidence and a stab incision made through the vaginal epithelium at this site with a number 11 blade (Fig. 9.8). A long needle loaded with number 3 silk is introduced through the stab incision from the vagina and passes through the paraurethral attachment into the retropubic space where its further course is guided by the abdominal surgeon who grasps it and draws it into the suprapubic field (Fig. 9.9). Next, a slender grasping instrument is inserted through this paraurethral site using the silk for traction and guidance; the silk is then discarded (Fig. 9.10). The fascial strip on that side is grasped by the instrument (Fig. 9.11), drawn through the paraurethral attachment and into the vagina (Fig. 9.12) where it is fixed with number 0 monofilament nylon, the fixation being effected by a deep paraurethral bite whilst the urethra is protected by the metal catheter. Before fixing the band in position, any slackness in the band is eliminated. The band does not need to be fixed under tension; there merely needs to be no slack, and this is not critical. While the vaginal incision is closed with several interrupted mattress sutures, the defect in the abdominal wall aponeurosis is repaired with interrupted sutures which add slight tension to the fascial bands. Three vacuum drains are placed in the

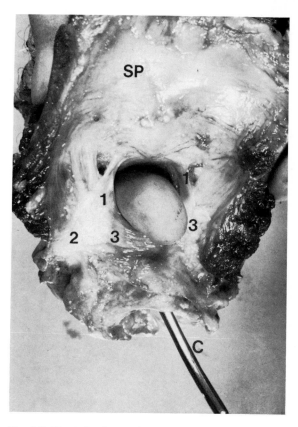

Fig. 9.7. The index finger of the perineal surgeon enters the retropubic space, through a space outlined by the subpubic arch, the posterior ligaments and the upper urethra. The sharp free medial border of each posterior ligament may be identified with ease. *SP*, symphysis pubis; *C*, catheter. Numbers as in Fig. 9.1a.

retropubic space, beneath the sheath and in the fat, and a supraurethral Penrose drain is placed beneath the subpubic arch. A number 12 Foley catheter is then inserted.

Post-operative Management

The catheter drains freely for 3 days, then is clipped and released for 24 hours and removed. Voiding usually poses no problem and providing 200 cc is voided on each occasion, no residual urine measurement is necessary. The suction drains continue until drainage ceases, then each is shortened by several centimetres daily until removed. The supraurethral drain is shortened at 48 hours and removed at 72 hours.

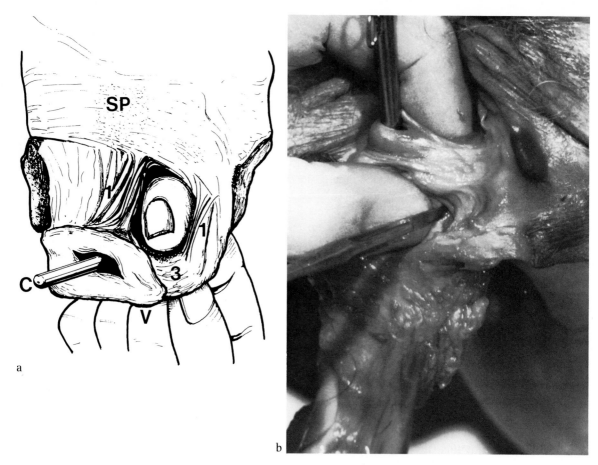

Fig. 9.8a,b. With the index finger in the supraurethral space, the thumb in the vagina, and the metal catheter in the urethra, the paraurethral attachment of the posterior pubourethral ligament can be palpated with accuracy and a stab incision is made in the vagina at this site. **a** Line drawing of the situation. **b** Stab incision performed on the cadaver. *SP*, symphysis pubis; *C*, catheter. Numbers as in Fig. 9.1a.

Complications

After previous abdominal surgery, the cutting of the fascial bands can be difficult, but is resolved by taking them from a paramedian position, lateral to the midline. Sheath closure can be helped by relaxing incisions, but any greater defects require the use of mersilene mesh. Incisional hernia has been a rare late complication, but not after the use of mersilene mesh.

In the patient with previous retropubic surgery, marked adhesions between the pubic bone and bladder is the rule. Sharp dissection by the abdominal surgeon adjacent to the pubic bone, guided by the finger of the perineal surgeon in the supraurethral space, usually solves this problem without bladder entry. If bladder injury should occur, the defect is carefully closed and the dissection continued.

Haematoma formation is the greatest potential problem, so numerous drains are necessary.

Early and late complications are almost unknown—there are no problems with voiding. There have been no urinary fistulas in 235 procedures, but six small incisional hernias have occurred. In one patient, recurrence of stress incontinence followed the development of a unilateral incisional hernia and continence was restored by its correction.

Follow-up Assessment

Patients have continued to be followed up since 1965 when the first procedure was carried out, either by direct interview or questionnaire (Zacharin 1977b, 1983). Assessment of urinary

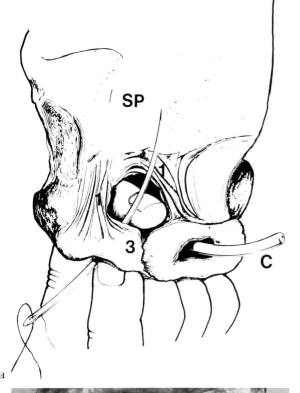

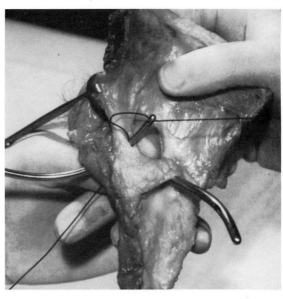

Fig. 9.10. The grasping instrument is drawn through the paraurethral attachment of the posterior pubourethral ligament by traction on the silk suture. Following this step the silk is discarded and plays no further role in the procedure.

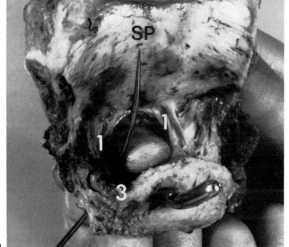

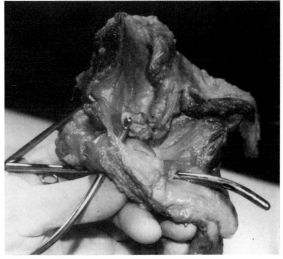

Fig. 9.9a,b. The long needle loaded with number 3 silk passes from the vaginal stab incision through the paraurethral attachment of the posterior pubourethral ligament and into the retropubic space. **a** line drawing. **b** cadaver specimen. *SP*, symphysis pubis; *C*, catheter. Numbers as in Fig. 9.1a.

Fig. 9.11. The aponeurotic strip is received by the jaws of the grasping instrument.

Results

control is made by the patient according to her own particular level of normal control. Three grades are recognised—normal control, improvement in control and failure (i.e. the same control level that existed before surgery).

During a 15-year period (1965–1980) 194 women were treated by abdominoperineal urethral suspension. Of these, 160 have been contacted and the outcome is given here (Table 9.2). One hundred and fifty-six of these women had already experienced

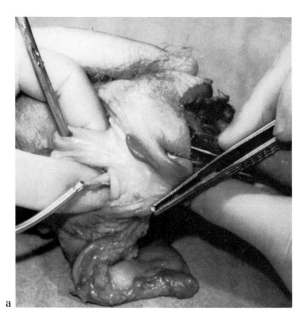
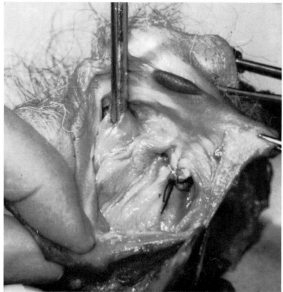

a   b

Fig. 9.12. a The strip is drawn through the paraurethral attachment of the posterior pubourethal ligament and into the vagina. b The strip is drawn down to eliminate any slack and fixed with a transfixion suture of number 0 nylon which also closes the stab wound.

one or more attempts at surgical correction of their incontinence; a wide spectrum of techniques had been used which included vaginal repair with or without hysterectomy, Marshall–Marchetti–Krantz procedure, Burch colposuspension and suburethral slings.

Of the 160 women contacted for follow-up, 124 were cured, 11 improved and 25 were failures. The cure rate, therefore, was 78%, rising to 84% if the improved cases are included. At 5 years, the cure rate was 66%, rising to 76% if the improved cases were included. At 10 years, the cure rate was 67% rising to 73% if the improved group was again included (Table 9.3). Although the rate declines slightly with time, the cure rate remains quite good at 10 years, suggesting that the long-term benefit of abdominoperineal urethral suspension continues, provided simple rules relating to obesity, exercise and cigarette smoking are observed.

Mechanism of Failure

Operating on women with urge incontinence will certainly be unsuccessful, but this is a failure of selection, not a failure in technique. Technical failure has been noted with weight increase, resumption of smoking and the cessation of muscle exercises leading to a deterioration in muscle excellence. Reversal of these traits has led to renewed continence control. Incisional hernia has produced recurrence, which is cured by repairing the hernia. Excessive or repeated heavy lifting has been noted in several females with recurrence. Whilst the aponeurotic bands will withstand most normal activities, including tennis and golf, they will not tolerate excessive mistreatment. Repeat surgery has been successfully performed on several of these women whose bands failed.

Conclusions

Stress incontinence in the absence of prolapse is a mechanically produced symptom with three important associations: obesity, smoking and poor muscle activity. Conservative treatment must be completed prior to surgery. The procedure is applicable no matter what previous surgery has been performed, big advantages being that the supraurethral area is always virgin territory and that suburethral dissection is not required. Careful surgery can produce a high rate of long-term cures, which will be maintained providing the patient continues with the peroperative conservative management.

Table 9.2. Fifteen-year experience with abdominoperineal urethral suspension

Year	No. of patients	Cured		Failed		Improved		Lost to follow-up
		1975	1980	1975	1980	1975	1980	
1965	5	3	3	2	2			
1966	1	1	1					
1967	6	5	4	1	1			1
1968	9	6	5	2	2	1	2	
1969	14	11	7	1	2	2		5
1970	4	2	2	2	2			
1971	7	5	4	2	2			1
1972	2	1	1	1	1			
1973	10	6	5	1	3	3	1	1
1974	10	6	5			4	3	2
1975	12	12	8		1			3
1976	19		12		2		1	4
1977	22		19		1			2
1978	26		15		3		2	6
1979	24		16		1		1	6
1980	23		17		2		1	3
Total	194		124 (78%)[a]		25 (16%)[a]		11 (6%)[a]	34

[a] Among the 160 cases available for follow-up.

Table 9.3. Treatment results with abdominoperineal urethral suspension

Follow-up period (yr)	No. of cases	Lost to follow-up	Traced	Cured	Improved	Failed	Cured*	Improved
10 (1965–1970)	39	6	33	22	2	9	67%	73%
5 (1970–1975)	45	7	38	25	4	9	66%	76%
Total (1965–1980)	194	34	160	124	11	25	78%	84%

References

Bhatia WN, Ostergard DR (1982) Urodynamics in women with stress urinary incontinence. Obstet Gynecol 60:552–559

Cardozo LD, Stanton SL (1980) Genuine stress incontinence and detrusor instability—A review of 200 patients. Br J Obstet Gynaecol 87:184–190

Hodgkinson CP, Stanton SL (1980) Retropubic urethropexy or colposuspension. In: Stanton SL,Tanagho EA (eds) Surgery of female incontinence, 1st edn. Springer, Berlin Heidelberg New York, pp 55–68

Turner Warwick R, Brown ADG (1979) A urodynamic evaluation of urinary incontinence in the female and its treatment. Urol Clin North Am 6:203–216

Zacharin RF (1963) The suspensory mechanism of the female urethra. J Anat 97:423–427

Zacharin RF (1968) The anatomic supports of the female urethra. Obstet Gynecol 32:754–759

Zacharin RF (1977a) "A Chinese anatomy". The pelvic supporting tissues of the Chinese and Occidental female compared and contrasted. Aust NZ J Obstet Gynaecol 17:1–11

Zacharin RF (1977b) Abdominoperineal urethral suspension: A ten year experience in the management of recurrent stress incontinence of urine. Obstet Gynecol 50:1–8

Zacharin RF (1983) Abdominoperineal urethral suspension in the management of recurrent stress incontinence of urine. Obstet Gynecol 62:644–654

10 Neourethra: Rationale, Surgical Technique and Indications*

Emil A. Tanagho

Introduction

In women it is the urethra as a whole—about 4 cm long—that acts as a sphincteric unit providing enough outlet resistance to maintain urinary continence. Authorities agree that no anatomical entity that may be called a "sphincter" can be isolated and dissected. The urethral muscular tube with its two coats—one, inner longitudinal and the other, outer semi-circular—provides sphincteric function. The outer muscular coat of the urethra originates in the outer longitudinal coat of the bladder, the fibres of which loop around the urethra: urethral sphincteric function is attributed to these abundant circularly orientated fibres. Myogenically, neurologically and histologically, this muscular sphincteric unit is identical to the detrusor and is, in fact, in direct continuity with it.

Complete urinary incontinence, whether of congenital, traumatic, iatrogenic or even neuropathic aetiology, may be managed via construction of a sphincteric tube similar to the urethra. A mechanism of control not too different from that of the normal sphincteric unit may thus be provided. A scarred, fibrotic, damaged urethral tube may be replaced. A sphincteric unit absent because of developmental reasons, traumatised or iatrogenically damaged may also be created or re-created.

Anatomical Considerations and Rationale for Operation

A segment of the anterior bladder wall situated just above the internal meatus is ideal for such a reconstructive procedure. It is one of the heaviest segments of the bladder wall: its musculature is arranged in an outer longitudinal coat, a middle coat of heavily condensed circular fibres and a weak inner longitudinal coat. The heavy circular fibre condensation is limited to a segment 2–2.5 cm long just above the internal meatus.

---

* The reference list at the end of this chapter is intended as a guide to further reading, not as a comprehensive set of references to the original literature

About 1970, we envisaged the possibility of raising this segment of the anterior bladder wall as a flap, then fashioning it into a tube. This tube would, of course, contain the heavy middle circular coat with thin delicate longitudinal fibres on either side. We proceeded to study the occlusive effect of this circular coat in such a reconstructed tube to see whether it could exert enough compression through centrally orientated force to close its lumen and thus provide sphincteric control. A canine experimental model was developed in which, after radical prostatectomy, an anterior flap about 2.5 cm wide and 2.5 cm long was fashioned from the bladder wall, then formed into a tube and anastomosed to the distal end of the urethra (Fig. 10.1). Radiological studies and urodynamic evaluation proved without a doubt that this reconstructed tube was acting as a sphincter and generating adequate closure pressure to keep the dog continent. Encouraged by these results, we applied the same principle to humans, both male and female. In men we used it commonly for management of incontinence to provide adequate urinary control after radical prostatectomy for prostatic carcinoma. In a like manner, we

repaired serious injuries to the posterior-urethra—with complete disruption or destruction of the sphincteric prostatic segment—by developing a tube from the anterior bladder wall and re-anastomosing it to the distal urethra. This neourethra functioned satisfactorily. When the same principle of repair is applied to women, it is much easier to accomplish and can be valuable as a bridge or as a substitute for a damaged or absent sphincteric unit.

Indications

The neourethra technique of operation should not be adopted lightly. It should be reserved for patients with complete urinary incontinence. Fortunately, most female patients with urinary incontinence, however severe (if it is not of the neuropathic or urge variety), may usually be helped with much simpler procedures. These cases are related to anatomical distortion of the vesicourethral relationship, primarily abnormal position and weakened support.

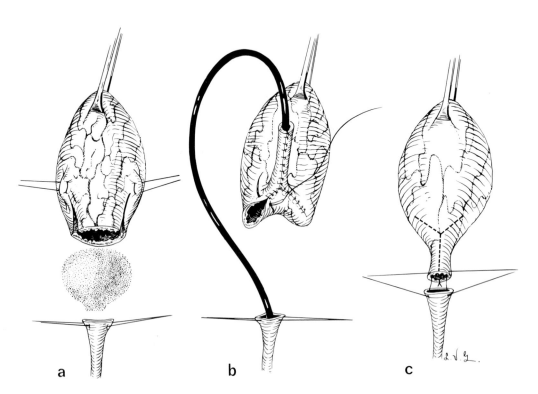

Fig. 10.1 a–c. Surgical experimental model for testing the procedure. The 2.5 cm square flap is raised (a), then formed into a tube around a catheter (b). The bladder outlet is reconstructed by bringing the apex of the trigone to the base of the tube. Finally the reconstructed tube is anastomosed to the distal end of the urethra (c).

By restoration of vesicourethral support and position, most of the sphincteric activity is usually regained, so that construction of a new sphincteric unit is not necessary.

Sometimes, however, we encounter a patient whose urethra has already lost all sphincteric function as a result of intrinsic weakness of the sphincteric elements—from repeated operations and scarring, from resection for urethral, vulval or vaginal tumours, from extensive urethrovaginal fistula formation and, occasionally, from complete disruption and destruction of the sphincteric segment due to serious pelvic fractures. A few rare congenital lesions might be encountered—either complete lack of development of the urethra or presence of a rudimentary urethra, especially in association with persistent urogenital sinus—that would require the construction of a neourethra. In this situation the technique described above has been quite satisfactory.

Female epispadias is a classic example for the Leadbetter operation. The urethra is very short and shows impaired sphincteric function. Most of the time, there is associated bilateral vesicoureteral reflux, for which bilateral reimplantation is indicated. Consequently, this reconstruction for a neourethra becomes a procedure of choice.

Pre-operative Evaluation

A full history and clinical examination are necessary and urodynamic studies include a mid-stream specimen of urine for culture and sensitivity, simultaneous urethral and bladder pressure measurements during progressive bladder filling and urine flow rate recording and endoscopy.

Operative Technique

Tanagho Technique (Anterior Bladder Flap)

The surgical procedure is relatively simple: its main feature is transection of the bladder wall at exactly the level of the internal meatus, separating the bladder on one side from the urethra on the other. Before this transection is attempted, the bladder is half distended and the outlines of the flap to be raised from its anterior wall are marked by four stay sutures

2.5 cm apart in either direction. The result is a 2.5×2.5 cm square flap still attached to the anterior bladder wall by its base (Fig. 10.2). After the flap is outlined, the anterior bladder wall is cut at the level of the internal meatus until the lumen of the proximal urethra is entered. This incision is then carried from inside to complete the separation of the bladder from the distal urethra. After the bladder is completely isolated, it is slightly dissected around its base. The two lateral incisions to complete the development of the flap are made. A 12F or 14F Foley catheter is passed through the urethra and pulled in the wound and the flap is folded around it, incorporating the heavily condensed circular fibres of the anterior bladder wall. An interrupted 3–0 Dexon suture at the base of the tube and another at its apex, together with a one-layer closure, are used. To reconstitute the normal anatomical relationship between the bladder cavity and the neourethra, the apex of the trigone is secured by a mattress suture to the base of the flap—this results in a V-shaped incision in the base of the bladder. Each side of this incision is now closed by interrupted 3–0 Dexon sutures. Usually, the bladder is drained by a suprapubic tube, and the neourethra is supported by the urethral catheter used as a stent. After complete closure of the bladder base, the reconstructed tube is anastomosed by four or five interrupted 3–0 Dexon sutures to the cut end of the urethra. If there is no urethral canal, that end of the tube can be brought out to the vaginal vestibule just below the pubic arch. This will either establish direct continuity between the bladder and the residual segment of the urethra, or create a completely new urethra with its outside opening into the vaginal vestibule. Both ways have been tried in women and both have been successful.

At completion of reconstruction and establishment of anastomosis, it is advisable to support the new vesicourethral junction to avoid collapse of the neourethra under the weight of the mobilised bladder. Two sutures are attached from the vesicourethral junction to the back of the rectus muscles to provide minimum stretch with no tension.

Leadbetter Technique (Trigonal Tube)

In 1964, Leadbetter described a technique comparable to ours to construct an absent urethra, or to lengthen a previously existing urethra, a short urethra or a damaged sphincteric unit. Instead of

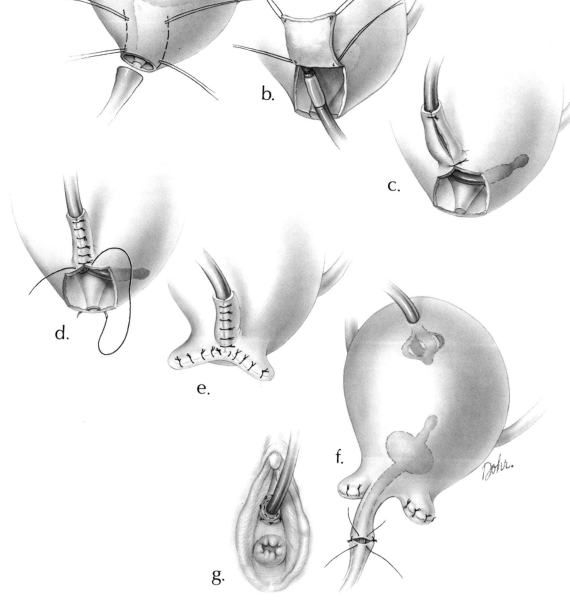

Fig. 10.2. a Four stay sutures are inserted to mark the outline of the anterior wall bladder flap. **b** Bladder flap raised and attached to the anterior bladder wall by its base. **c** Anterior flap formed into a tube around a 12F or 14F catheter. **d** One-layer closure to reconstruct bladder outlet. **e** Bladder closed and ready for an anastomosis to the distal urethra. **f** Urethral anastomosis. **g** Neourethra in position with indwelling urethral catheter.

using an anterior bladder flap, a trigonal tube is constructed by using the base of the bladder to form the neourethra. It is effective inasmuch as it maintains continuity between the urethral canal and the bladder base. However, it lacks the mobility, elasticity and versatility of a neourethra fashioned from an anterior bladder flap. In addition, this technique requires bilateral reimplantation of the ureter at a higher point in the bladder base to give adequate space below the ureteral orifice, incorporating the entire trigone, which can be fashioned into a tube to form the sphincteric unit.

After complete mobilisation of the bladder neck and urethra, a mid-line incision is done all the way down to the internal meatus. After bilateral ureteral reimplantation at a higher level from inside the bladder is completed, the intended posterior flap is outlined by stay sutures which are usually placed up to the level of the interureteric ridge and all the way down to the apex and trigone. They form a 1–1.5-cm wide strip of trigonal and detrusor musculature in the bladder base. The mid-line incision is then curved downwards around the internal meatus and directed posteriorly to be extended along the marked stay sutures in the base of the bladder. The full segment of the bladder is cut, leaving behind another strip 1.5 cm wide, attached to the anterior vaginal wall and the urethral vaginal septum. These two lateral flaps with the anterior bladder wall are raised, then the posterior trigone and flap are shaped into a tube wrapped around a small catheter or stent of calibre 8F or 10F. This is done in either one or two layers, but we usually find it extremely difficult to use two layers; we are satisfied with one layer interrupted closure with 3–0 Dexon sutures. The most proximal end of the tube will be the new site of the internal meatus. The two flaps of the bladder wall are then sutured in the mid-line in a continuous line with the anterior incision in the bladder wall. Suprapubic drainage is established and the urethral catheter is left as a stent. After this operation a certain degree of support should be provided, as is done in vesicourethral colpopexy.

This procedure lends itself well to reconstruction in women because the urethra itself can be easily moulded around to flow into the reconstructed tube, maintaining its continuity with the base of the bladder. It does require, however, the existence of a urethral tube and bilateral ureteral reimplantation, which adds to its magnitude and concomitantly introduces potential complications and morbidity.

Nevertheless, when a case requires both reimplantation and a neourethra, this technique is ideal. We have applied it in neourethral reconstruction for congenital anomalies, as well as in iatrogenic cases, and we have had a high rate of success, approximately 80%.

Post-operative Management

If a suprapubic Penrose drain is used, it is removed at 3 days. The urethral catheter is removed between 5 and 6 days. No antibiotics are employed unless infection develops. The total stay in hospital is 8–10 days.

The patient is seen again after 2 weeks for symptom review and culture and sensitivity of urine. She attends next at 3 months and then at 6 months for a symptom review, physical examination and repeat culture and sensitivity of urine. If any problem is encountered, urodynamic assessment and endoscopy are performed.

Complications

If the operation is carried out according to indications for complete urinary incontinence, no patient will be made worse.

In case a fistula develops with delayed healing, the urethral and suprapubic catheters should be left in for an additional week, at which time the patient's condition should be reviewed. If the catheters have been removed, urethral catheterisation should be reinstituted for 1–2 additional weeks.

Stricture at the site of anastomosis after the anterior bladder flap has been created may occur 2–3 months after operation. It should be treated by urethral dilatation.

Case Examples

Case 1. A 17-year-old woman had severe pain at her first attempt at sexual intercourse. She did not complain of urinary incontinence which, however, had been a lifelong problem, and for which she had to wear nappies (diapers) at all times. The external genitalia appeared normal, but when the labia were spread only one large opening could be seen. This opening was at first taken to be the vaginal canal. Pelvic examination allowed insertion of one finger into a huge cavity that proved later to be the bladder cavity. Endoscopic examination revealed that the opening at the depth of the vaginal vestibule was actually the bladder neck. A normal left ureteral orifice and left hemitrigone were observed. However, there was no right ureteral orifice. In its place was a puckered opening which, when catheterised and filled with dye, proved to be the vaginal canal ending in a small uterus. It became clear that this young woman lacked a urethra and had a vaginal canal ectopically opening into the base of the bladder, as well as a left solitary kidney and lack of development of the right nephric system (Fig. 10.3).

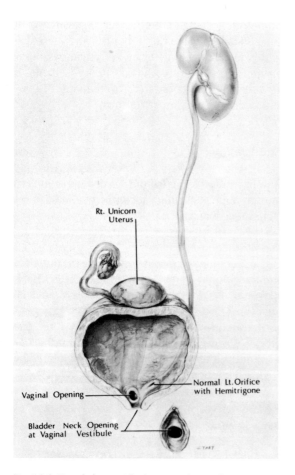

Fig. 10.3. Female born with absent urethra and ectopic vagina opening into the base of the bladder. A widely open internal meatus occupies the vaginal vestibule, with normal external genitalia. Endoscopically, only a left ureteral orifice with hemitrigone is seen. Inside the right orifice, there is a gaping opening of the ectopic vaginal canal leading to a small uterus with fallopian tube and ovary.

We were thus confronted with complete lack of development of the urethral canal, but with a normal vaginal vestibule and normally developed labia majora and minora and a diminutive and rudimentary vagina opening ectopically into the bladder base. Surgical reconstruction was attempted. Through a vaginal approach the bladder neck was circumscribed and dissected from its connection to the vaginal vestibule. The dissection was extended posteriorly and retrotrigonally until the vaginal canal was freed all around and transected from the bladder wall. The bladder was mobilised freely and displaced upward, while the vaginal canal was also dissected, mobilised and pulled downward to replace the bladder. Its opening was sutured to the vaginal vestibule in the position previously occupied by the bladder neck (Fig. 10.4). Through a suprapubic exposure, the mobilised bladder was freed further and repositioned more cranially.

Along the principles of the technique previously described, the square flap from the anterior bladder wall, just above the internal meatus, was shaped into a tube for the reconstruction of a 3.5 cm long urethral canal. The apex of the trigone was then sutured to the base of the reconstructed tube and the bladder closure was completed. Through a stab wound incision below the pubic arch and anterior to the repositioned vaginal canal, a pathway was created in which the neourethra could lie. The end of this reconstructed tube was then sutured vaginally to the vestibule just below the clitoris. The bladder was drained through a suprapubic cystostomy and a urethral catheter.

Convalescence was uneventful. Suprapubic drainage was maintained for a total of 6 weeks because of some retraction of the internal meatus which required dilatation. After removal of the suprapubic tube, the patient was completely dry and voided with an adequate stream. When she attempted sexual activity shortly thereafter, she experienced some urine leakage. She was then advised to abstain from sexual intercourse for at least 3 more months. During this time she regained urinary control and had no incontinence problems when she resumed sexual activity. She is currently happily married. She is able to keep completely dry and has an active sexual life.

This particular case exemplifies the most stringent test in the sphincteric activity of a reconstructed neourethra developed from the anterior bladder wall. The patient has no other means but this reconstructed tube for her sphincteric function. It

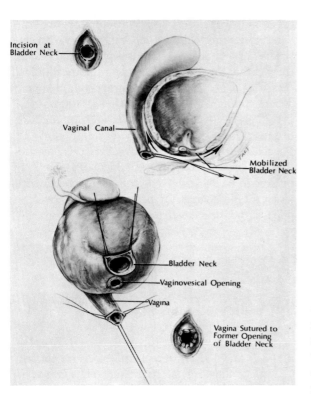

Incision at Bladder Neck

Vaginal Canal

Mobilized Bladder Neck

Bladder Neck

Vaginovesical Opening

Vagina

Vagina Sutured to Former Opening of Bladder Neck

Fig. 10.4. Steps in surgical repair. Circumscribing the internal meatus opening in the vaginal vestibule, progressive mobilisation of the bladder outlet is carried out until connection between vaginal and bladder base is reached. The original site of the vesicovaginal opening is closed and the vaginal end is brought out into the vaginal vestibule to replace the original bladder outlet opening.

has been totally adequate, permitting free urinary flow, yet complete control. Excretory urograms obtained after operation revealed a well-preserved upper urinary tract, as well as complete bladder emptying.

Case 2. The same technique was applied to another patient who had sustained a serious pelvic injury with complete disruption and destruction of the urethral segment. Suprapubic cystoscopy was instituted immediately. The patient then developed a vesicourethrovaginal fistula (which was actually at the bladder neck since the urethra itself had already been seriously damaged and torn). After mobilisation of the bladder neck, an anterior flap was reconstructed. It was anastomosed to the remaining external meatus and the bladder base was reconstructed on the same principles. The patient had a complete and uneventful recovery, with total sphincteric control.

Results

Rate of Success

During the last 12–15 years, we have performed over 50 bladder neck reconstructions with formation of a new urethra, using the anterior bladder flap technique and trigonal tubularisation in about equal numbers. More than 50% of these patients had multiple congenital anomalies, including simple female epispadias, lack of urethral development, high persistent urogenital sinus, cloacal malformations and several other bizarre congenital anomalies in a variety of combinations. Most of the remaining cases resulted from trauma and iatrogenic damage: severe pelvic fractures and lacerations of the urethra; extensive internal urethrotomy or transurethral resection; inadvertent extensive meatotomy in what was mistaken for a vaginal septum rather than the urethral floor; and extensive urethrovesicovaginal fistula after attempted repair of a pre-existing diverticulum or after complicated neglected labour. In a few instances, the neourethra was built on top of the existing urethra in order to develop increased outlet resistance in the neuropathic bladder, to allow intermittent catheterisation and to provide a means of management because of the difficulty of handling complete urinary incontinence. In all our patients urinary incontinence was complete. Only complete reconstruction with a neourethra and a new sphincteric mechanism would have been of any value to them.

It is our philosophy to embark on this approach before attempting any artificial sphincter implantation. With these reconstructive procedures, our overall success rate is 75%–80%, which makes it much more attractive to us than risking the inherent morbidity of a mechanical device. When construction of a neourethra is successful, the continence gained is permanent. The artificial sphincter is almost always liable to future setbacks and the need for repair. (This issue is discussed in more detail in Chap. 11.)

We classify our results as excellent, good, fair and failure. Patients with an excellent result are those who attain complete control with no need for protection and can achieve complete bladder emptying with an adequate flow rate and no evidence of obstruction. Those with good results show remarkable improvement. They might lose a few drops of urine with full distension under stress and may need minimal protection during activity, but they are for all practical purposes socially dry and are generally quite satisfied with the result. However, they might have to empty the bladder more frequently, and may need to be careful with activity, especially when the bladder is full.

Patients with fair results improve somewhat, yet still have to rely on protective means to keep dry. Incontinence is a relative issue: instead of using ten pads per day, they might use one, two or three per day. These patients have improved and are happy; however, we consider these fair results inadequate.

Of course, the failures are straightforward—either failure to regain control or failure to empty the bladder because of increased outlet resistance. In some of these patients, especially those with neuropathic dysfunction, we were aware pre-operatively that they would have to rely on intermittent catheterisation. Even though the surgical outcome was expected, we still classify these patients among the failures.

The success rate included both the excellent and good results, which constituted over 75%. The failure rate included patients with fair results as well as the failures, and accounted for the approximately 25% remaining.

Mechanism of Failure

It is interesting to note that most failures were anticipated, either pre- or peri-operatively. The commonest cause of failure was the poor quality of musculature used to reconstruct the sphincteric mechanism. This sometimes was quite clear pre-operatively, but we attempted reconstruction out of desperation. Most of the time, however, this was not apparent until the time of surgery, when the bladder wall was seen to be quite attenuated, scarred, fibrosed and lacking in muscular activity. Most of these patients remained wet. Invariably they did regain a bit of control, but this could not qualify the reconstruction to be considered other than a failure.

Although poor musculature was most common, one failure resulted from the iatrogenic development of a urethrovaginal fistula caused by vaginal injury during the freeing and mobilisation of the bladder outlet for reconstruction in a post-traumatic case. This necessitated another attempt at repair. In another failure, the neourethra was under some tension that resulted in meatal retraction, which necessitated another procedure to advance the external meatus to the outside. One patient with epispadias was unable to void post-operatively, despite the fact that there was no demonstrable mechanical obstruction or neuropathic disorder. She is totally dependent upon intermittent catheterisation.

It is apparent from the results and the analysis of the cause of failure that the basic rationale for the procedure is sound. What will defeat reconstruction will be either a technical problem or an intrinsic muscular weakness. From this experience, more stringent guidelines for patient selection will be applied and the incidence of failure will be markedly reduced.

Summary

In 1969 and 1972, we reported experimental and clinical studies of a technique of sphincteric reconstruction for treatment of complete urinary incontinence. The rationale of operation is that the anterior bladder wall above the internal meatus has an abundance of transverse fibres, and that a flap of this segment, when shaped into a tube, will amply provide circularly orientated fibres capable of exerting an occlusive effect on this tube, thus supplying sphincteric function. In the posterior flap, the transverse fibres at the interureteric ridge, as well as some of the detrusor circular fibres from behind the trigone, will provide the circularly orientated muscular coat of the reconstituted tube. Experimental and urodynamic evaluations proved the correctness of this rationale. In properly selected cases, this operation offers a success rate of about 80%. The same principle applied to a variety of congenital anomalies associated with absence or incomplete development of the urethra, as well as after traumatic rupture or iatrogenic damage and scarring, has proved equally successful. Results depend entirely on the reconstructed sphincteric tube, which usually provides control without any help from the voluntary component. This procedure should not be attempted lightly, even in cases of total urinary incontinence. In women, a certain degree of control can usually be regained with much less extensive surgical reconstruction.

In specific cases—mainly when both ureteral reimplantation and neourethra are needed, as in female epispadias—the Leadbetter technique presented in 1964 is advisable and successful.

References

Gross RE, Cresson SL (1952) Treatment of epispadias: A report of 18 cases. J Urol 68:477–488

Lapides J (1965) Surgical therapy for abnormalities of the urinary sphincter in the female. Br J Urol 37:609–619

Leadbetter GW Jr (1964) Surgical correction of total urinary incontinence. J Urol 91:261–266

Leadbetter GW Jr, Fraley EE (1968) Surgical correction for total urinary incontinence: 5 years after. J Urol 97:869–873

Tanagho EA (1975) Anatomy and physiology of the urethra. In: Caldwell KPS (ed) Urinary incontinence. Sector, London

Tanagho EA (1976) Urethrosphincteric reconstruction for congenitally absent urethra. J Urol 116:237–242

Tanagho EA (1978) The anatomy and physiology of micturition. In: Stanton SL (ed) Clinics in obstetrics and gynaecology, pp 3–26. Saunders, London

Tanagho EA, Smith DR (1968) Mechanism of urinary continence. I. Embryologic, anatomic and pathologic considerations. J Urol 100:640–646

Tanagho, EA, Smith DR (1972) Clinical evaluation of a surgical technique for the correction of complete urinary incontinence. J Urol 107:402–411

Tanagho EA, Smith DR, Meyers FH, Fisher R (1969a) Mechanism of urinary continence. II. Technique for surgical correction of incontinence. J Urol 101:305–318

Tanagho EA, Meyers FH, Smith DR (1969b) Urethral resistance: Its components and implications. I. Smooth muscle component. Invest Urol 7:136–149

Tanagho EA, Meyers FH, Smith DR (1969c) Urethral resistance: Its components and implications. II. Striated muscle component. Invest Urol 7:195–205

11 Artificial Sphincter

William L. Furlow

Introduction

The development of a totally implantable, externally controllable artificial urinary sphincter by Scott et al. (1973) has had a profound effect on men, women and children with urinary incontinence. From its inception, the bold concept of re-establishing volitional control of micturition through the use of an implantable device has stimulated the imagination of those of us who, over the years, have continued to search for new and improved methods whereby our patients can regain continence.

Patients with total urinary incontinence, whatever the cause, seem to have a predictable pattern of behaviour, which is generally self-inflicted as the result of their constant leakage. They are frequently withdrawn, depressed, disinclined to travel or visit friends, ill-tempered and difficult to live with. Their life-styles may be significantly affected. Their confidence in holding down responsible jobs is frequently eroded, and not infrequently they choose early retirement rather than risk the profound embarrassment that results from the odour of urine in wet clothing. Black is often the predominant colour worn by males and females because, wet or dry, black appears the same.

The artificial urinary sphincter appears to offer two important advantages over past methods of treating urinary incontinence: the device is applicable to males and females, and voiding is not obstructed. Therefore, it is not only appropriate but also essential that an up-to-date work on urinary incontinence should include a description of the artificial urinary sphincter.

The artificial urinary sphincter and its surgical method of implantation, as well as the urodynamic methods for patient study and selection, have been in a continuous state of evolution. This chapter follows closely the changes associated with device designs, surgical techniques, and patient investigation and selection that have evolved since the initial introduction of the device. The material in this chapter is both subjective and objective, being based principally on the author's experience but also on that of others whose experience is available for critical review.

Developmental History

The artificial urinary sphincter, as conceived by Scott et al. (1973) and first developed by American Medical Systems, was first implanted in humans in June 1972, and was known as model AS 721. Historically, the concept of a pressurised cuff encircling the urethra and effecting circular compression of the urethra for the purpose of maintaining urinary control must be credited to Foley (1947). In this device (Fig. 11.1), a syringe-like mechanism attached to a segment of exteriorised tubing connected to the urethral cuff was used to inflate the cuff with air. However, the device did not receive widespread acceptance by the medical profession.

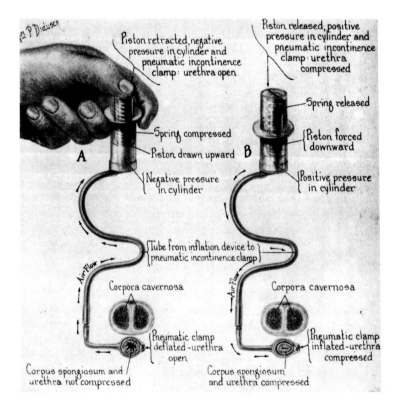

Fig. 11.1. Foley incontinence device.

The First Model, AS 721 (Fig. 11.2)

In this form, the artificial sphincter was designed to close the urethra by means of a hydraulically operated cuff encircling the urethra. The reservoir holding the fluid used to inflate the cuff was placed inside the abdominal cavity. The two pumping mechanisms, which inflated and deflated the cuff, each consisted of a bulb and two valves. The valves controlled the direction of the flow of fluid inside the prosthesis and, more importantly, were designed to set the precise pressure inside the cuff. The inflating mechanism and its two valves controlled the transfer of fluid from the reservoir into the inflatable cuff (Fig. 11.3a); the deflating mechanism, which also consisted of a pump and two valves, reversed the direction of flow, pumping fluid from the cuff into the reservoir (Fig. 11.3b) when activated. A more important part of the deflating mechanism was the V-4 valve positioned between the deflating pump and the reservoir; it controlled the pressure applied to the urethra through precise setting of the pressure inside the cuff. In this way, regardless of the number of times the inflating bulb was squeezed, the cuff would reach a predetermined pressure equilibrium. Pressure settings for the various valves were established through investigational research in the laboratory so that cuff pressures would be compatible with tissue survival. Medical-grade silicone elastomer was used for the basic construction of this prosthetic device.

Sphincter with Pressure-Regulation Balloon, AS 761 (Fig. 11.4)

Experience showed that the main problem associated with model AS 721 was the potential failure of the valve critical for the effective maintenance of cuff pressure—the V-4 valve (Furlow 1976, 1979). Therefore, an alternative means of controlling cuff pressure was developed, and in October 1976, model AS 761 was introduced. This model represented an effort to simplify the surgical procedure and to increase the mechanical reliability of the system. Model AS 761 was essentially the same as model AS 721, except for the addition of a pressure-regulating balloon positioned between the cuff and the deflating bulb. With this design, when fluid was pumped into the cuff and balloon combination, the balloon regulated the cuff pressure and thus eliminated the need for critical dependence on the pressure-regulating effects of the V-4 valve.

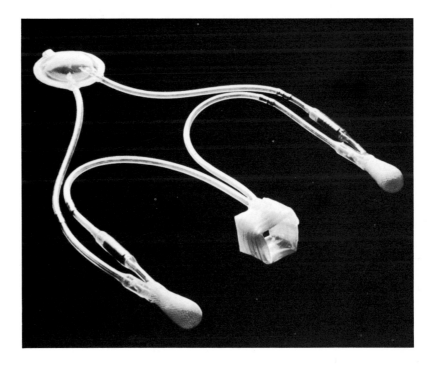

Fig. 11.2. Artificial sphincter model AS 721.

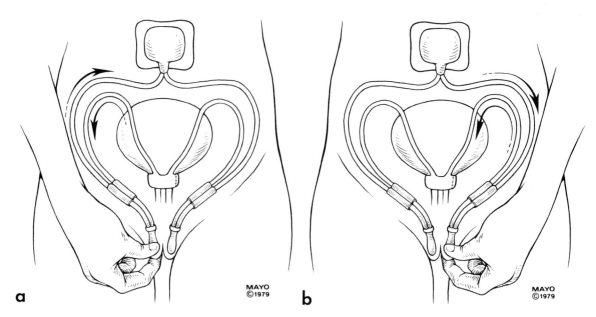

Fig. 11.3. a Inflation of artificial sphincter model AS 721. (By permission of Mayo Foundation). **b** Deflation of artificial sphincter model AS 721. (By permission of Mayo Foundation).

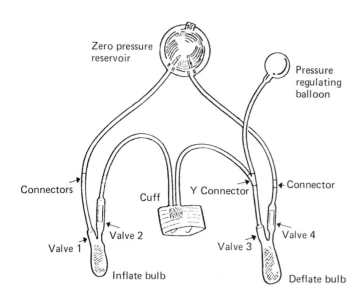

Fig. 11.4. Artificial sphincter model AS 761.

Before model AS 761 was released for general use, it was evaluated by the Balloon Sphincter Clinical Study Group (1977). This group consisted of 25 surgeons from the United States, Canada and Germany. During that time, 82 model AS 761 artificial urinary sphincters were implanted. Of the 82 patients, 47 (57.3%) had successful initial implantations resulting in continence, 2 (2.4%) had implantations that improved their conditions and 33 (40.2%) had unsuccessful implantations. In addition, 21 patients who had had model AS 721 implanted had a change to model AS 761 by the addition of the pressure-regulating balloon. Of these 21, 4 had successful restoration of continence and 17 did not. Thus, the overall success rate with model AS 761 was 49.5% (51 patients). Two patients (2%) had improvement, and 50 patients (48.5%) had failures.

In the analysis of this device by the Clinical Study Group, the failures were divided into three major groups: those due to patient selection, those due to errors in surgical technique and those resulting from mechanical failure of the device itself. Of the 50 failures, 25 resulted from mechanical complications, such as valve failure, reservoir leakage and faulty inflating bulbs; 13 from surgical complications, such as infection and urethral erosion; 7 from errors in patient selection (patients with detrusor hyperreflexia and uninhibited detrusor contractions); and 5 from unknown causes.

Thus, model AS 761 was considered by the Clinical Study Group to be useful only in rare situations in which the urethral tissues would require the lowest possible pressures for continence, such as in patients with urethral tissues that were ischaemic from radiation or with very thin-walled urethras or in the atherosclerotic elderly male. This device is no longer being produced.

Automatic Reflation Sphincter AS 742 (Fig. 11.5)

Model AS 742 differed significantly from both model AS 761 and model AS 721 because the cuff was inflated automatically by the pressure in the pressure-regulating balloon, which forced fluid through a fluid resistor at a controlled rate. This device consisted of a single deflating bulb that, when activated, pumped fluid from the cuff into the balloon until the bulb collapsed. Collapse indicated depressurisation of the cuff. Once the cuff was depressurised, it remained so for between 90 s and 2 min, until fluid flowing from the balloon through the fluid resistor refilled the bulb and began to repressurise the cuff. Because of the automatic re-inflation built into the design of this device, the cuff could not be left in the deflated position.

This device, as with the earlier devices, underwent critical evaluation by the Balloon Sphincter Clinical Study Group (1978). Model AS 742 was implanted in 90 patients, both male and female. Of the 41 patients who received model AS 742 as the original implant, 28 (68.3%) had successful restoration of control, 2 (4.9%) had improvement in urinary control and 11 (26.8%) had implantations that

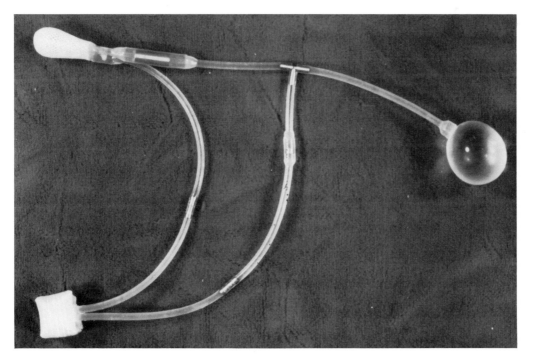

Fig. 11.5. Artificial sphincter model AS 742.

failed. An additional 49 patients underwent conversion to model AS 742 from other models. Of these 49 patients, 42 (85.7%) became totally continent, 1 (2.0%) was improved, and 6 (12.3%) had results that failed. Thus, the overall success rate for model AS 742 was 78% (70 of the 90 patients), whereas 3 (3%) were improved and 17 (19%) had implantations that failed.

The causes of failure were similar to those for model AS 761. Of the 20 instances in which implantation was not successful, 3 were due to patient selection, 11 were due to surgical error, 1 was due to mechanical failure and 5 were due to unknown causes.

On the basis of these results, the Clinical Study Group considered model AS 742 the preferred device. The main advantages of this device were ease of implantation and ease of operation by the patient. Also, fewer parts were involved, so that chances for mechanical complications were reduced. The main disadvantage with model AS 742 was that it did not provide any mechanism that would allow the cuff to be left in an open position during healing. Thus, the fitting of the appropriate cuff size might be more critical with model AS 742 than with model AS 721. An additional concern with this model was the lack of any supportive mechanism to prevent stress incontinence. Subsequent follow-up of these patients, as well as the implantation of a large number of additional devices of model AS 742, has shown that stress incontinence is not a problem.

Automatic Reflation Sphincter AS 791/792 (Fig. 11.6)

After our experience with model AS 742, a significant design improvement in the automatic reflation device took place with the development of the model AS 791/792 automatic reflation device. Changes in device design consisted of the development of an inflatable snap-on cuff. This eliminated the use of suture material for placing the cuff around the bladder neck or bulbous urethra, and thus simplified the application of the inflatable cuff surgically. In addition, the number of connections was reduced from six to three, by the development of a stainless steel control block assembly that incorporated the delayed fill resistor and directional fluid transfer valves within the assembly. Thus, some of the tubing required for the model AS 742 was eliminated. Similarly, the pump design was changed somewhat to simplify implantation of the pump into the female labium or the male scrotum.

The basic components of the model AS 791/792 were a balloon pressure reservoir, a stainless steel

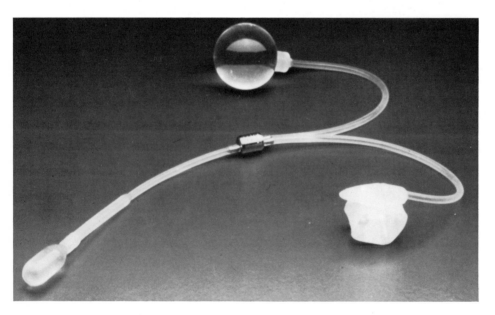

Fig. 11.6. Model AS 791/792.

control block assembly, a deflate pump mechanism and an inflatable snap-on cuff. The basic function of the device was similar to that of the AS 742, inasmuch as when all the components were implanted and connected in the proper manner the device was a semi-automatic reflation mechanism. As with the AS 742, this device did not provide any means for leaving the cuff in the deflated state and could not be turned on or off at the discretion of the physician.

For this reason, the author (Furlow 1981) introduced a new concept of delayed activation for implantation of the semi-automatic artificial sphincter models AS 742 and AS 791/792 in an effort to minimise vesical neck erosion in female patients who had undergone multiple previous operations to correct their urinary incontinence. In the initial experience in this group of patients (four women and seven girls), cuff placement was achieved around the bladder neck, the pressure-regulating reservoir was implanted in the prevesical space, and the tubing from the cuff and the reservoir was brought subcutaneously through Hesselbach's triangle into the region of the external inguinal ring. The cuff tubing was plugged with a stainless steel plug and the cuff was left in the deflated mode. The balloon pressure reservoir was filled in the manner described under "Operative Technique", and also was plugged with a stainless steel plug. The deflating pump was positioned in the right labium subcutaneously, and its tubing was positioned adjacent to the other tubes and was capped with a stainless steel plug. The final resting place of all three tubes was, therefore, subcutaneous in the region of the right external inguinal ring. The key to this deactivation concept was that the control block, which provides for activation of the device, was not implanted at that time, so that the cuff remained deflated. During the 3-month follow-up period, the patient therefore remained incontinent. Before activation of the device, the urethra and bladder neck were carefully inspected cystoscopically and urographically. Activation was accomplished during a second operative procedure in which a small transverse incision over the subcutaneously placed tubes allowed for exposure of the tubes, pressurisation of the cuff, filling of the balloon pressure reservoir with the proper volume of fluid and attachment of the control block assembly. Once the control block assembly was connected to the tubes, the device was fully activated. Initial experience with the use of this concept was most favourable, not only in females but also in males with bulbous urethral cuff placement (Barrett and Furlow 1981).

Model AS 800: Controlled Activation and Deactivation

The newest design modifications of the artificial urinary sphincter represent a major breakthrough in device operation. The model AS 800 (Fig. 11.7a), like its predecessors, models AS 742 and 791/792, has a pressure-regulating balloon mechanism and an inflatable snap-on cuff. However, a pump control assembly directly incorporated within the deflate pump obviates the stainless steel control block assembly and, more importantly, provides a pressable button in the pump and a controllable "on-off" function (Fig. 11.7b). Therefore, primary deactivation in one operative procedure and secondary activation with another operative procedure are no longer necessary. The development of the new model AS 800 artificial urinary sphincter allows for a single-stage total implantation of the prosthetic device and the option for activation or deactivation whenever clinically indicated.

Indications

Early in our experience, the artificial genitourinary sphincter was considered only for patients in whom the surgical treatment of choice was urinary diversion by ureterosigmoidostomy or ileal conduit, but who preferred an alternative in an effort to achieve volitional urinary control. At present, the artificial sphincter is used in both males and females for various types of urinary incontinence, including incontinence after prostatectomy, stress incontinence, epispadias incontinence, incontinence after urethral replacement by bladder flap reconstruction, neuropathic bladder dysfunction secondary to meningomyelocele, spinal cord injury, multiple sclerosis, sacral agenesis, or spinal cord tumours, and isolated, rare types of urinary incontinence secondary to operative procedures. The proper application of the prosthesis requires urodynamic evaluation of the patient.

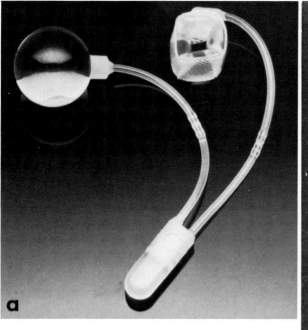
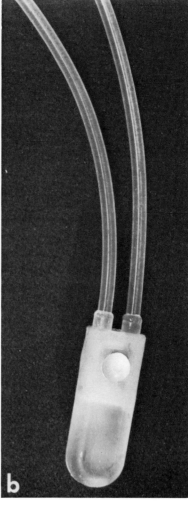

Fig. 11.7. a Model AS 800. **b** Pump control assembly.

Pre-operative Evaluation

The pre-operative testing of the incontinent female to be evaluated for suitability for a sphincter implantation should consist of the following investigations.

1. Uroflowmetry is done in all patients. Flow rates greater than 15 ml/s should be obtained to rule out any form of obstructive uropathy.

2. Cystometry is done in all patients to exclude the presence of detrusor hyperreflexia or to determine whether it can be controlled medically. When detrusor hyperreflexia is present, a concomitant sphincter electromyographic study is necessary to rule out detrusor-sphincter dyssynergia. A patient with uncontrollable detrusor hyperreflexia is not a candidate for implantation of an artificial genitourinary sphincter, because the intravesical pressure generated by the contracting detrusor usually exceeds the cuff pressure and causes leakage of urine.

3. The urethral pressure profile study has been used pre-operatively, intra-operatively and post-operatively for various reasons. Pre-operatively, urethral profilometry gives the physician an opportunity to demonstrate the inadequate closing pressures in the urethra, as well as rather high pressures that might necessitate pharmacological treatment. Excessively

high pressures that cannot be treated medically are often overcome by a preliminary operative procedure, such as a bladder flap urethroplasty or sphincterotomy, that reduces high resistance before the sphincter is implanted. Urethral pressure profilometry is also helpful intra-operatively to measure the closing pressures obtained at implantation, although these values are not absolute indicators of the subsequent success or failure of the device. Postoperatively, urethral profilometry is useful in determining the function of the artificial sphincter in comparison with the intra-operative result at implantation.

Other tests that may be performed include a residual urine test, sphincter electromyography and pressure-flow study.

In addition to these studies, cinefluorography may be considered useful in detecting abnormalities created by strictures and reflux. All patients should have a careful urinalysis, including a Gram stain, culture and sensitivity study of the urine, to select the antibiotic of choice in treating any infection. Panendoscopy should be done in all patients, both pre-operatively and post-operatively. In the pre-operative evaluation, endoscopy is useful in ruling out other pathological causes of the patient's urinary incontinence. It also serves as a useful aid in estimating the potential cuff size to be used. Postoperatively, endoscopy may be helpful in the evaluation of the operative result and in assessing the cause of some post-operative symptoms that may arise.

Selection of Model

At present, the model AS 800 is the preferred device for implantation in both adults and children. This device allows for both primary deactivation and secondary deactivation without necessitating a second surgical procedure. The surgeon has the option of selecting from a broad range of available balloon pressure reservoirs and from a wide range of cuff sizes. The rationale behind the appropriate selection of these components will be discussed as part of "Operative Technique".

Operative Technique

Aseptic Technique

The single most important consideration in the implantation of an artificial urinary sphincter is strict aseptic technique. Superficial and deep wound infections are a serious hazard with any prosthetic implant and almost always require total removal of the device to achieve clearing of the infection.

Asepsis begins with the pre-operative preparation of the patient. The patient scheduled to undergo implant surgery should have sterile urine for at least 48 hours before surgery. If the patient's urine is sterile pre-operatively, prophylactic antibiotic coverage is begun 24 hours before surgery and is continued post-operatively for between 7 and 10 days. A third-generation cephalosporin is generally used in a dosage of 250 mg every 6 h by mouth. The night before surgery, the patient is given a shower during which a preparation containing hexachlorophene or iodoform is used, with special emphasis on the abdomen, pubic area, genitalia and perineum. The actual preparation of the skin by shaving is deferred until surgery, at which time the abdomen, pubic area, genitalia, perineum and upper portions of the thighs are shaved. The patient is scrubbed for 15 min with an iodoform soap and painted with an iodoform solution. Fitzgerald and Washington (1975) demonstrated that patients prepared in this manner had a mean of 17 colony-forming units (cfu)/m² at closure of the incision, whereas 43 cfu/m² was achieved when an iodoform preparation was supplemented by alcohol and Freon and 96 cfu/m² when the iodoform solution was omitted and Merthiolate was added to the alcohol and Freon.

Staff members participating directly in the procedure should scrub their hands and arms for 10 min with an iodoform preparation. The wearing of a gown that has a water-repellent front and sleeves prevents contamination from saturation. Traffic should be kept to a minimum by bold, eye-catching signs at the entrances to the operating room—signs that state, "Artificial Sphincter Implant. Do Not Enter". Packing soaked with a povidone–iodine solution (Betadine) is used in the vagina to maintain sterile conditions and also to allow palpation of the vagina relative to the urethra. Periodically during the procedure, a solution of 1 g kanamycin and 50 000 units of bacitracin in

500 ml of normal saline (Schuster 1976) or 1 g neomycin and 50 000 units of bacitracin in 500 ml of normal saline (Furlow 1976) is sprayed into the wound.

Patient Position

Implantation of the artificial sphincter in women is carried out with the patient in the lithotomy positon. This position is modified so that, although the legs are spread, the knee crutches are lowered to place the level of the knees on the same plane as the surface of the abdomen. In this manner, the legs do not interfere with access to either the abdomen or the vagina and the position allows for help by surgical assistants.

Instrumentation

The instruments and supplies suggested for the implantation of an artificial genitourinary sphincter are shown in Table 11.1. Some special instruments have been designed by Scott especially for this type of urological prosthetic surgery, including the Scott dissecting scissors and right-angled scissors. However, these special instruments are not essential for successful implantation.

Surgical Procedure

A transverse suprapubic incision is made immediately above the symphysis to expose the urethra and bladder neck (Fig. 11.8). In some female patients,

Table 11.1. Suggested list of instruments and supplies for implantation of artificial urinary sphincter

Pack and supplies
Laparotomy pack, gown, gloves (dual finish)
2 10-ml syringes, 2 20- or 30-ml syringes
Raytex sponges, lap sponges, Kuettner dissector, nerve tape
Deseret prep pack, needle pack
No. 10 and 20 blades, bayonet cautery
Portovac and connector tubing, 0.25-in. Penrose drain
Foley catheter (12F or 14F)
Betadine solution
Solution of 0·1% neomycin and 50 000 units of bacitracin in 1000 ml of saline, 60-ml catheter, tipped syringe
Sphincter kit, 200 ml of 25% Hypaque, no. 22 spinal needle

Sutures
Routine abdominal sutures
3–0 Prolene (for sewing pocket around bulbs and tacking in reservoir; also, cut off needle and use as ties for fastening connectors)
1–0 Tevdek (for drains and for closure, sometimes)
1–0 chromic (for closure)
4–0 Vicryl

Dressing
Gauze
Tape (3-in. microfoam)

Instruments
Haemostats or clamps
    4 short
    4 Kocher
    4 6-in. Carmalt
    4 8-in. Carmalt
    4 Shallcross (right-angled)
    2 Adson (right-angled)
    2 Pean (curved)
    3 Harrington (right-angled)
    12 mosquitos with shods (6 curved and 6 straight)

Ruler (centimeter)

Retractors
Balfour
Israel and Murphy
3 Deaver (2 broad and 1 narrow)
2 Harrington
2 Bernatz
2 Stratte (not hinged)

Scissors
Mayo
Metzenbaum
Lillie
Suture

Forceps
3 Russian
2 Kelly
2 Adson (with teeth)
2 vascular (without teeth)

Needle holders
2 7-in. and 2 9-in. vascular
2 Hegar
3 6-in. diamond jawed (not hinged)
2 Stratte (not hinged)

Other
1000-ml graduate
500-ml graduate
Suction tubing and tonsil tip (plastic)
1-in. malleable retractor
1 straight scissors
Extra-long scissors
4 long Allis clamps

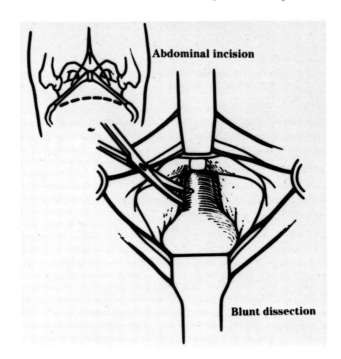

Fig. 11.8. Exposure of bladder neck and proximal urethra. (Courtesy of American Medical Systems, Inc, Minnetonka, MN)

transection of the rectus muscles better enables the surgeon to dissect behind the bladder neck. A tight pack within the vagina and a Foley catheter within the urethra provide for better determination of the position of the bladder neck and aid in avoiding entry into the vagina during the dissection behind the bladder neck (Fig. 11.9). Opening the bladder immediately above the bladder neck increases the accuracy of dissection behind the bladder neck. However, this portion of the procedure may carry increased morbidity with an increased chance of infection.

Dissection around the bladder neck begins on one side and then on the other and continues until only a fine, thin septum remains in the midline. The position of the bladder neck in relation to the vagina and the integrity of the posterior bladder neck and urethra are assessed at this time.

One should attempt to control venous bleeding now before dissecting through the vesicovaginal septum. The dissection is completed around the vesical neck and urethra, and a tunnel long enough to accept a cuff 2 cm in width is developed. Scott (1978, personal communication) has indicated that such a tunnel will barely accept the first phalange of the index finger. Further assessment and control of venous bleeding should be carried out before

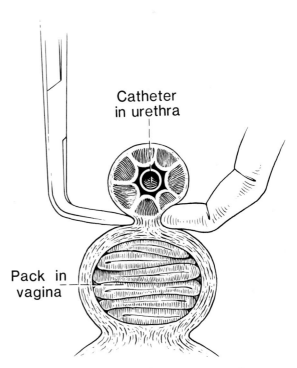

Fig. 11.9. Tight-fitting vagina pack allows accurate dissection between vagina and bladder neck.

placement of the cuff. This bleeding should be stopped by use of suture ligature, preferably 3–0 chromic catgut.

If careful inspection reveals that the vaginal wall and vagina have been injured on entry, the damage should be repaired by a running horizontal mattress absorbable suture; penetration of the vaginal epithelium must be avoided. Injury to the urethra or bladder should be similarly repaired. If there is watertight closure of the urethra or bladder neck, it is probably safe to proceed with placement of the inflatable cuff; however, if the surgeon has any doubt about satisfactory closure, the procedure should be stopped and allowance should be made for healing. In this situation, the operation may be attempted again in 6 months. However, if, in the surgeon's judgment, the closure is a satisfactory one, the procedure may be continued, although activation of the sphincter should not be attempted for at least 4–6 weeks. I prefer to delay activation for 6–12 weeks in patients in whom the urethra has required repair.

Most authors probably would concur with Scott (personal communication) in the statement that: "This procedure up to this point requires the utmost in judgment, skill and patience of the surgeon, relying on wisdom gained from past surgical experiences to complete this part of the surgery successfully."

Selection of Cuff Size

Passage of a right-angled Harrington clamp through the tunnel behind the bladder neck is used to draw the cuff sizer behind the bladder neck so that the urethral circumference can be measured (Fig. 11.10). It is best to err in selecting the larger size, because cuffs less than 7.5 cm long generally close completely when fully inflated. For example,

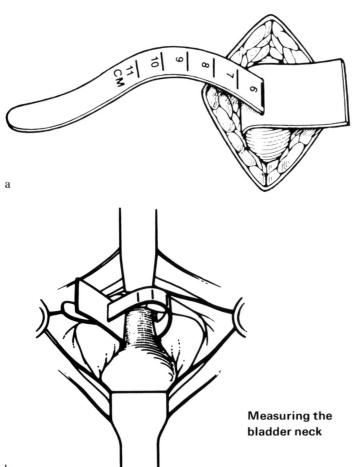

a

**Measuring the
bladder neck**

b

Fig. 11.10. a American Medical Systems cuff sizer. b Initial insertion of cuff sizer around bladder neck permits circumference measurements for cuff size selection.

if the appropriate cuff size is 4.5 cm, a 5- or 5.5-cm cuff should be selected to accommodate post-operative oedema without compromising continence.

Cuff Implantation

Once chosen, the snap-on cuff is filled with fluid and all air bubbles are evacuated. Silicone-shod clamps are used to occlude the tubing. The cuff is oriented so that the inflatable portion faces the urethra once the cuff is pulled through the tunnel behind the bladder neck (Fig. 11.11).

The external inguinal ring is identified; the tubing needle is inserted into it superficial to the external oblique fascia and through the inguinal canal and internal inguinal ring into the suprapubic space. The tubing needle accepts and occludes the ends of the tubing coming from the cuff, and is then used

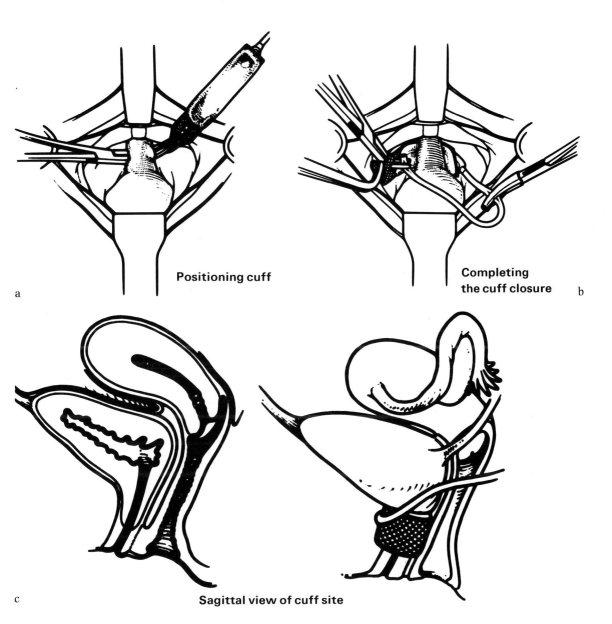

Positioning cuff

Completing the cuff closure

Sagittal view of cuff site

Fig. 11.11. a Tab end of snap-on cuff is grasped with right-angled clamp for posterior placement. **b** Cuff closure is completed by insertion of tubing into tab opening and locking of tab end of cuff to hub of tubing on opposite end of cuff. **c** Proper cuff position at female bladder neck.

to draw the tubing through the inguinal canal
(Fig. 11.12).

Selection of Balloon Pressure Reservoir

The balloon pressure reservoir is placed in the
prevesical space, and the tubing needle is again used
to draw the reservoir tubing through the inguinal
canal and out through the external ring on the same
side adjacent to the cuff tubing. In my opinion, selection of the balloon pressure reservoir range is critical
to a successful result and the minimising of subsequent urethral cuff erosion. In general, in all
female patients who have the inflatable snap-on cuff
positioned around the bladder neck and who have
not undergone previous pelvic surgery in and
around the bladder neck, the highest range of
reservoir pressure that should be selected is 60–
70 cmH$_2$O. Ranges higher than 70 cmH$_2$O are
seldom indicated and, from previous experience,
have a much higher risk of erosion. On the other
hand, from time to time it may be necessary to select
lower balloon pressure ranges, either 50–60 cmH$_2$O
pressure or, on rare occasions, 40–50 cmH$_2$O (Barrett and Furlow 1981).

The pump control assembly (Fig. 11.13) is placed
superficially within the labium. The bulb should be
positioned low within the labium but not too
superficially.

The superficial tunnel created within the labium
is best developed with a cervical curved dilator. Usually, the pump is placed in the right labium. The
redundant tubing is tailored for length and the
various tubing ends are matched and connected
over plastic connectors. After the connector is

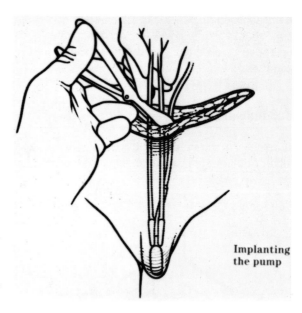

Fig. 11.13. Positioning of pump control assembly within labium.

inserted into one end of the tubing, air and blood
are displaced by injection of fluid into the tubing end
and the connector end through a blunt 22-gauge
needle (Fig. 11.14). The opposing end of the tubing
is then placed over the connector, and the two ends
are tied to the connector with 3–0 Prolene suture
material. All connections are made subcutaneously
(Fig. 11.15).

Before wound closure, the hydraulic function of
the device should be tested first by inflating and
deflating the cuff and then by filling the bladder with
sterile saline while the cuff is deflated and, once it
is filled, by inflating the cuff and withdrawing the
catheter. Light suprapubic pressure is then applied

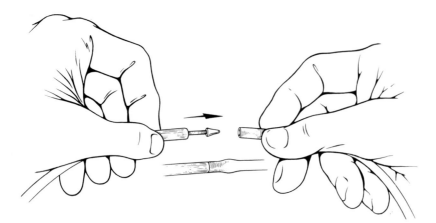

Fig. 11.12. Tubing is passed through inguinal canals by tubing passer needle to which tubing is attached.

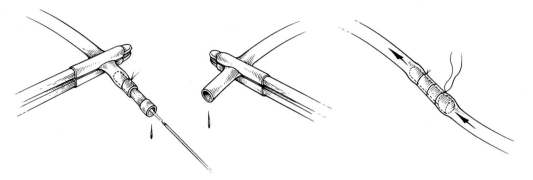

Fig. 11.14. Tubing lumens are flushed and filled with fluid to eliminate air and blood before connections are made.

to the bladder to determine the competency of the sphincter device. Intra-operative urethral pressure profile studies may be used to determine the closing pressure around the urethra and bladder neck, for comparison with closing pressures obtained pre-operatively. There is some question about the validity of this method of measurement intra-operatively, and the surgeon should not rely too much on the measurements as an indicator of the success or failure of the operative procedure. Generally, urethral pressure profilometry shows occlusion of the urethra for pressures ranging from 60–90 cmH$_2$O; however, post-operative urinary continence has been achieved with pressures as low as 30 cmH$_2$O. The wound is closed with interrupted 1–0 Prolene in the fascia and interrupted 3–0 chromic catgut in the subcutaneous tissue. The subcutaneous tissue is best closed in several layers to protect the device against contamination should a superficial wound infection develop. The skin is closed with a subcuticular suture of 4–0 Vicryl. No drains are used. A 12F Silastic Foley urethral catheter is left indwelling, with 5 ml of sterile saline inflating the balloon.

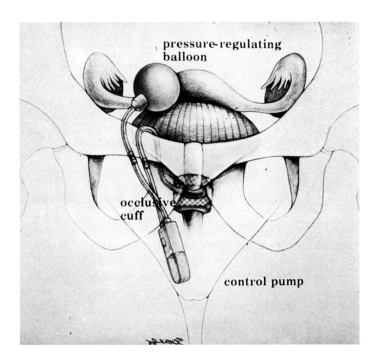

Fig. 11.15. Completed implantation of model AS 800 sphincter in female.

Post-operative Management

The patient is placed in the Trendelenburg position for the first 18–24 h after surgery to reduce the oedema that may result from the labial dissection. In addition, ice packs applied to the genitalia may be helpful during the first 2 or 3 days. After model AS 800 implantation, the cuff is left open (deactivated) at all times during the first 3–4 post-operative days.

If the bladder or urethra has not been opened during the dissection, the catheter may then be removed and the patient permitted to use the device. The patient should be instructed to open the cuff every 2 h during the day, and is to be awakened twice at night to open the cuff to permit voiding. After dismissal on the 7th post-operative day, the patient is permitted to retain urine for longer periods until normal voiding patterns are established. In selected patients, we are using nocturnal deactivation to reduce the time of cuff compression in a 24-hour period. I believe it is entirely possible that reduced compression time will further minimise the risk of erosion.

If the bladder has been opened, the cuff should be left open for at least 3–4 weeks post-operatively, to allow for adequate bladder healing before voiding is begun by activation of the pump control assembly. At times with the model AS 800, it is desirable to leave the cuff open for an extended time; to do so is entirely practical because of the deactivation button on the pump control assembly. In point of practice, my recommendation in female bladder neck sphincter implantations is that the cuff be left deactivated for up to 4 weeks before activation.

Results and Discussion

The implantable artificial urinary sphincter, although undergoing the usual changes in design associated with any artificial device, has withstood the test of time and implantation has proved to be an accepted treatment alternative in the management of urinary incontinence in both males and females. As of May 1978, 288 model AS 721 artificial sphincters had been implanted in the United States. The overall success rates with implantation of this device were approximately 60% in males and 50% in females. Results were slightly better in female patients who had not undergone associated bladder flap urethroplasty.

The main complications associated with the artificial sphincter have been infection and urethral erosion. Infection in the area of the prosthesis can seldom, if ever, be treated with antibiotic therapy and usually requires removal of the prosthesis. Generally, in most patients with a prosthesis-associated infection, the infection appears early, usually within 2–3 weeks after implantation.

Urethral erosion may be attributed to several surgical and mechanical factors associated with the device. Improper handling of tissue, improper selection of cuff size or balloon pressure range, and tubing kinks may be responsible for the onset of ischaemia of the urethral wall and subsequent erosion of the cuff through the urethral wall. In a series reported by Scott (1978), 18 patients had stress incontinence that was unresponsive to the usual operative procedures, each patient having undergone at least three operations in the treatment of stress incontinence. One patient had undergone nine operative procedures without success. In this group, 14 of the 18 patients achieved an excellent result with implantation of model AS 721. Females with neuropathic bladder dysfunction are excellent candidates for implantation of the artificial urinary sphincter, provided there is no evidence of detrusor hyperreflexia or the hyperreflexia is controlled by medication. Scott's overall success rate in females was 67.5%.

As of May 1978, the model AS 742 had been implanted in 148 patients. The overall success rate with this group (males and females) was 69% (102 of 148 patients). In females, the operation was considered successful only if there was no urinary leakage. Females with model AS 721 or model AS 761 in whom implantation failed and in whom model AS 742 was subsequently implanted had a success rate of 77% (17 of 22 patients). When model AS 742 was implanted initially in females with urinary incontinence, the overall success rate was 50% (9 of 18 patients). The overall success rate with original implantation of model AS 742 in males was 77% (24 of 31 patients) when the cuff was implanted around the bulbous urethra, and 77% (17 of 22 patients) when the cuff was placed around the bladder neck. Improvements in overall success were in part attributed to our use of the primary deactivation technique.

My experience (Furlow 1976, 1979, 1981; Barrett and Furlow 1981, 1983; Furlow and Barrett, to be published) with the implantation of the artificial genitourinary sphincter includes the implantation of 38 model AS 721, 31 model AS 742, 140 model AS 791/792, and 80 model AS 800 artificial sphincters.

To date, we have implanted the model AS 791/792 and model AS 800 artificial urinary sphincters in 31 females (Donovan et al., to be published). Previously, the model AS 721 and the model AS 742 had been implanted in seven females. Of the seven, two had neuropathic vesical dysfunction, and the model AS 721 was used. In each patient, the cuff was placed around the bladder neck and urethra. The device worked satisfactorily, maintaining continence for as long as 7 months. In one patient, however, urethral erosion developed 7 months postoperatively and an associated infection of the device required total removal. Later, this patient underwent ileal conduit urinary diversion. Urethral erosion developed in the other patient 9 months postoperatively, and she elected to have the device removed and to undergo an ileal conduit urinary diversion.

Since that time, another five patients who had stress incontinence associated with multiple previous operations have had sphincter AS 742 implanted. The follow-up at that time was only 6 months; all five were symptomatically improved and there were no complications.

Scott (1978) has had the most extensive experience with the earlier designs of the artificial urinary sphincter in females; his initial overall success rate was 67.5%. With the introduction of the model AS 742, I believe that a significant advance was made in the artificial sphincter. My experience with the model AS 742 has been highly favourable. Elimination of the critical valve settings in model AS 721 and the ease of implantation of this device have increased its adaptability to both female and male patients. Scott (1981, personal communication) reported a success rate of 90% using model AS 742 in females with stress incontinence.

Evaluation of the patient who has sphincter implantation associated with bladder flap urethroplasty indicates that the surgeon takes a higher risk of failure if the inflatable cuff is implanted at the same time as urethroplasty is done. Sphincter implantation should be deferred for 3–6 months after bladder flap urethroplasty, although dissection around the bladder neck may be more difficult as a result of post-operative scarring associated with the urethroplasty. However, the risks of contamination secondary to opening the bladder and leakage through the suture line into the vicinity of the cuff seem to be higher than the risks associated with subsequent dissection of the vesical neck and urethra after urethroplasty.

Patients with total urinary incontinence secondary to neuropathic vesical dysfunction are excellent candidates for implantation of the artificial genitourinary sphincter. Before development of the AS 800, children with meningomyelocele and sacral agenesis who were leaking required careful evaluation for the choice between model AS 721 and model AS 742. With model AS 800, this evaluation is no longer a factor, since the physician may leave the cuff in the open position at any time should the situation require it. This was not possible with models AS 742 and AS 791/792.

Models AS 791/792 and AS 800 were implanted in 31 female patients at the Mayo Clinic from December 1978 through December 1983. The ages of the patients ranged from 6 to 73 years. Incontinence in this group of female patients included 15 with neurological disease, 9 with recurrent stress incontinence, 5 with incontinence secondary to spinal cord trauma and 2 who had pelvic trauma with sphincteric involvement. The follow-up in this group ranged from 2 to 59 months, with the mean of 24.5 months. Of the 31 female patients who had implantation, 21 became continent or were greatly improved. It is important to note that 20 patients in this group had had previous anti-incontinence procedures. In 13 of these 20 patients, continence was re-established. Of the 10 patients in whom no improvement was shown, 7 had undergone previous surgery around the bladder neck. The primary cause of failure in nine of these patients was vesical neck erosion, which usually occurred between $1\frac{1}{2}$ weeks and 9 months post-operatively.

In the 21 patients in whom continence was successfully restored, 52 operative procedures, or 2.5 procedures per patient, were necessary. It should be pointed out that in only 5 of the 21 patients was primary activation carried out. Hence, seven patients had 14 procedures to achieve final activation of the device, and only nine patients had to have additional surgery to maintain continence. All the additional procedures were due to remediable mechanical problems. Six cuffs were replaced because of tissue atrophy around the bladder neck that required cuff resizing. Cuff leaks occurred in seven patients and required cuff replacement, and tubing kinks were found in two patients.

Although technically the implantation of an artificial urinary sphincter model AS 800 in the female patient is more difficult for anatomical reasons, the reason for the difficulty (in our experience) is that most of these patients have had previous surgical procedures. Of our nine patients with erosion, seven had had previous surgery and the remaining two had contributory factors that we believed led to erosion. Only 12 of our patients in whom implantation was successful had undergone previous surgery out of the total of 21. There is no question that previous surgery on and around the bladder neck has a negative influence on the survival of the urinary sphincter, because of the higher potential risk of cuff erosion. For this reason, I recommend that the devices in these patients be primarily deactivated for at least 4 weeks and preferably for up to 12 weeks post-operatively.

In the patients with model AS 791/792, most of whom had primary deactivation and required a second operation to activate the sphincter, the procedure rate of 2.5 per patient was acceptable. Obviously, introduction of model AS 800 now circumvents that necessity for a second operation, and the cuff can be simply deactivated by pressure on the deactivation button located on the pump. This leaves the cuff deflated and in the open position, until the physician determines that the time is right for activation of the device.

In one patient who underwent implantation of the model AS 791 and re-establishment of urinary control, development of pregnancy necessitated a third operative procedure to deactivate the device during the last trimester, followed by postpartum reactivation of her device surgically. Implantation of the model AS 800 would have circumvented this need, but this newest device design was not available at the time of her implantation.

Summary

Except for the technically exacting dissection around the bladder neck and urethra, implantation of the artificial genitourinary sphincter is a relatively simple surgical procedure. This is especially true with the introduction of model AS 800. At present, this device appears to meet the essential objectives for the development and application of an artificial prosthesis (Scott 1978).

1. The prosthesis can be used in both males and females.

2. The prosthesis produces urethral occlusion that is effective for urinary control and opens to allow free voiding with no interference of flow.

3. The prosthesis automatically opens if unphysiological bladder pressure develops or detrusor contractions occur and automatically increases the occlusion on physical effort or stress.

4. The occlusion mechanism and the pressures applied are automatic and inherent within the prosthetic design.

5. If the prosthesis fails, the patient is no worse off than before implantation.

6. Implantation does not require extensive alteration of the urinary tract.

7. The prosthesis allows subsequent repeated endoscopic procedures, if necessary.

8. The prosthesis does not interfere with sexual function in either male or female.

9. The prosthesis is dependable for the lifetime of the patient.

The long-term results with these devices are yet to be determined. Test cycling of the prosthetic device by the manufacturer indicates that the prosthesis can be cycled more than 80 000 times without deterioration of its function. This is equivalent to the patient urinating four times a day for more than 50 years. The experience of both Scott (1981, personal communication) and myself involves patients who now have had the device implanted for 4–5 years without any evidence of urethral necrosis or urethral obstruction. As the device is made of medical-grade silicone rubber (which is relatively inert and has been used in other prosthetic implants for nearly 20 years), it should function properly almost indefinitely, except for the possibility of a mechanical complication.

The artificial genitourinary sphincter will probably never entirely replace the operations devised for the treatment of female urinary stress incontinence. However, the device is an excellent alternative to treatment when all other methods of repair have failed. Because model AS 800 does not require two surgical procedures for primary deactivation and secondary activation, yet retains the intrinsically beneficial features of cuff pressure regulation, the problem of urethral erosion continues to be reduced as a complication of this device. The current design of model AS 800 provides for highly individualised management of patients in whom the artificial urinary sphincter is implanted relative to the selection of activation and deactivation as clinically indicated by the physician. Urethral erosion will be seen from time to time but probably will be the result of the surgical techniques rather than of a faulty mechanism associated with the device. The careful selection and evaluation of patients in conjunction with the proper selection of device, pressure-regulating balloon and cuff size, as well as skilful surgical techniques, should significantly increase the overall success rate with the use of the artificial genitourinary sphincter.

References

Balloon Sphincter Clinical Study Group (1977) American Medical Systems, Minneapolis

Balloon Sphincter Clinical Study Group (1978) American Medical Systems, Minneapolis

Barrett DM, Furlow WL (1981) Implantation of new semi-automatic artificial genitourinary sphincter: experience with patients utilizing a new concept of primary and secondary activation. Prog Clin Biol Res 78:375–386

Barrett DM, Furlow WL (1983) Artificial urinary sphincter in the management of female incontinence. In: Raz S (ed) Female urology. Saunders, Philadelphia, pp 284–292

Donovan MG, Barrett DM, Furlow WL (1985) Use of the artificial urinary sphincter in the management of severe incontinence in females. Surg Gynecol Obstet 161:17–20

Fitzgerald RH Jr, Washington JA II (1975) Contamination of the operative wound. Orthop Clin North Am 6:1105–1114

Foley FEB (1947) An artificial sphincter: a new device and operation for control of enuresis and urinary incontinence. J Urol 58:250–259

Furlow WL (1976) The implantable artificial genitourinary sphincter in the management of total urinary incontinence. Mayo Clin Proc 51:341–345

Furlow WL (1979) Advances and treatment. II. The artificial genitourinary sphincter. In: Proceedings of the 8th International Congress of Nephrology. Montreal, Canada, June 18–23 1978

Furlow WL (1981) Implantation of a new semiautomatic artificial genitourinary sphincter: experience with primary activation and deactivation in 47 patients. J Urol 126:741–744

Furlow WL, Barrett DM (1985) The artificial urinary sphincter: experience with the AS 800 pump-control assembly for single-stage primary deactivation and activation—a preliminary report. Mayo Clin Proc 60:255–258

Schuster K (1976) Operating room protocol in implantation of the inflatable penile prosthesis. Mayo Clin Proc 51:339–340

Scott FB (1978) The artificial sphincter in the management of incontinence in the male. Urol Clin North Am 5:375–391

Scott FB, Bradley WE, Timm GW (1973) Treatment of urinary incontinence by implantable prosthetic sphincter. Urology 1:252–259

12 Urinary Diversion

Peter R. Riddle*

Introduction

Urinary diversion as a permanent or temporary measure has been practised for a considerable time. However, it is only in the last one to two decades that it has become an acceptable practice in managing the intractably incontinent female patient.

The thought of a wet stoma once held untold horrors for a vast majority of patients and clinicians alike, but with the advent of modern totally dry adhesive appliances it is coming more and more into use.

There are, of course, only very limited numbers of incontinent patients suitable for diversion. They basically fall into two categories.

Classification of Patients

The first group comprises paraplegics and patients with a neuropathic bladder from any other cause. In this group, the radiological state of the upper tracts is of great importance; clearly, patients with grossly distended upper tracts can really only be managed with a skin diversion. The alternative management, with a permanent indwelling catheter, is very unsatisfactory and will lead to a lot of "urinary misery". There is no doubt that in this category of patient, i.e. those with spina bifida, sacral agenesis, spinal dysraphysism and allied problems, the clinician often waits far too long before referring the patient for diversion. In patients with intact upper tracts in whom the situation is mainly a retention with overflow problem, intermittent self-catheterisation is a useful procedure which, when tolerated, is preferable to skin diversion.

If there is obviously no hope of obtaining reasonable continence, then skin diversion should be undertaken before school age. A large number of these patients are eternally grateful, finding themselves dry and socially acceptable with this technique.

*I am grateful to Freda Wadsworth, MBE, for the illustrations.

In this first category of patient, diversion to the skin is almost mandatory; this is particularly so in the younger age group with a long life expectancy. In the severely disabled with disseminated (multiple) sclerosis, one must bear in mind the risk of exacerbating the disease, but this is usually outweighed by the great benefits of urinary diversion.

The second group of patients suitable for urinary diversion are those in whom multiple procedures have failed to cure non-neuropathic incontinence. Before embarking on surgery in such a patient, one must be certain that all other avenues, including artificial urinary sphincter, have been explored and that both the patient and clinician are satisfied that surgery is the only course left open.

In this group the upper urinary tracts are usually intact, as is the anal sphincter. For this reason, a ureterocolic diversion can be considered, so leaving the patient a "clean abdomen".

This type of diversion, provided the patient's upper tracts are normal and the bowel satisfactory, gives excellent results. It has the advantage that it can be converted into a conduit skin diversion if problems occur during ensuing years.

Having decided that urinary diversion is necessary, the type of procedure must be chosen.

Choice of Diversion

Broadly speaking, there are few contraindications to conduit skin diversion. Severe incapacity resulting from the neurological disease and rendering the patients themselves incapable of looking after their stomas is unhelpful but not insuperable. Bedridden patients who have a good, easy-to-look-after stoma are a much lighter nursing problem than bedridden incontinent patients. One should not be deterred by the severity of their disease. If the abdominal wall is so disfigured by the spinal abnormality that the fitting of a urostomy bag is impossible, skin diversion is, of course, contraindicated. There are, however, definite contraindications to a ureterosigmoid diversion. It cannot be contemplated with dilated or damaged upper urinary tracts, nor with severe diverticular disease of the colon or any degree of proctocolitis. Anal sphincter weakness is again a bar to this type of surgery. Heavy irradiation to the "whole pelvis" renders this type of operation more hazardous, and skin diversion is preferable in such patients.

In all cases of incontinence, when one is considering urinary diversion it is essential to bear in mind the age and possible life expectancy of the patient; one is looking for a long, dry life and it must be remembered that the prime objective of surgery is to overcome the patient's incontinence problems.

There are many types of skin or bowel diversion. They all revolve around the same theme. There have been attempts to develop a continent vesicostomy (Turner-Warwick 1976) and similar ideas with a continent urinary ileostomy (Ashken 1974). These, however, have yet to withstand the test of time. I cannot stress too strongly that these patients wish to be dry and this can be achieved with a good ileal, or colonic, loop diversion, or alternatively with a ureterocolic anastomosis. Therefore, these are the two procedures I shall describe in this chapter.

Ileal Loop

Pre-operative Management

Although full bowel preparation is probably unnecessary, I think it should be carried out. There is no doubt that the creation of an ileal loop is a major abdominal procedure, followed by an "ileus" for a variable time. For this reason, mechanical preparation of the bowel with aperients, enemas, and washouts, coupled with a low-residue diet, is very helpful. "Bowel sterilisation" with the standard preparations should also be combined with this mechanical preparation. This is particularly so if one may have to consider a colonic loop, or even a ureterocolic anastomosis, once having performed the preliminary laparotomy. Siting of the ileostomy stoma pre-operatively is helpful, and if the patient can manage to walk around the ward with a urostomy bag applied, full of water, it will give her great confidence for the future.

Technique

The patient should be placed on the operating table, with the head of the table slightly lowered. The operation should be performed from the patient's left side. Intravenous infusion should be started and a nasogastric suction tube passed. Access to the abdomen is afforded through a long left paraumbilical paramedian incision, the length varying according to the patient's build. After a preliminary laparotomy, a self-retaining retractor is inserted and the abdominal contents packed, so leaving the pelvis and pelvic brim clear. It may be necessary to mobilise the sigmoid colon and the terminal ileum if these are tethered with congenital bands (Fig. 12.1). The next step is to pick up the posterior abdominal wall peritoneum over the bifurcation of the right common iliac artery and incise it longitudinally over 2–3 cm (Fig. 12.2). This will identify the ureter, which will be seen as a whitish vermicular tube. The ureter is gently picked up with blunt-nosed dissecting forceps, and broad curved artery forceps inserted under it. The ureter will readily lift up and one can then hook the forefinger under it, so lifting the ureter free. The ureter is freed up and down for about 6–7 cm in total; it will free easily. The lower end is clamped and divided, and the proximal end left to drain freely into the peritoneal cavity. The lower end is tied with suitable catgut (Fig. 12.3).

The left ureter is approached by dividing the peritoneal attachment on the lateral border of the sigmoid colon, again approximately at the pelvic brim level. By mobilising the colon medially, the bifurcation of the left common iliac artery is found, and with it the ureter. The left ureter is freed in a similar fashion as described before, but in this instance greater length should be obtained distally.

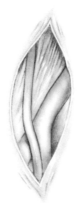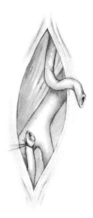

Fig. 12.2. (*Left*) Ileal loop. Exposure of the right ureter crossing bifurcation of common iliac artery.

Fig. 12.3. (*Right*) Ileal loop. Division of the right ureter.

It should be freed to a higher level than on the right so as to avoid any kinking as it crosses the mid-line. The ureter is clamped distally and divided, the distal end being tied as before.

Next the mobilised sigmoid colon is lifted with the left hand and the right forefinger is used to burrow under the mesentery, freeing a tunnel between the two peritoneal incisions. The left ureter will be easily passed along this tunnel, so that it will eventually lie in proximity to the divided upper end of the right one (Figs. 12.4, 12.5). The choice must now be made as to which of the two varieties of anastomosis described by Wallace (1966, 1970) is the more suitable.

The divided ureters will be found to lie comfortably in one of two directions, either side by side horizontally, or vertically. The lower ends should be spatulated for a suitable distance, usually 2 cm for normal-sized ureters, so as to form a common stoma. The adjacent borders are approximated with 4–0 polyglycolic acid or catgut sutures, either as a continuous approximation or with interrupted sutures, according to their size (Fig. 12.6). Each end of this approximation has an anchoring suture left behind. The ureters are now left and the conduit fashioned.

Leaving the terminal 15–20 cm of the ileum intact, a 20-cm segment is isolated, great care being taken to preserve the vascular arcades to this segment. The mesentery is divided to a slightly deeper

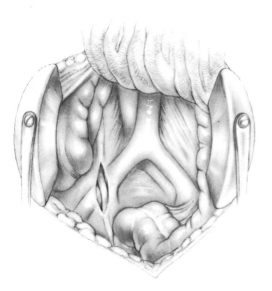

Fig. 12.1. Ileal loop. Incision of posterior wall peritoneum to display right ureter.

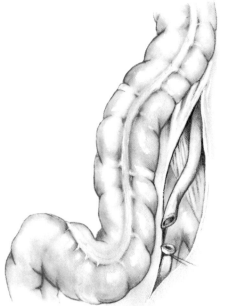

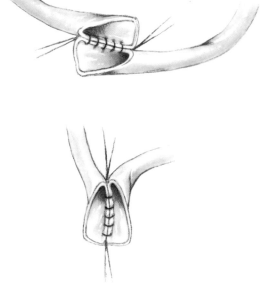

Fig. 12.4. Ileal loop. Freeing and division of the left ureter.   **Fig. 12.6.** Ileal loop. Suturing of ureters.

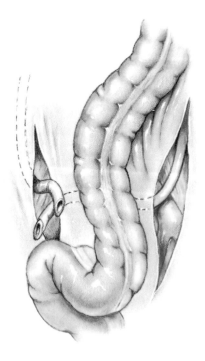

Fig. 12.5. Ileal loop. Positioning left ureter under mesenteric tunnel to lie alongside right ureter.

level on the distal side, as this is the end to protrude through the abdominal wall (Fig. 12.7).

The conduit is now dropped inferiorly, the bowel being reconstructed above (Fig. 12.8). The enteroanastomosis re-establishing bowel continuity is best performed with a continuous all coats 2–0 chromic catgut suture, with a seromuscular interrupted layer of black silk sutures. The various techniques for enteroanastomosis are well described in texts of general surgery. The mesenteric border is next closed with interrupted 2–0 catgut sutures, care being taken to avoid the vessels running in the adjacent borders. The anastomosis between the proximal end of the ileal conduit and the conjoined ends of the ureters is now established. This is best performed over splints, utilising either separate splints for each ureter, in which case no. 8 Levine nasogastric tubes are highly suitable for normal-sized ureters, or else a suitably sized T tube, the limbs of the T passing into both ureters and the stem of the T coming out through the conduit. Whichever splinting technique is used, long broad-based blunt artery forceps are passed proximally along the con-

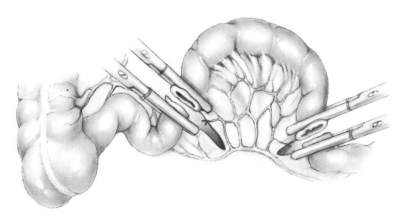

Fig. 12.7. Ileal loop. Isolation of ileal loop and its mesentery.

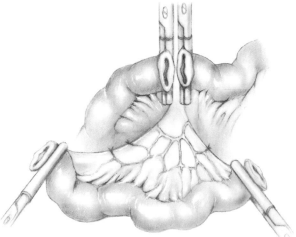

Fig. 12.8. Ileal loop. Reconstruction of the ileum.

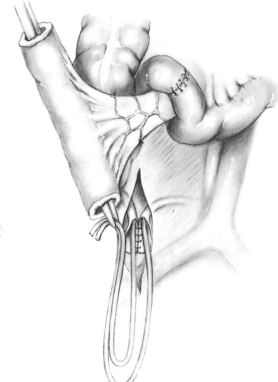

Fig. 12.9. Ileal loop. Withdrawal of the splints.

duit to grasp the distal end(s) of the splints. By with-drawing the forceps, the splint(s) are brought out through the conduit (Fig. 12.9). The anastomosis between the conduit and the ureters is made with 4–0 polyglycolic acid or chromic catgut, using either interrupted or continuous sutures (Fig. 12.10). The peritoneal edges surrounding the anastomosis are now tacked on to the proximal end of the conduit, so anchoring it to the posterior abdominal wall. The conduit is now ready to be brought out to the exterior. This is best done directly through the abdominal cavity, without trying to bring it out extraperitoneally.

The self-retaining retractor is released so that the abdominal incision falls together. Tissue forceps are applied to the skin edge on the right border, and also clips to the anterior sheath and peritoneal edge on that side. By pulling medially on these, the abdominal wall can be brought back into a relatively normal position. Now it is possible to make a correct tunnel through the abdominal wall for the conduit

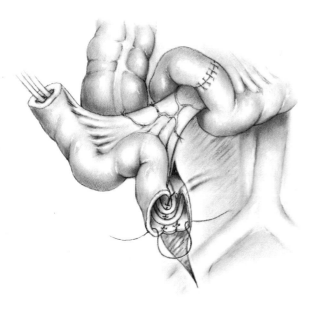

Fig. 12.10. Ileal loop. Fashioning the anastomosis between conduit and ureters.

to pass along. A circular disc of skin and subcutaneous tissue 2–3 cm in diameter is removed down to the external oblique aponeurosis. This is performed by tenting-up the centre of the skin disc with tissue forceps and amputating the tent with a sharp knife (Fig. 12.11a). After stopping any bleeding in this fatty tunnel, the external oblique muscle is divided in a cruciate fashion and the apices removed (Fig. 12.11b). The underlying muscle, either external oblique and transversus or rectus muscle, is now exposed. With dissecting scissors, the muscle is split in the line of its fibres and the peritoneal cavity entered. It is important that at least two fingers can pass through this tunnel.

By passing in tissue forceps from outside, the end of the conduit can be grasped and gently eased out along with the splint(s). Approximately 5–6 cm of bowel should protrude in order to fashion a satisfactory spout. Light tissue forceps are passed down the lumen of the extruding bowel and the inside of the conduit firmly grasped about 2–3 cm down (Fig. 12.11c). Next, using blunt-nosed long-toothed

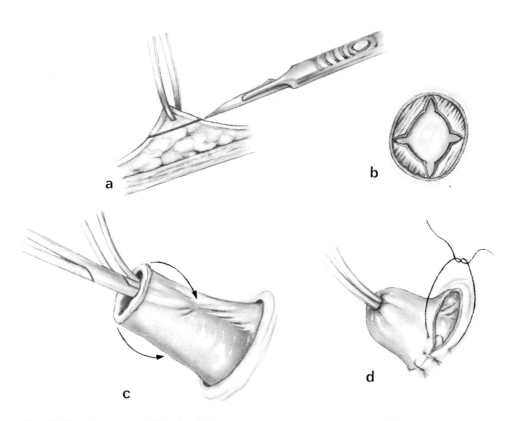

Fig. 12.11. a Amputation of skin disc. **b** Trimming opening in aponeurosis. **c** Withdrawing conduit through opening. **d** Forming the ileostomy spout.

dissecting forceps, the bowel is eased opening back over itself, so forming a satisfactory ileostomy spout (Fig. 12.11d). A mucocutaneous approximation is now made with interrupted 2–0 chromic catgut sutures. Some of these pick up the serosal surface of the bowel, so preventing subsequent retraction or prolapse of the stoma. The abdominal wall is now closed using a standard technique. A drain is brought out from around the anastomosis site, either through the wound or through a separate stab incision. The ileostomy appliance of one's choice is now carefully fitted.

Post-operative

Care

Induced diuresis is now important, along with antibiotic cover, again of one's own personal preference. Nasogastric suction and intravenous infusion are continued until satisfactory bowel movements are established, at which time the patient can be fully mobilised. A permanent urinary ileostomy appliance can be fitted, usually around the tenth post-operative day when the sutures are removed, care being taken to instruct the patient on the technique of its appliance.

Complications

Problems due to the technique itself are few and are best described under the headings of early and late. The two main early complications are urinary or faecal leakage, and a somewhat protracted "ileus". If there has been no previous irradiation, urinary leakage is very uncommon and, provided a satisfactory drain is in situ, it will usually dry spontaneously. If, however, in this situation the vascularity of the loop is questionable, as can be judged by the colour of the stoma, then re-exploration should be carried out in order to establish a new loop. Small bowel leakage is a far more serious complication, particularly if there has been previous irradiation. It usually does not settle down spontaneously and re-exploration is necessary. In this situation it is important not to wait until the patient's condition has deteriorated; in other words, early rather than late re-exploration is preferable. Prolonged ileus

must be borne with patience, and correct maintenance of fluid and electrolyte balance should be ensured.

The most important late complication is obstruction to the ureters, as they join the loop. On the left side, the ureter may obstruct as it passes under the mesentery. Fortunately this complication is rare and virtually confined to cases where irradiation has been used previously. Re-exploration is, of course, necessary, but it is difficult, and no hard and fast rules can be laid down as to what should be done. Much will depend on the operative findings. To safeguard against gross obstruction occurring without the clinician being aware of it, routine modified intravenous urograms are essential. A 20-min urogram approximately 6–8 weeks after the operation is helpful. Following this, similar single pictures at 3 and 6 months are all that is necessary. If these are normal then probably nothing further should be done. There is little doubt that there are a number of cases, particularly those where the upper tracts are already damaged, in which continued deterioration of the upper tracts will occur. Where infections occur, it is essential to obtain proximal loop urine, by passing a catheter down the loop, in order to obtain uncontaminated urine from the skin diversion.

As the very long-term follow-up of children with ileal conduits brought to light the deteriorating situation, so the use of colonic conduits came into vogue. However, the same long-term results were obtained, and there is probably little to choose between these two methods.

Ureterocolic Anastomosis

Pre-operative Management

The bowel preparation is the same as for the ileal loop. The patient is positioned on the operating table as for an ileal conduit procedure. An intravenous infusion is started and a nasogastric tube passed. The thighs are abducted and the perineum is cleaned so that at a suitable time during the operation, a large rectal tube can be passed.

Technique

The abdomen is opened with a long left paramedian incision. The abdominal contents are packed off so that the pelvis is empty apart from the rectosigmoid colon. The ureters are exposed as before, but in this instance they are freed inferiorly as far as is possible before division and tying of the distal ureter. This allows plenty of ureter for the anastomosis. The freed right ureter is brought across to lie alongside the lower sigmoid colon so that a suitable position can be found for anastomosis (Fig. 12.12). The left ureter will be found to lie comfortably at a higher level.

There are a variety of techniques for anastomosing the ureter to the colon and the majority of these are now historical. The one described by Leadbetter (1950) is virtually universally practised.

Having ascertained the level of anastomosis of the right ureter, the anterior tinea coli is picked up with fine tissue forceps just below the anastomosis point and again 6 cm proximal to this. Using a fine knife, an incision is made in the line of the longitudinal muscle between these forceps (Fig. 12.13). With an assistant gently holding one edge of this incision with fine forceps, the opposite edge is picked up and, with gentle blunt and sharp dissection, the muscle is completely divided until the mucosa protrudes.

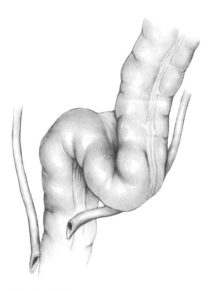

Fig. 12.12. Ureterocolic anastomosis. Positioning ureters alongside the lower sigmoid colon.

One then incises the proximal end of the muscle cut laterally on the right side (Fig. 12.14).

At this stage of the operation, an assistant insinuates an arm under the drapes and introduces a large Depezzar catheter, with the top of the mushroom amputated, into the rectum. This can easily be felt by the operator and the head of the catheter can be manipulated up to the site of the anastomosis. A small nick is made in the mucosa at the distal end of the muscle spit, so opening into the lumen of the bowel. The distal end of a no. 8 Levine tube or other suitable splint is now thread down through this mucosal incision and into the open end of the Depezzar catheter and out through the anus (Fig. 12.15). The proximal end of this splint is thread into the spatulated lower end of the right ureter and so into the pelvis of the kidney. The spatulated lower end of the ureter is anastomosed end-to-side through the mucosal opening in the bowel using interrupted 4–0 catgut sutures (Fig. 12.16).

Once the anastomosis is complete, the ureter is laid along the muscle tunnel and the muscle approximated over the ureter with fine interrupted catgut sutures (Fig. 12.17). The ureter should be anchored for about 2 cm outside the tunnel to prevent kinking as it enters the tunnel.

A similar anastomosis is now made with the left ureter into the colon, but at a slightly higher level. Once both anastomoses are completed, a comfortable position is found for the rectosigmoid colon to lie so that neither ureter is under tension. The bowel is anchored in this position with a few interrupted catgut sutures.

The abdomen is closed in the standard fashion. A pelvic drain brought out either through the end of the wound or through a separate stab incision may be used, according to the operator's preference. The rectal drain is securely sutured to the perineum. The two splints will pass comfortably down a urinary bag drainage tube, the nozzle of which secures the splints issuing from the Depezzar catheter (Fig. 12.18).

Post-operative

Care

Diuresis and antibiotic cover are instituted in the immediate post-operative period. Intravenous fluids

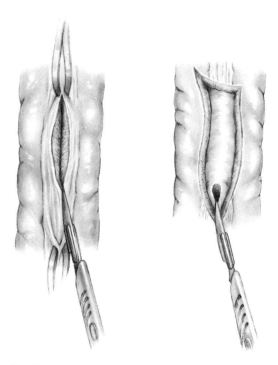

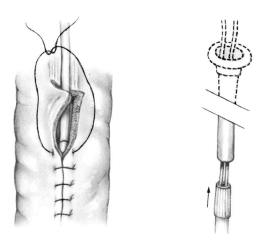

Fig. 12.17. (*Left*) Ureterocolic anastomosis. Closure of the longitudinal muscle over the ureter.

Fig. 12.18. (*Right*) Ureterocolic anastomosis. Passage of the splints into the urinary bag drainage tube.

Fig. 12.13. (*Left*) Ureterocolic anastomosis. Incision of the longitudinal muscle of colon.

Fig. 12.14. (*Right*) Ureterocolic anastomosis. Incision of the proximal end of the muscle and of intestinal mucosa.

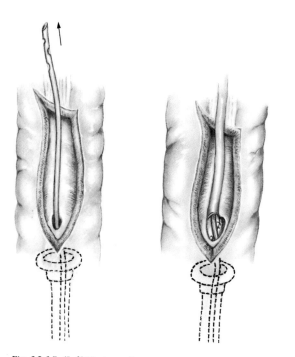

Fig. 12.15. (*Left*) Ureterocolic anastomosis. Threading the splint into colon.

Fig. 12.16. (*Right*) Fashioning the ureterocolic anastomosis.

are continued until bowel sounds occur, which they do reasonably early (round about the fourth or fifth day). When flatus is passed, the rectal tube and splints are removed. Bowel actions are encouraged four to five times a day and once or twice at night. Because of the risk of hyperchloraemic acidosis and hypokalaemia, the routine use of 2–4 g sodium bicarbonate daily and potassium supplements is recommended.

Complications

Complications directly related to the anastomosis are ascending infection, hyperchloraemic acidosis and hypokalaemia. These can be suitably corrected by the appropriate treatment. If, however, they prove troublesome, then conversion of the diversion to a conduit may be necessary.

A troublesome complication is nocturnal incontinence; the use of the rectal plug stimulator at night is helpful in combatting this. A more serious complication is the development of a "colitis" in the long-term case, and here again resistance to treatment may necessitate conversion to a conduit. By far the most serious complication, fortunately rare, is the development of an adenocarcinoma at the site of the ureteric implant; here, clearly, conversion and bowel resection are necessary.

Continent Ileal Pouch

The development of an appliance-free urinary diversion has long been the dream of the urologist. Many attempts have been made dating from the latter part of the last century (Mauclaire 1895). The early attempts at continent stomas through the anal sphincter, although still tried, have largely given way to continent ileal pouches (Kock et al. 1982) and ileo-caecal reservoirs (Ashken 1974, 1982).

The indications for these must be strict, as the re-operation rate is exceedingly high. It would appear that stomal siting in the severely deformed patient may be so difficult as to be almost impossible, and that this would constitute a valid reason for adopting a continent ileal diversion. Again, where cultural or religious fetishes preclude a wet stoma, this alternative should be considered.

These appliance-free urinary skin diversions have been in existence for a very long time, but are only in their surgical infancy. They have not stood the test of time and still have no place in the routine urinary diversion.

References

Ashken MH (1974) An appliance-free ileocaecal urinary diversion: preliminary communication. Br J Urol 46:631–638

Ashken MH (1982) Urinary reservoirs. In: Ashken MH (ed) Urinary diversion. Springer, Berlin Heidelberg New York pp 112–139

Kock NG, Nilson AE, Nilsson LO, Norlen LJ, Philipson BM (1982) Urinary diversion via a continent ileal reservoir: Clinical results in 12 patients. J Urol 128:469–475

Leadbetter WF (1950) Transactions of American Association of General Surgeons 42:39–51

Mauclaire M (1895) De quelques essais de chirurgie experimentale applicables au traitement de l'exstrophie de la vessie et des anus contre nature complexes. Ann Mal Org Genito-Urin 13:1080–1086

Turner-Warwick R (1976) Leak-proof cystostomy. J Urol Nephrol (Paris) [Suppl 8] 2:405–413

Wallace DM (1966) Ureteric diversion using a conduit, a simplified technique. Br J Urol 38:522–527

Wallace DM (1970) Uretero-ileostomy. Br J Urol 42:529–534

13 Urethrotomy

Peter H. L. Worth

Introduction

In a book primarily concerned with the management of urinary incontinence it may seem out of place to have a chapter describing procedures specifically designed to reduce urethral resistance. These may be necessary in two situations: (a) when urinary infection is a recurring problem and (b) when incomplete bladder emptying occurs, which may also be associated with incontinence. Recurring infections may result from either inefficient but compete emptying, or incomplete emptying resulting from a decompensated detrusor—that is, one which produces a good contraction to initiate voiding but is unable to maintain its contraction. In these cases urethral resistance may be normal or raised. Neurological disease may affect both the detrusor and sphincter function, causing detrusor-sphincter dyssynergia which may result in incontinence although the urethral resistance may be higher than normal.

Methods of Investigation

It is very important to try and define the pathophysiology exactly in terms of bladder (detrusor) function and urethral activity before deciding what action should be taken. This information is best obtained using the tests described in Chap. 2. In addition, an intravenous urogram will show if there is any upper tract abnormality. Information about the bladder is less reliable—the presence of residual urine may be misleading. It is also important to have some information about renal function such as the blood urea and creatinine.

The cystometrogram will give accurate information about detrusor function. The original type of urethral pressure profile demonstrated static urethral activity and how much squeeze could be produced, but was not particularly helpful in trying to demonstrate functional obstruction. However, with the new range of catheters with built-in transducers a much better picture of urethral activity is obtained, and computerisation allows areas of interest in the profile to be analysed in great detail. It is now possible to be more precise in deciding at what level obstruction is present and how best to deal with it. Most important of all is synchronous video pressure-flow cystourethrography (Bates et al. 1970), which enables one to see what is happening in terms of outlet appearance and detrusor function. One would hope to get the answers to the following questions: "What effect does the detrusor have on the bladder neck? Is there an area of narrowing in the urethra? Is there any prolapse present? What is the bladder capacity, how much is voided and how much residue remains at the end of voiding?"

If the presence of a neurological problem is suggested by the tests, the expertise of a neurologist must be sought. Abnormal bladder and sphincter function may be the first manifestation of a neurological disorder such as multiple sclerosis, and certainly a disc protusion or a spinal cord tumour must not be overlooked.

The decision to treat a patient may be difficult. Some patients can have large residues (over 300 ml) with a sterile urine, normal upper tracts and renal function. Any interference is likely to introduce infection and, unless good emptying is achieved as the result of treatment, it may be extremely difficult to get rid of the infection.

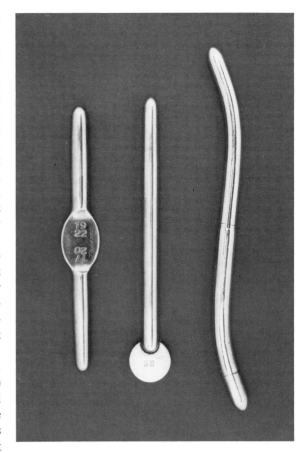

Fig. 13.1. Types of dilator. *Left to right:* Canny Ryall (measured in English gauge); Wynham Powell (measured in Charriere, French gauge, circumference in mm); Hegar.

Techniques

Urethral Dilatation

Urethral dilatation and internal urethrotomy are techniques designed to exert an effect on the urethra alone. The bladder neck is not affected unless it is very severely stenosed by scarring.

Urethral narrowing is a relative phenomenon, and before deciding how much dilatation is required it is important to know the initial diameter of the urethra. An ordinary metal dilator (Fig. 13.1) is not an accurate way to assess this. Bougies-à-boules were designed specifically for this purpose, but are rarely used nowadays since the urethrotome has gained popularity. These bougies will show the narrowest part of the urethra; the instrument is inserted into the urethra and then withdrawn, the process being repeated with increasing size of bougie until the instrument is felt to be firmly gripped.

Mechanical narrowing of the urethra is rare. It is usually at the external urinary meatus, but occasionally it is more extensive and results from previous anterior vaginal wall repair. More commonly, the obstruction is functional and cannot be calibrated by bougies-à-boules. The urethra may calibrate in excess of 20F and be functionally obstructed.

Once it has been established that urethral obstruction is present, urethral dilatation can be carried out. How much the urethra should be dilated is difficult to say, but I prefer to go 10 points on the French scale above the calibrated figure, for instance 20–30 or 25–35. Since urethral narrowing is relative, it is inappropriate to say that every urethra should be dilated to a specific size. If a poor result is obtained by this method it can be repeated going up a further 5 points, but it is infinitely better to do too little than too much.

What does urethral dilatation achieve? If there is organic narrowing, dilatation acts by stretching the tissues and probably tearing them, so that when healing has occurred the calibre of the urethra may again decrease, making it very likely that a single dilatation will not be effective in the long term. In the presence of functional obstruction—by far the most common case—slow, gradual and repeated dilations do not tear any tissues and have less harmful results.

Internal Urethrotomy

It was really in an attempt to improve the results of dilatation that new techniques were evolved and the urethrotome was developed. The old-fashioned urethrotomes were certainly more effective than dilatation in treating urethral strictures in the male, and so application of urethrotomy to the female seemed logical.

The Otis urethrotome has a blade which projects about 2 mm (Fig. 13.2). It will, therefore, not cut deeply into the wall of the urethra. It will cut the muscle lining the wall of the urethra, but it will not touch the striated component of the external sphincter and, as with dilatation, it will have no effect on the bladder neck unless it is very scarred.

Calibration with the urethrotome is easy. The wheel is turned and the instrument moved in and out until the urethra is felt to grip. The figure on the dial is noted and the blades opened a further 10 points on the scale. This will achieve adequate dilatation, but if it is decided to do a urethrotomy, the blade is withdrawn in the 12 o'clock position (Fig. 13.3). Additional cuts can be made at 3 and 9 o'clock, but it is unlikely that these will have any effect unless the instrument is opened a further 5 points on the scale before these cuts are made. A cut at 6 o'clock is inadvisable because of the risk of a urethrovaginal fistula. It is probably better to restrict the urethrotomy to one cut only. Patients are often more comfortable with an indwelling 20F urethral catheter kept on continuous drainage overnight, but it is not essential.

Internal urethrotomy rarely produces complications. Bleeding may occur, especially if there has been a previous anterior repair. It often stops spontaneously but it can be controlled either by applying local pressure to the urethra by inserting a vaginal pack, or by tying a swab round the catheter and pushing it against the external meatus, making sure that the balloon of the catheter is against the bladder neck.

If the patient has an incompetent bladder neck, or one that opens easily with involuntary detrusor contractions, slight leakage of urine may occur in the early post-operative period, but this usually stops quite quickly.

Provided organic obstruction has been adequately relieved, patients who present with recurrent infections will be cured; if symptoms persist or recur it can be shown that obstruction has not been adequately relieved or has recurred. These good results are what one can expect to achieve in women who have stable bladders, but in those who have confirmed detrusor instability, although the obstruction may have been adequately and successfully relieved, symptoms may persist in 66% of patients (Farrar et al. 1976). This is due to the fact that instability does not resolve and is contrary to what one finds in the male, when, if instability is secondary to obstruction, it will resolve in 60% of patients once the obstruction has been satisfactorily relieved.

There is unfortunately very little evidence to show that urethrotomy does in fact produce any better results than simple dilatation. In studying a group

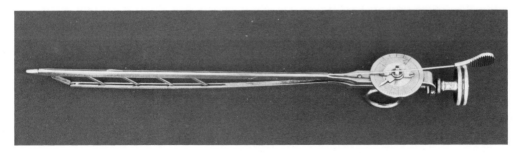

Fig. 13.2. The Otis urethrotome, showing the blade partially withdrawn.

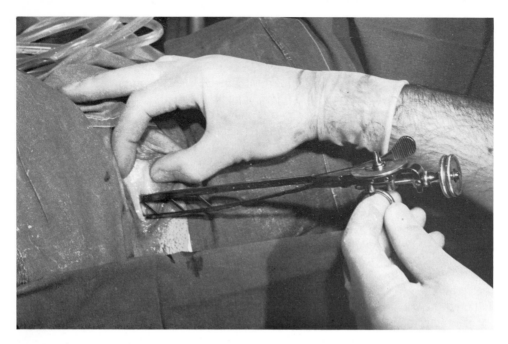

Fig. 13.3. The Otis urethrotome in situ prior to making an incision at 12 o'clock.

of women who had persistent urinary incontinence despite previous surgery, Moolgoaker et al. (1972) analysed their results and found a group who had urethral narrowing. In some it was an isolated finding, but in others there was, in addition, either sphincter weakness or detrusor instability. These women had a variety of treatments, but were eventually improved by internal urethrotomy, which was carried out to 45F empirically. If indicated, surgery for stress incontinence was carried out, but if detrusor instability was present this was treated with medication resulting in further improvement. In a further study (Moolgoaker et al. 1976) a quicker return to normal voiding with less infection was found in women who had an internal urethrotomy carried out routinely at the time of surgery for stress incontinence, compared with urethral dilatation; the results of both were very much better than with no urethral procedure.

Bladder Neck Procedures

Primary bladder neck obstruction in the female is very rare provided the diagnosis is based on strict urodynamic principles. Outlet obstruction as a whole is rare and in the majority of cases (90%) it is situated in the distal urethra. Primary obstruction

is usually due to dyssynergia, the bladder neck mechanism failing to relax when the detrusor contracts. A high pressure is therefore generated, but despite this there is a very poor flow rate.

Secondary bladder neck obstruction may develop as a result of relative inefficiency of the detrusor. In some situations the bladder neck opens adequately when the detrusor initially contracts, but the detrusor decompensates and the bladder neck closes, leaving a big residue. Occasionally, the detrusor may be truly atonic and is incapable of generating enough pressure to open the bladder neck. Obstruction is also found after cystoplasty, when the bowel pressure, despite augmentation with abdominal pressure, may be incapable of opening the bladder neck.

Before embarking on surgical treatment of bladder neck obstruction, it is important to try to determine whether the distal mechanism is reasonably competent. This can be done by observing how efficiently the individual can interrupt the stream during voiding, but also and more accurately, by detailed urodynamic studies and pressure profile measurements. Relieving bladder neck obstruction in the presence of a high detrusor pressure and a relatively incompetent distal mechanism may produce unsatisfactory results.

Provided the diagnosis has been established there

are several ways of treating the bladder neck surgically. Open surgery should be avoided although Y-V plasty was a popular method of treatment in the past, and in many cases it was done when there was no definite urodynamic evidence of obstruction; for instance, most children who had ureteric reimplantation for reflux had a Y-V plasty as well. Endoscopic bladder neck resection, although hardly ever indicated, will relieve bladder neck obstruction, but it is difficult and potentially dangerous in the female. It is very difficult to assess the thickness of the muscle and there is very little tissue between the bladder and the vagina.

Bladder neck incision, carried out under direct vision, can be accomplished by first adequately dilating the urethra and inserting a urethroplasty speculum (Fig. 13.4), and then incising the bladder neck muscle anteriorly with a small blade. This is probably more efficient than an endoscopic technique of the kind one uses in men (Turner Warwick et al. 1973). The problem always arises as to how deep to go because not only is it difficult to know how much muscle there is, but also it is impossible to know how much relaxation of the muscle is required. It is better to err on the cautious side and be prepared to repeat the procedure, rather than have an incontinent patient—a serious complication. However, by using this technique, if one has done too much, it is relatively easy to do an open operation and repair the bladder neck, something that cannot be done if too much tissue has been resected.

Alternative Techniques

Surgery

If the balance between satisfactory emptying and retention cannot be achieved by the techniques that have been mentioned what else is available to help the patient? If there is an element of prolapse present, which could be causing urethral distortion, then some sort of repair might be beneficial, provided one is satisfied that urethral obstruction has been relieved.

Intermittent Catheterisation

Clean self-catheterisation is a satisfactory technique which many patients find acceptable, but I would recommend that it should only be used when one is convinced that no other surgical methods are possible. By being cautious as well as aggressive in one's surgical approach one may be able to avoid catheterisation; and it is surprising how an internal urethrotomy carried out in the way already described may rid the patient of a residue and by so doing improve continence, avoiding the situation when catheterisation was considered essential or had already been established.

Lapides popularised the technique of intermittent catheterisation in 1972, and showed what good results could be obtained in terms of reduced urinary

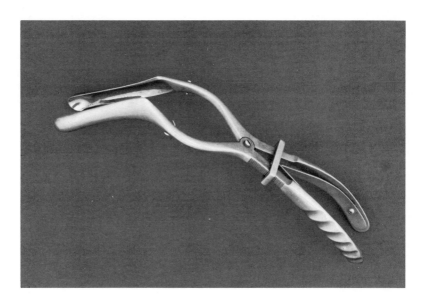

Fig. 13.4. The posterior urethroplasty speculum.

infection and patient improvement (Diokno et al. 1983). He felt that chronic overdistension of the bladder produced infection by impairing the blood supply and reversed this by keeping the bladder empty.

Medical Management

It is perhaps appropriate to mention at this stage medical methods of altering urethral function. By measuring the urethral pressure profile it is very easy to see what effect drugs may have on the various components of urethral resistance. It is sometimes possible to alter urethral resistance so that a patient's symptoms may be sufficiently improved for surgical treatment to become unnecessary. A full review of drug therapy is to be found in Chap. 16.

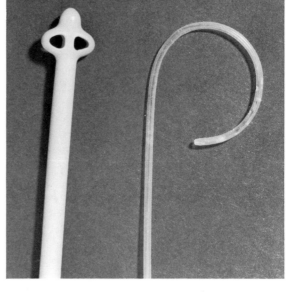

Fig. 13.5. Bonanno catheter (*right*) and Malecot catheter (*left*).

Bladder Drainage

In a patient with a significant pre-operative residue, it is very important to assess accurately the residual urine post-operatively. Rather than subject the patient to repeated urethral catheterisation, I would recommend putting in a suprapubic catheter at the time of the initial procedure. It is especially useful in the management of the patient who has a very big bladder, because even if the balance between detrusor and urethral resistance has been reached, it may take quite a long time to get the residue down to an acceptable level—less than 100 ml. With the suprapubic catheter in situ it can be clamped so that the bladder is able to work normally. The residue can be measured twice a day and by emptying the bladder in this way infection can be reduced or even eliminated.

Simple suprapubic stab catheters such as the Bonanno (Fig. 13.5) are easy to introduce and are very satisfactory for a short time, as required in the post-operative management of a vaginal repair. These catheters will probably last up to 3 weeks. As an alternative I would recommend the use of a Foley or Malecot catheter (Fig. 13.5), not greater than 20F, introduced through a small suprapubic incision. The technique is to introduce a dilator, which has a small hole drilled through the end, into the bladder via the urethra (Fig. 13.6). The bladder

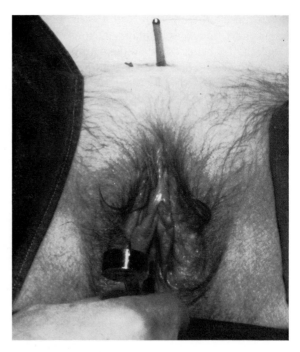

Fig. 13.6. Hey–Groves dilator which has been introduced into the bladder and then cut down on, so that the end appears out of a small suprapubic wound.

should first be filled with 200–300 ml of water. The dilator is then pushed up against the anterior abdominal wall and an incision made on to it through the skin, rectus sheath and bladder wall.

The catheter is then fixed to the dilator with a piece of nylon (Fig. 13.7), and pulled into the bladder. It is important to check that the catheter is in the bladder by exerting suprapubic pressure and seeing the catheter drain. Filling the bladder at the start of the procedure will reduce the chance of inserting the catheter into the peritoneal cavity—a distinct possibility when the patient has had a lot of lower abdominal and bladder surgery.

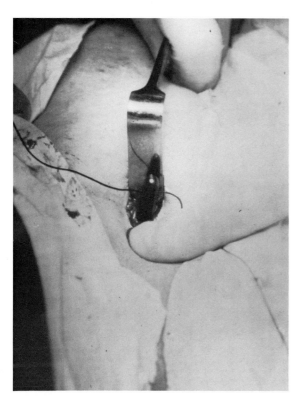

Fig. 13.7. A nylon thread being passed through the end of the Hey–Groves dilator prior to the attachment of a catheter.

Conclusions

There are a number of ways of approaching the management of urinary problems associated with outflow obstruction. Patients may present with urinary infection, difficulty in voiding or various types of incontinence. It is important to define the nature of the problem by urodynamic methods before deciding on the best management. This will vary depending on the requirements of the individual patient and the preferences of the individual surgeon.

References

Bates CP, Whiteside CG, Turner Warwick RT (1970) Synchronous cine pressure flow cystourethrography with special reference to stress and urge incontinence. Br J Urol 42:714–723

Diokno AC, Sonda LP, Hollander TB, Lapides J (1983) Fate of patients started on clean intermittent self-catheterisation therapy 10 years ago. J Urol 129:1120–1122

Farrar DJ, Osborne JL, Stephenson TP, Whiteside CG, Weir J, Berry J, Milroy EJG, Turner Warwick RT (1976) A urodynamic view of bladder outflow obstruction in the female: factors influencing the results of treatment. Br J Urol 47:815–822

Moolgoaker AS, Ardran GM, Smith JC, Stallworthy JA (1972) The diagnosis and management of urinary incontinence in the female. J Obstet Gynaecol Br Commonw 79:481–487

Moolgoaker AS, Rizvi JH, Payne PR, Parker JC (1976) The effect of internal urethrotomy and urethral dilatation on the post-operative course of patients undergoing surgery for stress incontinence, J. Obstet Gynaecol Br Commonw 83:484–488

Turner Warwick RT, Whiteside CG, Worth PHL, Milroy EJG, Bates CP (1973) A urodynamic view of bladder neck obstruction and its treatment by endoscopic incision. Br J Urol 45:44–59

14 The Management of Vesicovaginal and Urethral Fistulae

John B. Lawson and Christopher N. Hudson

Although at first sight the general principles of management of lower urinary tract fistulae might appear to be broadly uniform, in fact there are significant variations related to aetiology.

Aetiological Groups

Obstetric

Where maternity services are not fully developed and contracted pelvis is common, obstetric fistulae are the type most often seen. Because of this they constitute a major gynaecological and social problem in many developing countries (Lawson 1968; Editorial 1981; Harrison 1983). These fistulae are generally slough injuries following prolonged pressure from obstructed labour, compounded by infection. As a result, the size of the fistula is almost always a reflection of tissue loss, and scarring may be severe. Trauma sustained at the time of a difficult operative delivery may be an additional factor.

Surgical Trauma

Surgical and other direct trauma is the main cause of fistulae in communities where modern maternity care has largely eliminated obstetric injuries. In surgical cases, significant tissue loss is relatively uncommon. Therefore the type of defect, early management and definitive treatment all differ from those in obstetric injuries (Moir 1973).

Pelvic Malignancy

In patients with pelvic cancer, fistulae may follow treatment by irradiation either alone or combined with surgery. Local over-dosage, perhaps from a misplaced intracavity source, causes excessive tissue destruction and results in a fistula. Surgery in a previously irradiated field even many years later may be followed by fistula formation. Sometimes, when the tumour has penetrated the full thickness of the vesicovaginal septum, even successful local treatment will inevitably lead to a fistula. Occasionally, patients treated for pelvic cancer may present with an established malignant fistula.

Fistulae associated with cancer and its treatment form a small but important aspect of pelvic oncology and pose special difficulties (Ingelman-Sundberg 1953). Fistula formation may be a distressing phenomenon associated with the terminal phase of malignant disease. Compassionate and palliative management is required, but not necessarily a totally negative approach. These patients are as deserving of full expert consideration and treatment as other fistula patients with a normal life expectancy.

Clinical Presentation

Abnormal communications between the bladder and the female genital tract usually become apparent as incontinence. Very rarely, this symptom may be denied by a patient with a demonstrable fistula when the levator ani muscles are capable of completely occluding the vagina below a high fistula. A few patients with a fistula between the bladder and the uterine isthmus after lower segment caesarean section may be completely continent but complain of cyclical haematuria (Falk and Tancer 1956; Reece et al. 1982). Patients with a very small surgical fistula may give a confusing history if they are only incontinent when the bladder is full. Leakage may only occur at night or when the patient stands up after lying down. Although the symptom of continuous leakage without voluntary micturition is very characteristic, it will often not be obtained from patients with small fistulae. Patients with urinary fistulae, in whatever community they live, feel rejected by relatives and friends because they smell of urine, and they may therefore withdraw from society in their misery. Successful relief of these distressing symptoms must be one of the most rewarding results of pelvic surgery.

An accurate history is essential, and may have to include a careful search of past hospital records for details of surgical operations and other therapeutic procedures. For instance, a history of haematuria after hysterectomy may imply an unrecognised bladder injury during the operation, or pain and bleeding after the insertion of a radioactive source may suggest that it was misplaced.

Vaginal examination does not always reveal the origin of the urinary leakage. When the diagnosis is in doubt, a carefully conducted dye test is required. This entails filling the bladder with a coloured solution via a urethral catheter with the patient in the lithotomy position. The so-called three swab test may be misleading and direct observation of the leak is essential; multiple fistulae may be diagnosed in this way. Cystoscopy is only marginally helpful in locating a small vesicovaginal fistula. Often the fistula can only be seen from within the bladder by identifying a probe passed through a vaginal aperture. Cystoscopy may, however, disclose other vesical pathology.

The alternative diagnosis of ureteric fistula needs to be considered. Continued leakage of colourless urine per vaginam after methylene blue solution has been instilled into the bladder is very suspicious. A normal urogram does not exclude a uretero-vaginal fistula or a congenital ectopic ureter. Cystoscopy, ureteric catheterisation and retrograde radiography or dye tests with intravenous methylene blue or indigo carmine may be required.

A fistula between the small bowel and the genital tract may be mistaken for a urinary fistula, as fluid intestinal contents are usually odourless and closely resemble urine. It is quite possible for intestinal fistulae to open into the anterior fornix, so even fistulae in this situation are not necessarily connected to the urinary tract. Urethral fistulae which involve the bladder neck cause incontinence, but defects of the distal urethra do not. The latter may, however, be associated with other damage to the bladder neck closure mechanism.

Finally, some patients whose fistulae have been successfully closed may have such severe urethral incompetence that their symptoms mimic those of a persistent fistula.

Pre-operative Care

Early Management

The early management of a vesicovaginal fistula is very important and will clearly vary with the antecedent cause and underlying condition.

Surgical trauma to the bladder unrecognised during operation can usually be repaired within 24 h, provided extravasation of urine into the tissues has not been extensive.

However, post-operative fistulae usually develop between the 4th and 21st days, and these should be treated with continuous bladder drainage via a urethral catheter. Provided most of the urine drains through the catheter it is worth persisting with this treatment for 4–6 weeks in the hope that the defect will close spontaneously.

Obstetric slough injuries developing after obstructed labour should also be treated by continuous catheter drainage, combined with antibiotic therapy to limit tissue damage by infection. If sloughing of the rectal wall has also occurred and a rectovaginal fistula has formed, the flux of faeces through the vagina will adversely affect spontaneous healing. In these cases, therefore, a preliminary transverse colostomy should be performed: an iliac colostomy is undesirable as it may complicate subsequent abdominal operations performed to repair either the vesical or rectal defects.

All aspects of management, including the temporary nature of any colostomy, should be fully discussed with the patient. The assistance of a stoma therapist may be invoked (Stevens 1978). Attention to the patient's morale is particularly important, and introduction to a successfully treated patient gives valuable encouragement.

Other associated problems, such as obstetric nerve palsies, vulval excoriation and pelvic infection, must be treated vigorously. Improvement in the patient's general health will pay dividends when definitive repair is attempted at a later date.

In both obstetric and irradiation fistulae there is considerable sloughing of tissues. When the sloughs eventually separate there is a clear demarcation of relatively healthy tissue, and it is imperative that this process should have settled down before reparative surgery is undertaken. In obstetric cases a minimum of 3 months should be allowed to elapse, but in irradiation cases it may be necessary to wait for 12 months or more. This can be very trying for the patient, but partial continence may be achieved by Yeates' method, using a sponge tampon and Paul's tubing (Yeates 1959). In most surgical cases a 3-month delay is also advisable, despite the recent advocacy of earlier repair by Fourie (1983). When the bladder has been injured at abdominal hysterectomy some distance from the vaginal vault, the first event will have been extravasation of urine into the pelvic dead space, with the formation of an infected haematoma cavity contaminated by urine. This eventually discharges through the vaginal vault. The abscess cavity must be allowed to close in before attempting surgery, and a course of an appropriate antibiotic may help resolution.

If an operation for the repair of a fistula has been unsuccessful, an interval of at least 8 weeks must be allowed to elapse before a further attempt at closure is made. These are precisely the patients in whom pressure to operate too early has to be resisted.

Associated Conditions

Once the diagnosis of fistula has been established, it is essential to deal first with associated conditions which could influence management and outcome. Anaemia, for instance, obviously needs to be corrected. Urinary tract infection should be detected and treated appropriately before surgery, although the achievement of completely sterile urine may be impossible before closure of the fistula. If a catheter specimen of urine for culture cannot be obtained, it may be necessary to collect a "clean catch" specimen by dripping the urine into a sterile bedpan.

Excretory urography is essential; this must be recent as ureteric dilatation may only develop after progressive fibrosis. Preliminary radiography will also detect vesical or even vaginal calculi (Fig. 14.1), which must be removed before definitive repair (Raghavaiah and Devi 1980). Very rarely, there may be uraemia and electrolyte disturbance due to bilateral obstructive uropathy, which should be managed in consultation with a renal physician. Upper urinary tract decompression may be required

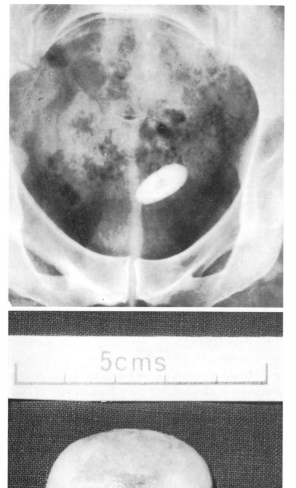

Fig. 14.1. Vesical calculus complicating radiation fistula of 5 years' duration. *Above*, X-ray; *below*, photograph.

(by needle nephrostomy or intubated ureterostomy), or even dialysis.

Locally, vulval excoriation should be cleared up with barrier cream. Occasionally, pre-operative nursing of the patient in a prone position on a Bradford frame or Stryker bed is necessary to get the skin to heal.

In malignant cases, life expectancy must be assessed. It is wise to consider whether the patient is likely to achieve voluntary control of micturition either after closure of her fistula or after urinary diversion,

as the prospects for this may be impaired by senility or neurological disease. Sometimes it may be best to help the patient to cope with the uncorrected disability by making use of the best available palliative measures.

Concurrent Rectovaginal Fistulae

Recto-vaginal fistulae commonly accompany vesicovaginal fistulae after obstructed labour. The temptation to close bladder and rectal defects at the same time should be resisted, as one or other repair will probably break down owing to tension. Usually after a preliminary transverse colostomy, the bladder fistula should be repaired first, as the reverse order will impair access. Only when the bladder fistula has been proved to be closed should the rectal defect be dealt with.

Local Assessment

Both the authors firmly believe that preliminary examination under anaesthesia is an essential step in the evaluation of a fistula preparatory to planning its treatment. At this procedure the exact site, size and relationship to other structures is determined (Fig. 14.2). In low fistulae, fixity to the pubic rami is common and involvement of the urethrovesical junction is important. In high fistulae the ureters may be involved. With very large defects of obstetric origin, the intramural portions of one or both ureters may have sloughed as well. In these circumstances the ureteric orifices may be found in the edges of the fistula, but occasionally a ureter may open separately into the vagina. Patency should be demonstrated by the passage of a probe or a ureteric catheter.

The condition of the tissues must be carefully assessed. Persistence of sloughs means that operation should be deferred, and this is particularly important in post-irradiation cases. Induration usually indicates inflammatory response: in surgical cases this may be caused by a non-absorbable suture, but in endemic areas schistosomiasis may be responsible. If there is any doubt, biopsy of the edge of the defect will be indicated, as secondary malignant change in a long-standing benign fistula has been described (Hudson 1968). After the treatment of malignant disease, a persistent tumour

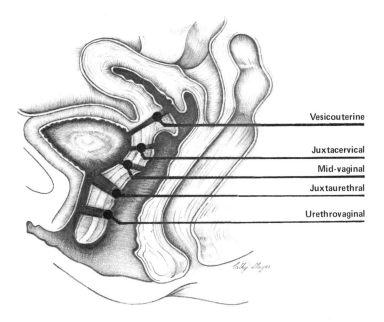

Fig. 14.2. Sites of genito-urinary fistulae.

obviously affects the prognosis, but not the need for relief of incontinence.

During the examination under anaesthesia, complicating factors such as vaginal stenosis or rectal fistulae may be found. In obstetric fistulae, extensive sloughing after obstructed labour often produces severe vaginal stricture, which will need to be divided during the repair to improve access. Vaginal strictures may also complicate surgical fistulae following prolapse repair.

Mention has already been made of associated rectovaginal fistulae, which may require diversion of the faecal stream by temporary transverse colostomy. It is important to realise that a posterior horseshoe-shaped stricture can occlude a small, high rectovaginal fistula so that faecal leakage does not occur until the stricture is divided. Careful digital examination is required to detect such a fistula: insufflation of air through a sigmoidoscope may produce a tell-tale leakage of gas into the vagina (Hudson 1970).

The final matter to be decided at the preliminary examination is the timing and route of repair. General considerations on timing have already been mentioned, but it must now be decided whether the local tissues are sufficiently quiescent.

If a fistula is to be successfully repaired, the choice of route will depend largely on access. Arguments between the protagonists of an abdominal or vaginal approach have little merit because both routes have their place (Lawson 1972). The best results may be expected from a versatile operator selecting the approach most suited to the individual case. In general, though bladder fistulae and those involving the urethra should be repaired per vaginam, most high fistulae can also be repaired by this route and the post-operative period is much more comfortable. But if access is poor and the fistula cannot be drawn down, an abdominal approach may be easier. Concurrent involvement of the ureter or bowel in a surgical fistula would suggest the abdominal route. Obesity greatly hampers surgery whichever approach is chosen, but is probably worse for the abdominal approach.

If the fistula is to be repaired by the vaginal route it is necessary to decide at the preliminary examination under anaesthesia whether the prone (knee-chest) or the lithotomy position gives the better access (Fig. 14.3). The lithotomy is preferred in most cases, but the prone position provides the best exposure to juxta-urethral fistulae adherent to the back of the pubis. It is also helpful in massive fistulae as it reduces prolapse of the posterior bladder wall through the defect.

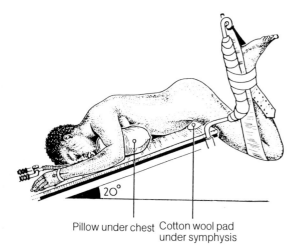

Pillow under chest   Cotton wool pad
under symphysis

Fig. 14.3. Knee-chest position. The flexed thighs hanging over the end of the table prevent the patient from sliding up it. The pillow under the chest facilitates abdominal respiratory movement. (Lawson 1967)

Surgical Repair

General

Surgery is needed for nearly all genital fistulae except those few uterine fistulae causing cyclical haematuria without urinary incontinence. For these, even drug-induced secondary amenorrhoea has proved successful (Rubino 1980). Diathermy coagulation of small tracks is not recommended. Very few vesicovaginal fistulae should be regarded as irreparable. Even fistulae complicated by advanced pelvic cancer may be better managed by low colpocleisis and catheter drainage than by urinary diversion. (Disentanglement of the ureters from pelvic growth only leads to prolongation of the act of dying and should be avoided.)

Certain complicating factors adversely affect the likelihood of successful closure and therefore require special care.

1. Vaginal stenosis, which may almost occlude the vagina after extensive pressure necrosis in obstructed labour, has to be opened up before repair per vaginam is practicable. Hour-glass contractions may be simply divided, but sometimes a Schuchardt incision, which is a deep episiotomy extending up to the cervix, is needed to give access. Relaxing incisions in the vagina should be left to granulate if closure would reform the contracture and put the

fistula repair under tension. They may need packing with absorbable haemostatic material such as Surgicel.

2. Local intrinsic bladder pathology also impairs the prognosis and should be treated before definitive repair. This includes periurethral abscesses and non-absorbable sutures inserted previously. In endemic areas, schistosomiasis may be responsible for extensive fibrosis in the bladder wall (Hassim and Lucas 1974). Biopsy of the fistula edge should establish the diagnosis. Pre-operative anti-schistosomal treatment is indicated: this will improve the prospects for healing but unfortunately will not alter established fibrosis. Tuberculous infection is a rare cause of urogenital fistula (Mohan et al. 1983).

3. Repeated attempts at repair gravely impair the prognosis, as each operation produces more fibrosis and further impairs the blood supply. The law of diminishing returns operates (Lawson 1980), so difficult or recurrent fistulae should be referred to centres of special expertise. A conference between a gynaecologist unfamiliar with the problem and an equally inexperienced urologist is not an adequate alternative, and failure is highly likely to culminate in a possibly unnecessary diversion procedure.

Various techniques for repairing fistulae will be described, but the success of any depends on accurate suturing without tension.

The authors consider that absorbable suture material should be used throughout all repairs, either extrachromic catgut 2–0 gauge or polyglycolic acid sutures 2–0 or 3–0 gauge. The use of non-absorbable materials such as nylon or silk in the bladder wall is contraindicated, as sutures left there will eventually extrude into the lumen, where calculi will form on them. The use of non-absorbable sutures to close the vaginal layer is permissible but their subsequent removal may be difficult.

Sutures must be placed with meticulous accuracy in the bladder wall, care being taken not to penetrate the mucosa. Interrupted stitches are best, about 3 mm apart and extending as far as possible away from the edges of the incision. Stitches that are too close together and the use of continuous or purse-string sutures tend to impair the blood supply and thus interfere with healing.

The bladder wall closure must be watertight, so it should be tested by instilling a coloured solution into the bladder before completing the repair. This procedure also sometimes reveals a previously unsuspected second fistula.

Vaginal Route

There are two basic techniques for closing fistulae per vaginam:

1. The most widely applicable is the Lawson-Tait method of flap dissection and closure in layers (Figs. 14.4, 14.5). Preliminary infiltration with a 1:200 000 solution of adrenalin facilitates dissection and reduces oozing.

2. Saucerisation, the classical method of Marion Sims developed by Moir (1967), is suitable for small residual fistulae which persist after incomplete closure of large defects (Figs. 14.6, 14.7).

These techniques are suitable for most mid-vaginal fistulae, but modifications are called for in special situations.

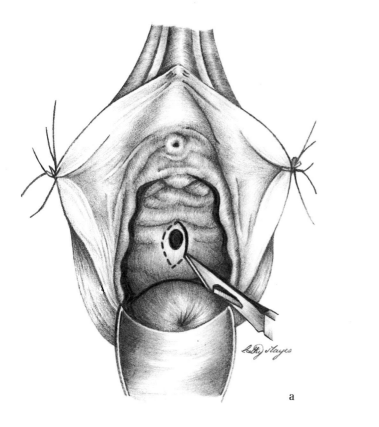

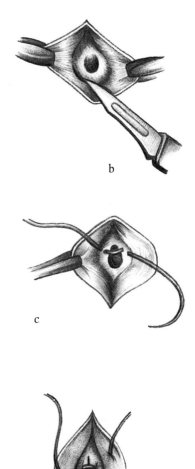

Fig. 14.4. a Healthy vagina is incised as an ellipse, the long axis of which corresponds to the long axis of the fistula. **b** Scar tissue is pared from the edges of the fistula. Dissection must be wide enough to mobilise the bladder defect to permit closure without tension. **c** First layer of the repair, inverting the edges of the defect towards the lumen of the bladder. **d** Second layer of the repair picks up the back of the vaginal flaps to obliterate the dead space and thus prevent haematoma.

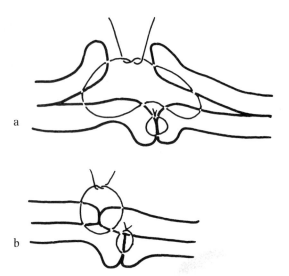

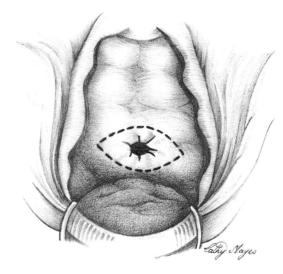

Fig. 14.5. a Second layer of sutures in the bladder wall picks up the back of the vaginal flaps to obliterate dead space and slide intact vaginal wall over bladder repair line. **b** Vaginal wall sutures consolidate the repair by picking up underlying bladder wall.

Fig. 14.6. The fistula is circumcised and scar tissue round the edge is excised to make a shallow saucer.

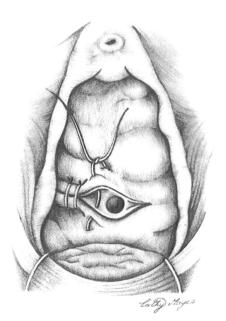

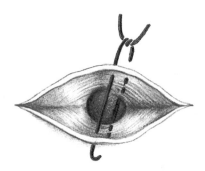

Fig. 14.7. The fistula is closed with a single layer of deep mattress sutures.

1. Juxtacervical fistulae in the anterior fornix, which mostly follow lower segment caesarean section, may be repaired per vaginam if the cervix can be drawn down to provide access. Dissection should include mobilisation of the bladder from the cervix. The repair must be transverse to reconstruct the underlying trigone; longitudinal repair would draw the ureteric orifices together and perhaps occlude them (Fig. 14.8).

2. Vault fistulae following hysterectomy can usually be reached per vaginam. The vaginal vault is incised transversely (Fig. 14.9). Mobilisation of the fistula is often facilitated by deliberately opening the pouch of Douglas behind it (Lawson 1977) (Fig. 14.10).

3. Juxta-urethral fistulae involving the bladder neck and proximal urethra may follow colporrhaphy. They are the commonest fistulae after obstructed labour, in which case tissue loss may be serious; fixity to the underlying pubis is a common problem. The lateral angles of the defect require careful mobilisation and closure to overcome any disproportion between the size of the hole in the bladder base and the urethral stump (Thomas 1947). A racquet-handle extension of the elliptical incision to expose the proximal end of the urethra facilitates closure in the mid-line (Lawson 1967). Transverse repair is usually necessary in obstetric cases, although longitudinal repair gives better prospects for urethral continence (Fig. 14.11).

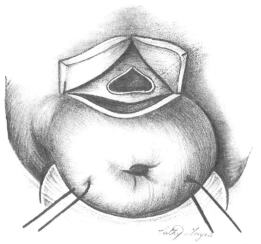

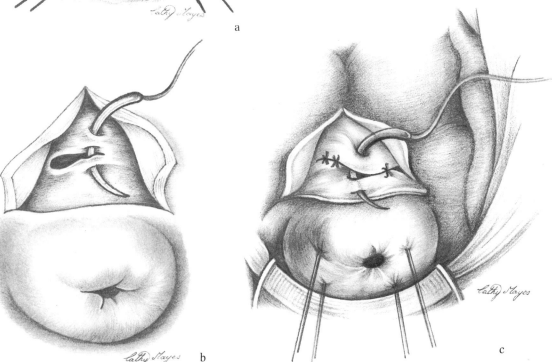

Fig. 14.8a–c. Repair of juxtacervical fistula. **a** Starting at the inferior margin, the fistula is mobilised to free the bladder from the underlying cervix. **b** The first layer of sutures inverts the edges of the defect towards the lumen of the bladder. **c** The second layer of sutures rolls the first layer against the intact cervix. Note the traction sutures on the cervix, which take up less space than a tenaculum.

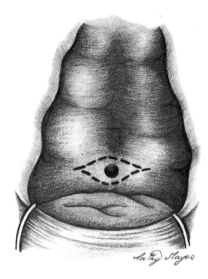

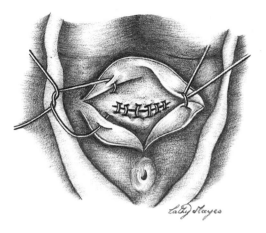

Fig. 14.11. Transverse repair of juxta-urethral fistula following obstructed labour. Patient in knee-chest position. Note the racquet-handle extension of the vaginal incision over the urethral stump.

Fig. 14.9. Post-hysterectomy vault fistula. A horizontal elliptical incision facilitates dissection.

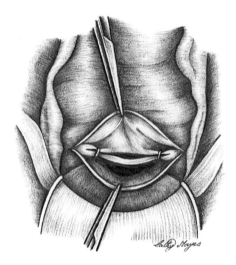

Fig. 14.10. Deliberate entry into the pouch of Douglas improves mobilisation.

4. Urethral loss, i.e. sloughing of the whole urethra, occasionally follows colporrhaphy, and for these cases the authors recommend Chassar Moir's modification of the Denis Browne operation (Moir 1964). A strip of anterior vaginal wall is made into a tube over a catheter (Fig. 14.12). It is most important to insert plication sutures behind the bladder neck if continence is to be achieved. The interposition of a Martius graft between the new urethra and the vaginal wall closure fills up the potential dead space and improves continence by ensuring

mobility of the bladder neck (Hassim and Lucas 1974). When the urethra has been destroyed by lymphogranuloma venereum the local blood supply is so seriously compromised that plastic procedures are doomed to failure. However, an acceptable degree of continence can sometimes be achieved by the simple expedient of creating a spout at the gaping internal meatus by means of two or three reefing sutures (Hudson et al. 1975) (Fig. 14.13).

5. Post-irradiation fistulae pose special problems. They are usually solidly fixed in hard scar tissue and obliterative endarteritis provoked by radiation produces a wide avascular zone round the defect. Post-irradiation fistulae cannot usually be mobilised, and flaps will slough because their blood supply is so poor and repair in layers will not heal. Closure of the vagina by colpocleisis is therefore necessary. Blaikley (1965) advocated total closure of the vaginal cavity after it had been denuded of epithelium. However, the authors have found that the residual dead space may be extremely rigid, and therefore not readily obliterated by sutures. We think it better to avoid mobilising the vault, merely closing off the upper vagina, which becomes a diverticulum of the bladder (Fig. 14.14). Dead space is filled in with a pedicle graft from a non-irradiated area (Lawson 1978).

Martius (1940) was the first to describe the pedicle graft of subcutaneous fat from the labium majus, which has an important place in fistula surgery. The

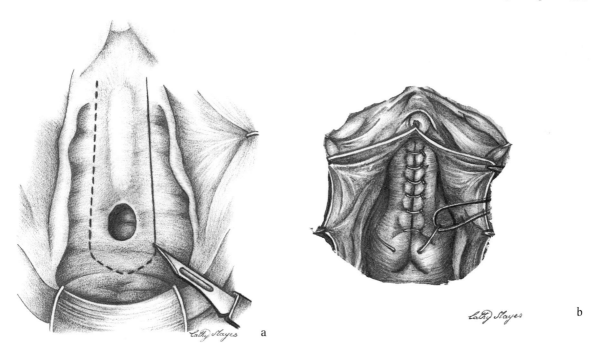

Fig. 14.12. a Reconstruction of lost urethra: parallel incisions 2 cm apart in the anterior vaginal wall. **b** New urethral tube fashioned from in-turned vaginal flaps. Note the plicating sutures at the bladder neck. A Martius graft should be interposed before repairing the vagina.

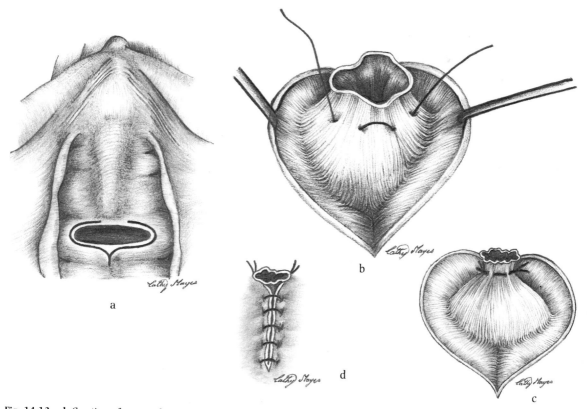

Fig. 14.13a–d. Creation of a meatal spout. **a** Racquet-shaped incision around the defect; **b** after mobilisation, insertion of reefing sutures; **c** creation of spout; **d** linear closure of vaginal defect up to the spout.

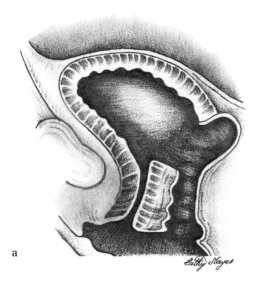

a

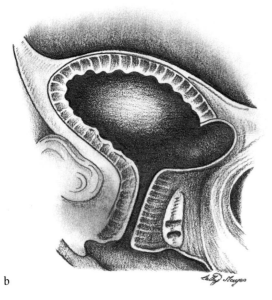

b

Fig. 14.14a,b. Post-irradiation fistula into the vaginal vault. **a** before and **b** after colpocleisis. The upper vagina has become a diverticulum of the bladder.

blood supply from the superficial external pudendal vessels is preserved when the graft is passed subcutaneously into the vagina to reinforce a repair or obliterate dead space (Fig. 14.15).

Ingelman-Sundberg (1953) introduced the gracilis graft to complete colpocleisis, drawing the inverted muscle into the vaginal cavity through the obturator foramen. Hamlin and Nicholson (1969)

have simplified the procedure by bringing the muscle across the pubic ramus through a subcutaneous tunnel. The gracilis muscle is supplied by two neurovascular bundles; normally the proximal leash is sufficient to maintain viability of the muscle if the gracilis is turned up at this point after division close to the knee (Fig. 14.16).

The concurrence of a rectal fistula does not preclude the use of the lower colpocleisis operation described above, provided the communication between the two fistulae would be large enough to permit free drainage per rectum. A colovaginal fistula must be recognised and free drainage established by rectal fenestration before colpocleisis, which will otherwise fail (Hudson 1984).

Abdominal Route

Repair by the abdominal route is indicated when high fistulae are fixed in the vault and are therefore inaccessible per vaginam.

1. Intravesical repair has the advantage of being entirely extraperitoneal, so the site of the causative pelvic operation does not have to be disturbed. The bladder is opened extraperitoneally, usually by a transverse incision. It is an advantage to elevate the fistula site by a tight vaginal pack, and the ureters should be catheterised under direct vision (Fig. 14.17). The technique of closure is similar to that of transvaginal flap repair except that for haemostasis the bladder mucosa is closed with a continuous suture, an exception to the general rule that it is better not to include the bladder mucosa in the suture lines of fistula repairs and to avoid continuous sutures.

2. There is little place for a simple intraperitoneal repair, but a combined intraperitoneal and transvesical repair is much favoured by urologists, and is particularly useful for vesico-uterine fistulae following caesarean section (Hudson 1962). Joly (quoted by Badenoch 1953) introduced the method, which consists essentially of a mid-line split of the peritoneal surface of the bladder: this is extended downwards in a racquet shape round the fistula (Fig. 14.18).

3. If there is a concomitant rectal fistula, interposition of an omental graft should be considered. Bastiaanse (1960) has emphasised its value in bringing fresh tissue with a good blood supply into

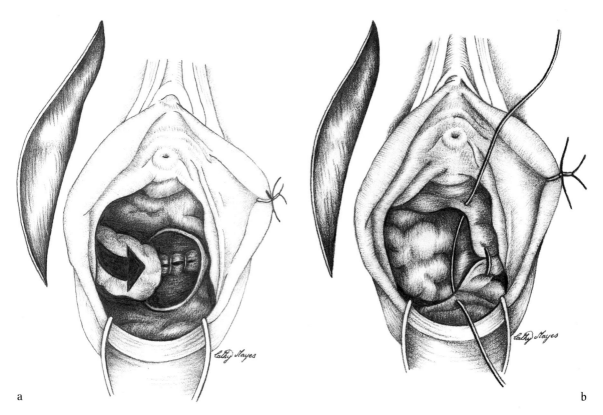

Fig. 14.15a,b. Martius graft of fat from the labium majus is passed subcutaneously into the vagina to obliterate dead space before completing the colpocleisis.

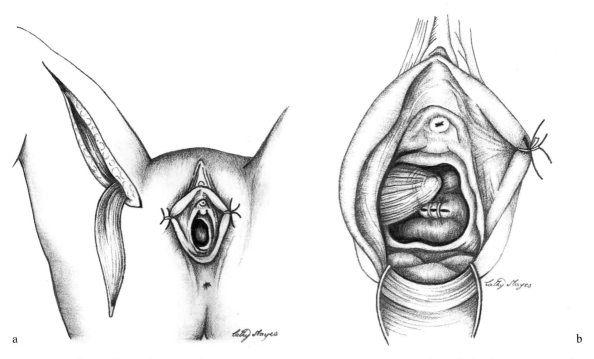

Fig. 14.16. a The gracilis muscle is divided close to the knee: during mobilisation its proximal vascular leash is preserved. **b** The distal end of the gracilis is brought subcutaneously over the inferior pubic ramus into the vagina (Hamlin-Nicholson technique).

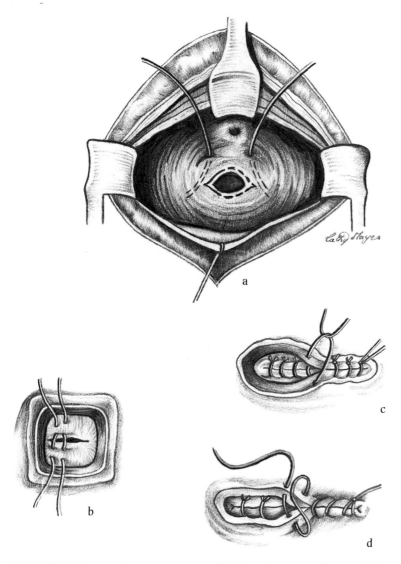

Fig. 14.17a–d. Intravesical repair. **a** Exposure of fistula: catheterisation of ureters. **b** Closure of vaginal defect after thorough mobilisation of overlying bladder. **c** Closure of muscle layer. **d** Closure of bladder mucosa by continuous haemostatic suture.

an irradiated area. Usually the intact omentum cannot be brought down low enough into the pelvis, so a pedicle graft has to be fashioned (Turner Warwick 1972) (Fig. 14.19).

Post-operative Management

Post-operative nursing care is almost as important as skilled surgery in the successful treatment of fistula cases. Continuous drainage of the bladder is essential. In ordinary circumstances this should be for 10–12 days, but 3–6 weeks is required for post-irradiation fistulae. The bladder is thus kept empty and at rest while the fistula heals: irrigation of the bladder should therefore be avoided if possible. The urinary output should be measured every hour so that interference with free drainage can be detected before any harm is done to the repair. The best way of preventing blockage of the catheter is to keep it continuously flushed with dilute urine, so a high fluid intake must be encouraged. Syphons and pumps are unnecessary.

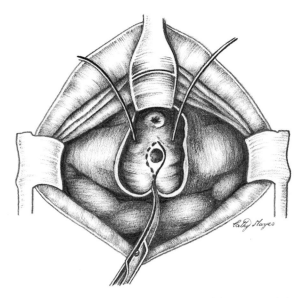

Fig. 14.18. Swift-Joly's mid-line hemisection of the posterior bladder wall which is extended round the fistula.

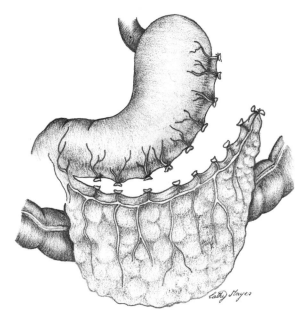

Fig. 14.19. Mobilisation of the greater omentum by separation from the colon and division along the greater curvature of the stomach. Note that the right gastro-epiploic vessels are preserved.

It is important to avoid infection by using a closed circuit system. Continuous drainage into a plastic bag incorporating a non-return valve is best. Urine samples should be collected daily from the closed circuit by syringe and needle puncture and sent to the laboratory for culture, so that appropriate antibiotic therapy can be instituted without delay.

When the catheter is removed the patient should be encouraged to micturate very frequently, as the bladder capacity will be found to be small at first and control may be defective.

The bladder may be drained through either an indwelling urethral catheter or a suprapubic cystostomy. For fistulae at or above the trigone, a Foley self-retaining urethral catheter is usually satisfactory. Pressure or traction on the fistula repair should be avoided, so suprapubic drainage is preferred for bladder neck or urethral fistulae.

After an abdominal repair, suprapubic drainage is always indicated. Any residual suprapubic sinus usually heals spontaneously, although occasionally a short period of continuous drainage per urethram may be required to achieve this.

The technique of inserting a suprapubic catheter by blind stab after distending the bladder, which is commonly used after routine vaginal surgery, is unwise after vaginal repair of mid-vaginal or vault fistulae: the freshly repaired bladder should not be distended in this fashion. This consideration is less important for juxta-urethral fistulae for which the stab technique may be used.

If the urine is heavily bloodstained during the immediate post-operative period, two-way bladder washouts may be required to prevent clot retention. A wide-bore suprapubic catheter and a Foley urethral catheter can be used if the repair-line is at or above the trigone. After juxta-urethral repairs a whistle-tip catheter is preferred to a Foley, held in place by a nylon stitch brought out through the abdominal wall over a Harris bar.

Complications

1. Vaginal bleeding in the immediate post-operative period is uncommon, and the authors therefore prefer to avoid vaginal packs if possible. Haemorrhage from divided strictures and relaxing incisions can usually be treated by evacuating the clot and laying in absorbable material such as Surgicel.

Post-operative haemorrhage into the bladder is particularly likely after suprapubic repair, and vigilance is required to prevent blockage of the catheter by the clot. Secondary haemorrhage into the bladder (usually about the sixth day) is of sinister significance as breakdown of the repair usually follows.

2. If urine ceases to flow through the catheter this usually indicates displacement of the catheter or blockage of its lumen. Urgent steps to re-establish free drainage are required if breakdown of the repair is to be prevented.

3. Leakage of urine per vaginam is usually due to failure of the repair (although the possibility of a ureterovaginal fistula should not be overlooked). The temptation to "cobble up" a leaking suture line in the early post-operative period must be resisted, as a larger fistula is likely to result. A wiser course is to persevere with continuous catheter drainage for up to 4 weeks, which may facilitate spontaneous closure.

4. One or even both ureters may be occluded in the repair of a fistula near the trigone. Confirmation of this complication may be obtained by intravenous urography. To release the obstruction it is not necessary to unpick an otherwise satisfactory repair. It is better to drain the affected ureter, as the obstruction may resolve with time or develop into a separate uterovaginal fistula which can be dealt with electively within a few weeks. Percutaneous nephrostomy is the best temporary expedient, a fine plastic tube being inserted into the renal pelvis under ultrasound control. If sophisticated medical imaging of this order is not available an intubated ureterostomy is a satisfactory alternative, a fine plastic tube being inserted by an extraperitoneal approach in the iliac fossa. Open nephrostomy should be avoided as it can damage the kidney and lead to its removal.

5. Urinary infection is rarely a serious problem if the method of closed circuit drainage described above is followed. However, occasionally gram-negative septicaemia occurs after very extensive surgery; this is much less likely if urinary tract infection has been eliminated before operation. Particular care should be taken to do this if renal function has been impaired by pre-operative obstructive uropathy.

Results

Mere closure is not the only criterion of success. If post-operative control of micturition is defective, clinical assessment may be difficult. All patients should therefore be submitted to a dye test in the lithotomy position 4–6 weeks after the repair; a general anaesthetic is not usually necessary.

Urethral incompetence should be reviewed at intervals of up to 6 months, at which stage further studies, including measurement of residual bladder capacity, may be required.

If there is any anxiety about the upper urinary tract, excretion urography should be repeated.

Patients with obstetric fistulae will already have lost vaginal tissue, and this is usually made worse by operative closure of the defect. The result may be severe stricture formation leading to apareunia. Forceful coitus may reopen the fistula, and plastic enlargement of the vagina may do likewise. In these circumstances, coital function may be restored by constructing a labial pouch (Williams 1964).

Results should be evaluated by success at the first attempt. In obstetric fistulae in developing countries, an experienced operator should be able to achieve 75% success at the first attempt, a further 15% being closed at a second attempt. The primary success rate for surgical fistulae should be over 90%, but with irradiation fistulae it may be as low as 60%.

These figures should not be confused with the operability rate, which should approach 100% in benign cases.

Management of Failure

The case for referral of difficult cases to special centres has already been made, but even there failure has sometimes to be admitted. Only in these circumstances should urinary diversion be undertaken.

The techniques of diversion available are described in Chap. 12, but some comment on choice of method for these patients is relevant.

For obstetric patients in developing countries one needs to balance a normal life expectancy with the unacceptability of an artifical stoma and the lack of adequate stoma after-care. The modern technique of reflux-preventing anastomosis probably means that implantation of ureters into the intact bowel is safe enough, as well as being more acceptable. In these cases the importance of establishing that there is no concomitant rectovaginal fistula cannot be over-emphasised, and the ability of the anal sphincter to preserve continence should be tested. This is likely to be impaired in lymphogranuloma venereum. Ureterocolic anastomosis may also be considered in older patients as being kinder than an abdominal stoma, but anal sphincter control may also be defective in this age group.

In conclusion we emphasise that permanent urinary diversion should only be considered as a last resort in the management of genital fistulae, to be used on the advice of an acknowledged expert when reparative treatment has failed.

References

Badenoch AW (1953) Manual of urology. Heinemann, London, p 411

Bastiaanse MA van B (1960) Surgical closure of very large irradiation fistulae of the bladder and rectum. In: Youssef AF (ed) Gynaecological urology. Thomas, Springfield, Ill, pp 280–297

Blaikley JB (1965) Colpocleisis for difficult vaginal fistulae of bladder and rectum. Proc R Soc Med 58:581–586

Editorial (1981) Obstetric fistula. Lancet I:1402–1403

Falk HC, Tancer ML (1956) Management of vesical fistulas after Caesarean section. Am J Obstet Gynecol 71:97–106

Fourie T (1983) Early repair of post-hysterectomy vesicovaginal fistula. S Afr Med J 63:889–890

Harrison KA (1983) Obstetric fistula: one social calamity too many. Br J Obstet Gynaecol 90:385–386

Hassim AM, Lucas C (1974) Reduction in the incidence of stress incontinence complicating fistula repair. Br J Surg 61:461–465

Hamlin RHJ, Nicholson EC (1969) Reconstruction of urethra totally destroyed in labour. Br Med J II:147–150

Hudson CN (1962) Vesico-uterine fistula following Caesarean section. J Obstet Gynaecol Br Commonw 69:121–124

Hudson CN (1968) Malignant change in an obstetric vesicovaginal fistula. Proc R Soc Med 61:1280–1281

Hudson CN (1970) Acquired fistulae between the intestine and the vagina. Ann R Coll Surg Engl 46:20–40

Hudson CN (1984) In: Todd IP, Field LP (eds) Rob and Smith's operative surgery, vol 3, 4th edn. Butterworths, London, pp 563–578

Hudson CN, Hendrickse JP de V, Ward A (1975) An operation for restoration of urinary continence following total loss of the urethra. Br J Obstet Gynaecol 82:501–504

Ingelman-Sundberg A (1953) Eine Methode zur operativen Behandlung von vesicovaginalen und rectovaginalen Fisteln im bestrahlten Gewebe. Arch Gynaekol 183:498–500

Lawson JB (1967) Injuries of the urinary tract. In: Lawson JB, Stewart DB (eds) Obstetrics and gynaecology in the tropics and developing countries. Arnold, London, pp 481–522

Lawson JB (1968) Birth-canal injuries. Proc R Soc Med 61:368–370

Lawson JB (1972) Vesical fistulae into the vaginal vault. Br J Urol 44:623–631

Lawson JB (1977) Vesico-vaginal fistulae. In: Roberts DWT (ed) Operative surgery—Gynaecology and obstetrics. Butterworths, London, pp 106–117

Lawson JB (1978) Management of genito-urinary fistulae. In: Clinics in obstetrics and gynaecology, vol 5. Saunders, London, pp 209–236

Lawson JB (1980) Vesico-vaginal fistulae. In: Proceedings of First International Conference of the Society of Gynecology and Obstetrics of Nigeria. Bröderna Ekstrands Tryckeri AB, Lund, pp 323–329

Martius H (1940) Fettlappenplastik aus dem Bulbokavernosusgebiet als Fistelnahtschutzoperation. Geburtshilfe Frauenheilkd 2:453–459

Mohan V, Gupta SM, Arora M (1983) Cysto-uterine fistula. Br J Urol 55:245–246

Moir J (1964) Reconstruction of the urethra. J Obstet Gynaecol Br Commonw 71:349–359

Moir J (1967) The vesico-vaginal fistula, 2nd ed. Bailliere, London

Moir J (1973) Vesico-vaginal fistulae as seen in Britain. J Obstet Gynaecol Br Commonw 80:598–602

Raghavaiah NV, Devi AI (1980) Primary vaginal stones. J Urol 123:771–772

Reece EA, Wible J, Gilhooly P, Tretter W, Crum C (1982) Congenital utero-vesical fistula. Diagn Gynecol Obstet 4:207–210

Rubino SM (1980) Vesico-uterine fistula treated by amenorrhoea induced with contraceptive steroids. Br J Obstet Gynaecol 87:343–344

Stevens P (1978) Stomatherapy in a developing society. In: Todd IP (ed) Intestinal stomas. Heinemann, London, pp 171–181

Thomas GB (1947) Treatment of a type of juxta-urethral vesicovaginal fistula. J Obstet Gynaecol Br Emp 54:665–671

Turner Warwick RT (1972) The use of pedicle grafts in the repair of urinary tract fistulae. Br J Urol 44:644

Williams EA (1964) Congenital absence of the vagina: a simple operation for its relief. J Obstet Gynaecol Br Commonw 71:511–516

Yeates WK (1959) Palliation of vaginal urinary fistulae. Lancet I:916

15 Ureterovaginal Fistulae

W. Keith Yeates

Introduction

The formation of a ureterovaginal fistula nearly always requires the combination of (a) an event that creates a communication between the vagina and the plane of the ureter; and (b) a lesion that sooner or later exposes the lumen of the ureter.

The commonest procedure that provides the potential pathway is a total hysterectomy; much less common circumstances are anterior exenteration (usually for carcinoma of the bladder), abdominoperineal excision of the rectum, obstetric injuries to the cervix and vault of the vagina, subtotal hysterectomy (the communication then being through the canal of the cervical stump), operative procedures on the vault of the vagina, including colporrhaphy, and intentional exposure of the ureter at vaginal ureterolithotomy.

Associated with the above, exposure of the lumen of the ureter can occur from a variety of causes.

Operative Injuries

Site

Operative ureteric injuries that result in ureterovaginal fistulae naturally occur below the pelvic brim, particularly in the juxtavesical part of the ureter—the point where the ureter is most difficult to identify and where it is most closely applied to structures that must be divided at total hysterectomy.

Types

Division. Accidental division can be partial, varying in extent, or complete, with or without ligation of the lower end of the ureter (Fig. 15.1a,b).

Excision. A length of ureter may be accidentally excised without ligation of the upper end. The lower end may or may not have been ligated (Fig. 15.1c).

Ischaemia. Sloughing is associated with ischaemia (Fig. 15.1d–g), which may be due to:

—Strangulation of part of the ureteric wall by partial ligation or transfixion with ligation

—Crushing of the ureteric wall from the temporary accidental application of a ligature (recognised and removed at operation) or a clamp
—Crushing by an encircling ligature with subsequent distension of the ureter above
—Removal of the periureteric tissues ("stripping the ureter")
—Radiation, which reduces the chances of incised wounds healing and increases the likelihood of necrosis after crushing injuries or stripping.

These mechanisms are often combined in the management of malignant disease in the pelvis, especially carcinoma of the cervix.

Intentional Incision. An incision may have occurred in the course of a ureterolithotomy procedure, or the ureters may have been intentionally divided at anterior exenteration with urinary diversion. The subsequent diversion may have been by ideal conduit or by ureterocolic anastomosis.

Obstetric Laceration

Some obstetric procedures, e.g. forceps delivery, may injure the cervix and upper vagina. Application of the forceps before full cervical dilatation may lacerate the cervix and careless use of a rotation forceps can traumatise the upper vagina.

Invasion by Growth

The ureteric lesions may be unilateral or bilateral (see p. 225).

Time of Occurrence

Depending on the mechanism, the leakage of urine may occur hours, days, weeks or months after the event—either operative or obstetric—that creates the potential fistulous track.

Early

From a few hours after operation, leakage is seen following unrecognised division (Fig. 15.1a, b) or excision (Fig. 15.1c) of the ureter. Urine formation may be in abeyance from hypotension at operation and leakage appears when the blood pressure rises.

Intermediate

Leakage appearing from a few days up to about 6 weeks after operation is due to sloughing of the

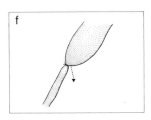

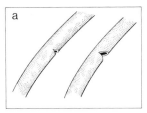

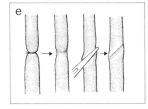

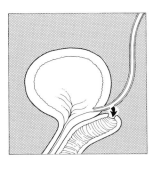

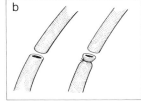

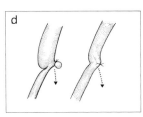

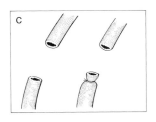

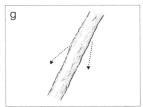

Fig. 15.1. Types of ureteric injury associated with ureterovaginal fistulae. **a, b** Division, **c** excision, **d–g** ischaemia.

ureteric wall from any of the causes of ischaemia mentioned (Fig. 15.1d–g).

It is very important to appreciate that ureterovaginal fistulae in this group are often associated with:

—Ureteric obstruction early in the clinical course by accidental ligature, periureteric oedema, haematoma or later by fibrosis, and/or
—Renal infection, which is particularly serious when obstruction is also present.

Late

Leakage appearing over 3 months after operation for a malignant lesion very often indicates a recurrence of growth in the pelvic cellular tissues.

Recognition of Fistulae

There are two parts to what is usually a straightforward diagnosis: proving that the fluid is urine and that it comes from the ureter.

A gauze pack is inserted into the vault of the vagina and a second one is placed below it to prevent it from being contaminated by any leakage of urine from the urethra.

Confirmation of Urinary Leakage

Intravenous indigo carmine is sometimes used as a urine label, but the renal function on the side of the ureteric injury is often deficient and a false-negative result may be obtained.

Pyridium (four tablets by mouth) is much less sensitive to decreased urinary concentration and will usually rapidly stain the pack orange.

The most reliable method, however, is to send the upper pack to the laboratory for testing for urea. Urine is the only fluid in the body where the urea concentration is high enough to give a crude positive test.

Confirmation of Ureteric Fistulae

Differentiation of the ureterovaginal fistula from a vesicovaginal fistula is most easily achieved in the ward by the standard procedure of passing a catheter and completely filling the bladder with indigo carmine solution (four ampoules of 4 ml in 500 ml water); after emptying the bladder the upper gauze is found to be wet but clear. Very rarely, reflux up a transected ureter will suggest the fistula is vesicovaginal, a misdiagnosis that will subsequently be corrected by cystoscopy and retrograde ureterography.

Spontaneous Closure of Fistulae

As in the case of fistulae elsewhere, spontaneous closure of a ureterovaginal fistula may be expected unless there is:

—Distal obstruction
—The intervention of other tissues (e.g. complete division)

—Ischaemia
—Persistent infection with or without the presence of a foreign body
—Neoplastic invasion.

The injury that is most likely to heal spontaneously is an incision with incomplete division of the ureter (see Fig. 15.1a). This type of injury is characterised clinically by very early appearance of the leakage, radiographically by minimal ureteric dilatation, and instrumentally by the ability to pass a ureteric catheter, or even just contrast medium (Figs. 15.2, 15.3) up to the kidney. In these circumstances spontaneous healing is a distinct possibility; it may take up to 2–3 weeks or a little longer.

In most cases the clinical course (later appearance of the leakage) and findings (dilatation of the upper urinary tract on intravenous urography and often obstruction to the passage of a ureteric catheter) indicate that there are factors preventing spontaneous closure and that operative treatment will be required.

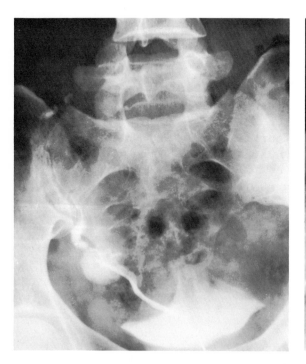

Fig. 15.2. Retrograde cystogram and right ureterogram showing extravasation of contrast around site of ureteric injury, but with passage up ureter indicating ureteric injury is incomplete. There is an impression of a haematoma on the bladder wall.

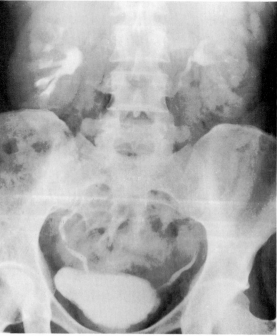

Fig. 15.3. Intravenous urogram of case in Fig. 15.2 3 months later, showing spontaneous healing of ureteric fistula. Site is indicated by a very minor degree of narrowing which is not causing obstruction.

Timing of Operative Intervention

Except in the incised wound (very early leakage) group there is often an ischaemic element and a few weeks' delay may increase the viability of the ureter immediately above the lesions.

About 4–6 weeks after operation is very often the most reasonable time to plan correction of a ureterovaginal fistula.

However, intervention should be brought forward when there is ureteric obstruction of an important degree (the intravenous urogram showing dilated calyces) and especially when there is fever probably referable to renal infection.

Adherence to the older policy of delaying repair for at least 3 months—until post-operative and post-irradiation reaction in the pelvic tissues has largely subsided—is unnecessary as these tissues can be left undisturbed by the use of a Boari flap (Fig. 15.16a) even when the lesion is in the juxtavesical part of the ureter.

Factors which may necessarily delay operation include the patient's general condition and the state of the abdominal wall.

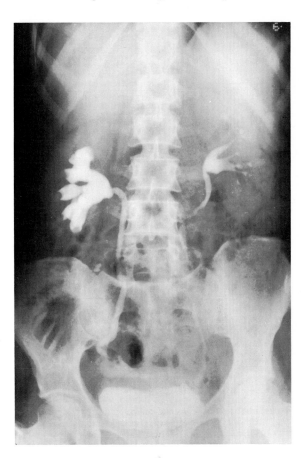

Fig. 15.4. Intravenous urogram showing moderate dilatation of the right upper urinary tract above ureteric injury in the pelvis. The contrast is seen extravasating particularly medially and into the vault of the vagina.

Pre-operative Investigation and Preparation

Identification of the Side of the Fistula

Because there is very frequently some obstruction at the site of the ureteric injury an intravenous urogram usually shows some dilatation of the ureter—and often of the calyces—on the side of the lesion (Fig. 15.4). If, however, there is no obstruction above the fistula, the ureter and kidney may look quite normal; sometimes (a trap for the unwary) the opposite ureter and kidney are dilated on account of slight ureteric compression from oedema or a pelvic haematoma (Fig. 15.5).

The most reliable method of identifying the injured side is cystoscopy and observation of the presence of efflux from the ureteric orifice of the intact side, and the absence of efflux on the injured side. This test is facilitated by adequate hydration by giving intravenous fluids and then an intravenous diuretic with or without indigo carmine.

Further confirmation of the side of the lesion may be obtained by attempting to pass a catheter up the non-effluxing side. There are four possible findings:

1. Usually the catheter is arrested at the site of the injury, most often 2–3 cm from the ureteric orifice. Injection of contrast medium through a bulb catheter may show that part of the ureteric wall is intact, the contrast passing through the fistula and up the ureter.

2. Sometimes the catheter passes up the full length of the ureter and drains clear urine rapidly, also indicating that part of the ureteric wall is intact.

3. Sometimes it apparently passes up the full length but does not drain urine, and a subsequent X-ray with the injection of contrast medium shows the catheter coiled up in a cavity in the pelvis (Fig. 15.6).

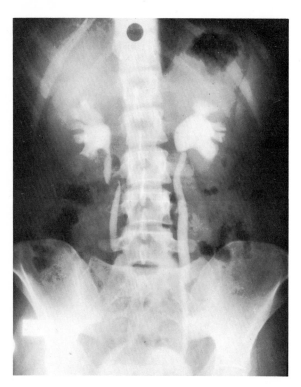

Fig. 15.5. Intravenous urogram showing moderate dilatation of the left ureter, renal pelvis and calyces in a case of a ureterovaginal fistula which was found to be arising from the right ureter. The dilatation of the left side was merely due to post-operative periureteric oedema.

4. Occasionally the catheter appears in the vault of the vagina having passed through a deficiency in the ureter close to the site of incision of the vaginal wall (Fig. 15.7).

Failure to pass the catheter up the ureter may be due just to the angle of the ureteric orifices or to a mucosal fold. It is therefore not so reliable a test as simply observing the absence of ureteric efflux from one side.

If, in spite of all the above investigations, there continues to be doubt as to the side of origin of the fistula, contrast should be injected through the opening of the fistula into the vault of the vagina by means of the bulb catheter (Figs. 15.8–15.11, a simple technique which should perhaps be used more often.

Case Report.

A nurse aged 41 years developed a uretero-vaginal fistula 5 days after a radical hysterectomy with node dissection for carcinoma of the cervix. Two months post-operatively, an intravenous urogram was performed which showed a duplex left kidney. The site of junction of the ureters was not demonstrated. The right kidney was normal. Cystoscopy showed no efflux from the right ureteric orifice. Ureteric catheters were passed easily up both ureters

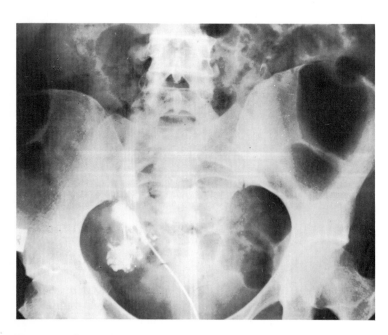

Fig. 15.6. Right ureteric injury showing catheter coiled up in a cavity outlined by injection of contrast. Some contrast has passed up the ureter indicating that the lesion was incomplete.

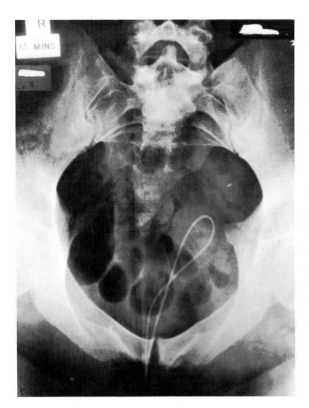

Fig. 15.7. Left ureterovaginal fistula. The left ureteric orifice did not discharge. The catheter passed through the left ureteric orifice and appeared in the vault of the vagina.

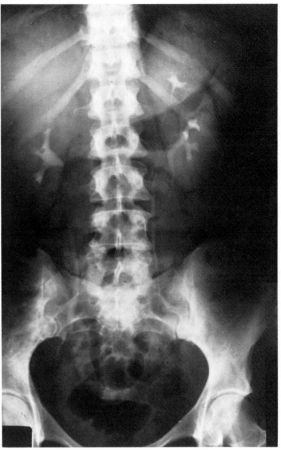

Fig. 15.8. Intravenous urogram showing the duplex left kidney. The site of junction of the ureters is not demonstrated. The right kidney is normal but the ureter is not fully demonstrated.

(Fig. 15.9): bilateral retro-ureterograms were performed using bulb catheters (Fig. 15.10). No fistula was demonstrated. Finally, a bulb catheter was passed into the opening of the fistula in the vaginal vault, and demonstrated the right urinary tract (Fig. 15.11). The right ureter was reimplanted with cure.

This was manifestly a case of partial ureteric wall deficiency without stenosis, with a valvular effect which allowed contrast to ascend without leakage, but urine descending was diverted into the vagina.

Recognition of Level

It is highly desirable that the level be recognised, particularly if the operator's ability is limited to direct reimplantation of the ureter into the bladder (see below)

The site of arrest of a ureteric catheter passed from below is, of course, only the lower level of the ureteric lesion. The site of leakage and level of viable ureter may be much higher, especially in fistulae from ischaemia.

A high-dose intravenous urogram with screening or delayed films will usually show the lower limit of intact ureter and will sometimes demonstrate the exact site of the leakage and show filling of the vagina (Fig. 15.12).

Operative Procedures

Objectives

Whenever the bladder function is normal, or can be restored, the affected ureter or ureters should be reimplanted into the urinary tract.

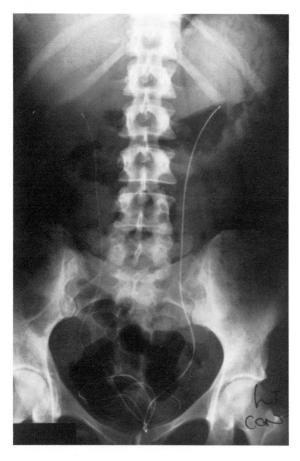

Fig. 15.9. Bilateral ureteric catheterisation.

Exploratory Laparotomy

An exploratory laparotomy should usually be immediately preceded by a cystoscopy to: (a) ascertain the state of the mucosa of the bladder; (b) note the bladder capacity (the larger this is, the easier it will be to make the bladder reach a high ureteric injury direct or to construct a Boari flap); (c) confirm the absence of efflux from the affected side and the inability to pass a ureteric catheter up the ureter.

A 22F Foley catheter is passed into the bladder, which is emptied. The catheter is spigotted and the end left accessible to the surgeon. The patient should be placed in a moderate head-down position.

The operator should be able to expose the whole of the pelvic ureter; usually this is relatively easy, but occasionally it is extremely difficult on account of distortion of the anatomy, fibrosis and vascularity of the tissues. It is advisable to carry out

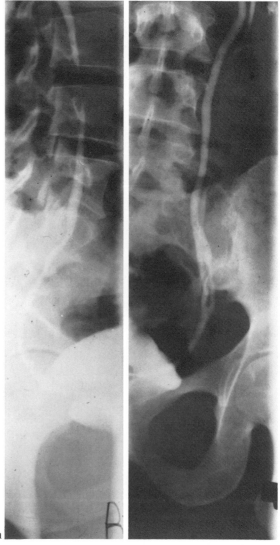

Fig. 15.10. Bilateral retro-ureterograms via bulb catheters showing **a** an apparently normal right ureter and **b** left duplex ureters joined just below the left sacroiliac joint. No fistula demonstrated by these means.

the exploration through a mid-line incision, ignoring the original incision, which has often been a Pfannenstiel.

Although lower lesions of the ureter can be approached extraperitoneally, in the vast majority of cases after hysterectomy the pelvic peritoneum is so adherent that it will be opened inadvertently in attempted extraperitoneal exposure.

It is therefore easier and more satisfactory to open the peritoneum intentionally and expose the ureter by incising the overlying peritoneum on the right side or by mobilising the pelvic colon on the left side.

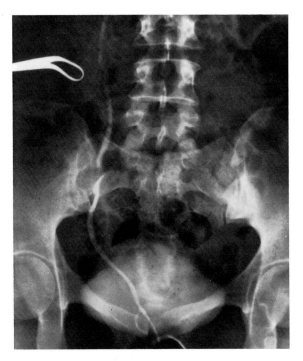

Fig. 15.11. Bulb catheter passed into opening of fistula in the vault of the vagina. Injection of contrast demonstrates whole of right upper urinary tract.

Fig. 15.12. Intravenous urogram of a right pelvic ureteric injury indicating lower level of intact ureter and extravasation of contrast into vagina.

It should be noted that, unlike the unoperated case, after pelvic operations on the ureter or radiation the ureters are usually adherent more to the pelvic wall or vessels than to the overlying peritoneum.

When the uterus has not been removed, e.g. in obstetric injuries, the pelvic ureter can be exposed by dividing the round ligament of the uterus and incising the peritoneum upwards lateral to the ovarian pedicle.

Once the ureter has been exposed at the pelvic brim it should be traced distally by incising the tissue over it without mobilising it more than is necessary. After a total hysterectomy there are usually no vessels of any size crossing the ureter above the site of the fistula.

The ureter should be divided through the lowest part of apparently viable wall. The viability at the site of section should be reappraised and if necessary the upper part of the divided ureter should be excised—repeatedly if necessary—until reasonably healthy ureter is found.

On some occasions the state of the tissues in the lower part of the pelvis is such that it is better to divide the ureter immediately above the involved area.

Selection of Procedure

Unless there are exceptional circumstances (as listed below) the primary objective is to reimplant a viable end of ureter into the bladder without tension, preferably by a technique designed to prevent ureteric reflux.

When the lower most viable part of the ureter cannot be reimplanted into the bladder direct in spite of its thorough mobilisation, the choice of method to bridge the gap lies between constructing a bladder flap (Boari) and implanting the ureter into the opposite ureter, or rarely via an ileal segment into the bladder.

Exceptional circumstances include:

1. The state of the pathological process in the pelvis, e.g. residual malignant disease with or without extensive radiation changes, may contraindicate a pelvic procedure, and nephrectomy would be the simplest, safest, and most reasonable choice.

2. The kidney of the affected ureter may be the site of extensive inflammatory changes, which are

unlikely to resolve with the relief of any ureteric obstruction; if the opposite kidney is normal a nephrectomy may be the procedure of choice.

3. Where there is a deficiency of ureter such as to require an ileal replacement on technical grounds, this may be contraindicated by the poor general condition or age of the patient, and a nephrectomy may clearly be the preferable procedure.

Urinary diversion is indicated in ureterovaginal fistulae only when for some local or neurological reason the bladder function cannot be restored.

A number of operative procedures are available for the correction of ureterovaginal fistulae. Some of these are discussed below.

Every surgeon who explores a ureteric injury should be capable of bridging a deficiency from the bladder to the level of the pelvic brim.

The procedures of extensively mobilising the bladder, performing a psoas hitch, and constructing a Boari flap (Ockerblad 1947), can all be easily practised in the post-mortem room, and are worthwhile experiences for all surgeons who operate in the pelvis.

Direct Reimplantation (Fig. 15.13)

If there is adequate length of ureter to reach the bladder, the ureter should be reimplanted into the bladder direct. An anti-reflux technique is preferable if there is adequate length available. Direct end-on anastomosis is a second-best choice. Fig. 15.14 illustrates the author's technique for reimplantation.

Psoas Hitch (Fig. 15.15)

When the selected site of division of the ureter can barely reach the bladder, ureteric reimplantation without tension can be facilitated by extensive mobilisation of the bladder on the contralateral side and fixing of the bladder above the new hiatus to the psoas muscle. Should the apex of the tented bladder not reach high enough, the curved incision on the upper part of the anterior wall can be converted into a Boari flap as described below.

When the site of division of the ureter is higher than can be reached easily by tenting-up the bladder

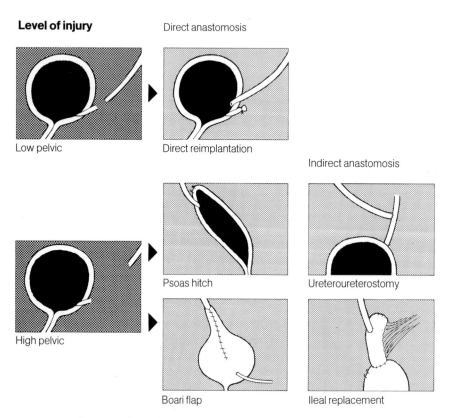

Fig. 15.13. Outline types of procedures for reimplanting the ureter into the bladder.

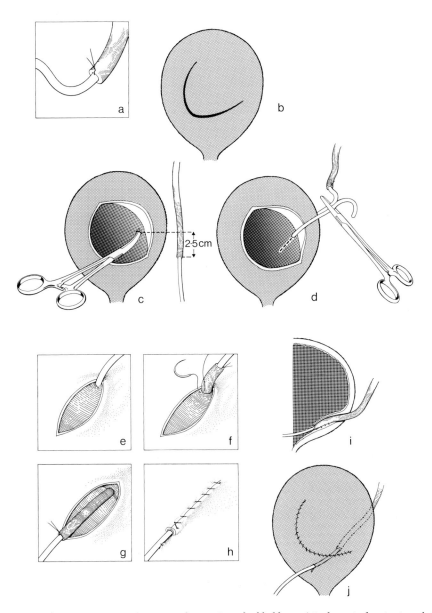

Fig. 15.14a–j. Direct reimplantation of ureter into the bladder. **a** Attachment of ureter to polythene tube by fine catgut. **b** Incision for opening anterior wall of bladder. **c** Tilting of bladder towards side of injury to identify site for reimplantation. **d** Use of loop of polythene tubing as retractor to tense bladder mucosa below site of new hiatus through muscular wall of bladder. **e** Incision and separation of mucosal flaps after raising mucosa with injection of saline. **f** Ureter drawn through new hiatus and fixed to underlying bladder muscle with 4–0 chromic catgut. **g** Ureter after fixation to underlying muscle. **h** Closure of overlying bladder mucosa. Note original transfixing suture through tube has been removed and new fixation suture through mucosa of trigone. **i,j** Closure of bladder after drawing polythene tube through anterior bladder wall.

as described, there is usually a choice between replacing its lower part by constructing a flap from the bladder and implanting the ureter into the side of the opposite ureter (transureteral ureterostomy).

Although protagonists of transureteral ureterostomy report the safety of the procedure even when there is manifest infection in the affected side,

most urologists would probably elect to confine the procedure to cases they considered sterile.

On the other hand, where there are technical problems in constructing a Boari flap, e.g. if the bladder capacity is unusually small, a minor degree of infection should not be regarded as an absolute contraindication to transureteral ureterostomy, as

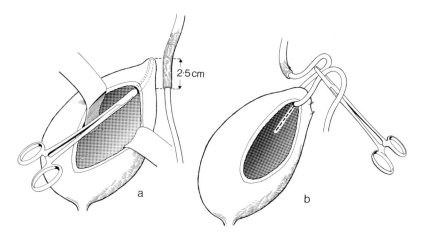

Fig. 15.15a,b. Psoas hitch for higher ureteric lesions. The technique is very similar to that shown in Fig. 15.14.

this is a much smaller procedure than the alternative sort of nephrectomy—ileal replacement.

Boari Flap (Fig. 15.16a, b)

The capacity of the average female bladder allows a bladder flap constructed from the dome of the bladder to reach above the pelvic brim without difficulty. The breadth of the flap should be great enough to ensure a satisfactory blood supply and to allow it to be wrapped round the lower two centimetres of the divided ureter. (If implantation without a flap is unexpectedly found to be possible the procedure previously described, usually combined with a psoas hitch, is carried out).

The flap is then constructed by dividing the bladder on each side as far as the posterolateral corner, making the ends of the incision diverge to provide a broad-based pedicle.

The ureter can be anastomosed to the upper end of the flap by placing it in a submucosal tunnel (Fig. 15.16c). The mucosa is raised by injecting a small amount of saline and then creating a tunnel with blunt-ended scissors, beginning at the cut edge, and perforating the mucosa about 2 cm further down.

A fine clip is then passed through the perforation and along the tunnel and grasps the free end of the tube attached to the ureter. The edges of the mucosa of the ureter and bladder are then sutured with 4–0 chromic catgut. The tube is brought across the bladder and then through a small stab incision as previously described. The back of the flap is fixed to the psoas. The free edges of the flap and the incision in

the fundus of the bladder are repaired by a continuous 2–0 chromic catgut suture.

The abdominal wound is closed with intraperitoneal tissue drainage; the bladder is drained by the Foley catheter.

Indirect Reimplantation

Transureteral Ureterostomy (Fig. 15.17)

The exploration and exposure is initially the same as previously described.

The ureter on the opposite side is exposed and mobilised towards the mid-line. The cut end of the affected ureter is then brought across the mid-line and the site for the ureterotomy in the normal ureter is selected. The normal ureter is opened longitudinally for a distance corresponding to the degree of dilatation of the affected ureter; if the affected ureter is not dilated the incision in the normal ureter should be about 1 cm long and the divided ureter should be slightly spatulated to allow a wide anastomosis.

Anastomosis is carried out with interrupted 4–0 chromic catgut sutures about 3 mm apart. Fortunately it appears to be unnecessary to intubate the anastomosis.

The wound is closed with one tissue drain. If this can be made to lie extraperitoneally by creating a subperitoneal tunnel, it is probably slightly preferable to the alternative of transperitoneal drainage.

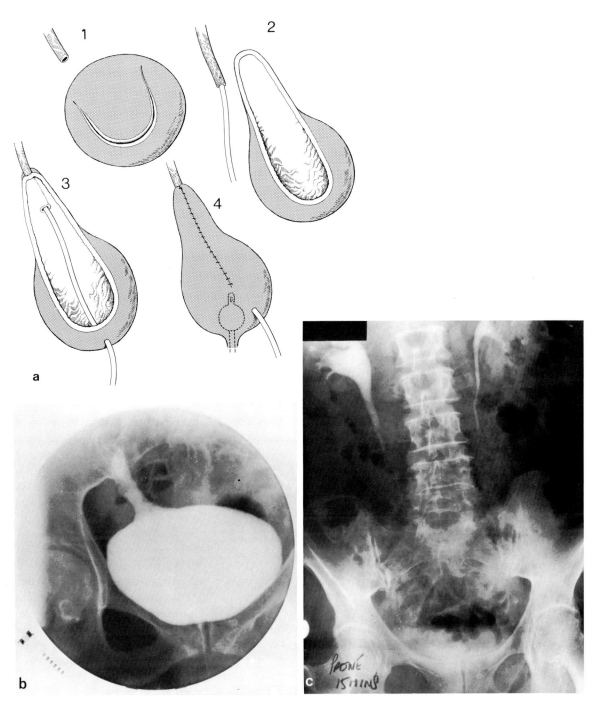

Fig. 15.16. a Construction of bladder flap with implantation of ureter through separate mucosal tunnel. **b** Cystogram. **c** Intravenous urogram 20 years after construction of bladder flap.

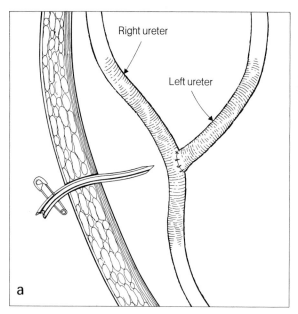

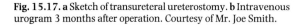

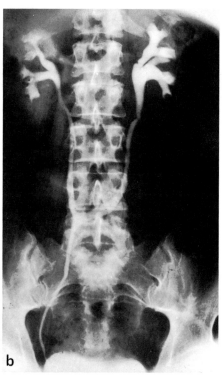

Fig. 15.17. a Sketch of transureteral ureterostomy. b Intravenous urogram 3 months after operation. Courtesy of Mr. Joe Smith.

In the rare circumstances of the patient having previously had a nephrectomy on the opposite side to the ureteric injury, the cut end of the affected ureter can be anastomosed to the residual ureter of the opposite side.

The vast majority of cases of ureterovaginal fistula can be managed by one of the above techniques.

Ileal Replacement (Fig. 15.18)

Ileal replacement of the ureter is of course a much more serious procedure than reimplantation of the ureter into the urinary tract direct. It is not to be considered when the function of the affected kidney is poor and the opposite kidney is normal; the correct treatment in these circumstances is a nephrectomy.

However, in the rare circumstances where the ureteric injury is too high for implantation into the bladder, and when the opposite kidney is not normal or is absent (and its ureter is not suitable for some reason for the affected ureter to be anastomosed to it), the lower part of the ureter should be replaced by a loop of ileum.

Following routine bowel preparation the affected ureter is exposed as previously described. The bladder is mobilised and displaced towards the side of the lesion, as in the direct implantation procedures, so as to minimise the length of ileum required. A suitable segment of terminal ileum with its attached mesentery is isolated as in the construction of an ileal conduit and continuity of the bowel is restored. The loop can easily be made to lie isoperistaltically. The upper end of the loop is closed. The ureter is intubated, the tube being fixed to the ureter about 0.75 cm from its cut edge, which allows this to remain free for anastomosis to the mucosa of the ileum (Fig. 15.18b).

The ileum is opened about 4 cm from its upper end and the ureter anastomosed to it using 4–0 chromic catgut. The bladder is then opened at its highest posterolateral point, and a disc about 2 cm in diameter is excised from its wall. Any excess of ileum and its mesentery is excised. The cut edge of the ileum is then anastomosed to the opening in the bladder by a continuous 3–0 chromic catgut suture. The polythene tube is brought out through the bladder as previously described and the bladder and abdominal wall closed with intraperitoneal tissue drainage (Fig. 15.18a). The bladder is drained by catheter.

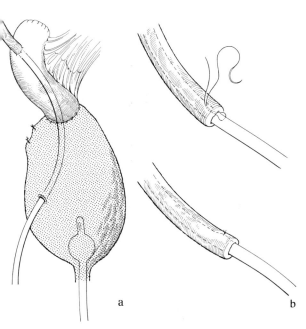

Fig. 15.18. a Method of fixing polyvinyl chloride tube to ureter.
b Replacement of lower part of right ureter with segment of ileum.

Particular care is required in the post-operative phase to ensure that there is no obstruction to the urethral catheter by mucus; it is advisable for the bladder to be gently irrigated 12-hourly—or more frequently if necessary—for the first week. In all these procedures the tissue drain should be shortened on the fourth and removed on the fifth day. The skin suture holding the polythene splint (stent) should be cut at the end of a week; the tube becomes loose within the next 3 days and is easily withdrawn. Closed catheter drainage is maintained for another 2 days.

Bilateral Ureteric Injuries

Any combination of a ureterovaginal fistula on one side and any type of ureteric injury—including a fistula—on the opposite side can occur.

The principle of their management is very similar to unilateral injuries. A particular feature is that the presence of obstruction in the opposite ureter may precipitate the necessity for earlier exploration than would normally be planned for the fistula on the other side.

The injuries may be repaired by; bilateral direct reimplantation; direct implantation and a Boari flap; bilateral implantation into a central Boari flap; bilateral Boari flaps; or a transureteral ureterostomy combined with a Boari flap (Fig. 15.19a–f).

In rare cases of bilateral high ureteral lesions, a loop of lieum, placed isoperistaltically, can be used to replace the pelvic parts of both ureters (Fig. 15.19g).

Primary Nephrectomy

Occasionally removal of the kidney is to be preferred to reimplantation of the ureter. There are no absolute rules. When, in the absence of gross correctable obstruction, the function of the affected kidney is poor (as judged by intravenous urography and sometimes isotope renography) and that of the other kidney normal, or there are radiation changes and residual malignant disease in the pelvis, the decision is easy; and in practice the indications for nephrectomy are fairly obvious in most cases.

In countries where medical services are well developed the combination of ureterovaginal fistula and vesicovaginal fistula is a rarity. The basic principles are similar, the combination of the procedures for a vesicovaginal fistula being combined with the procedures described above for ureterovaginal fistula.

Urinary Diversion

If for any reason the bladder function cannot be restored in a case of ureterovaginal fistula or fistulae, urinary diversion is required. The indications are, therefore, based on the state of the bladder rather than that of the ureter(s).

When (as is usually the case) the pelvic tissues have been irradiated, the only safe and satisfactory procedure is the construction of an ileal conduit.

In the rare circumstances when there has been no previous irradiation, the ureters are of reasonable calibre (e.g. in severe obstetric trauma) and the rectal function has been shown to be adequate by the ability to retain 200 ml urine for 2 h, a ureterocolic anastomosis is usually the procedure of choice (Chap. 12).

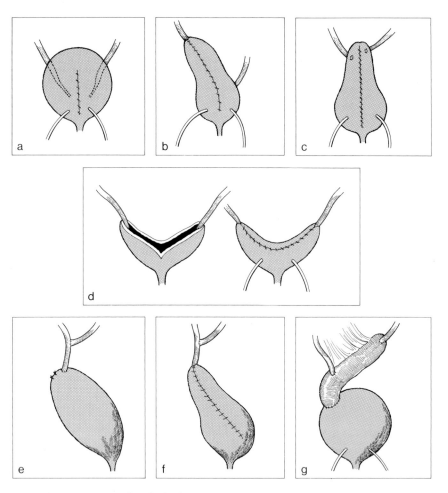

Fig. 15.19a–g. Diagrams of methods of reimplanting ureters in bilateral injuries. **a** Both direct. **b** One direct, other by bladder flap. **c** Both into central bladder flap. **d** Bilateral bladder flaps. **e** Ureteroureterostomy combined with psoas hitch. **f** Transureteral ureterostomy combined with bladder flap. **g** Ileal replacement of both lower ureters. Foley catheter has been omitted for clarity.

Post-operative Complications

Leakage

When a ureter has been divided through healthy tissue and reimplanted without tension, rapid healing without leakage is the usual course. Occasionally there may be slight leakage from the tissue drain or through the vaginal vault, but this will rapidly cease.

Especially if the ureter has been sectioned through irradiated tissue the anastomosis may completely break down, with leakage through the tissue drain or vaginal vault. Should this rare event occur when the opposite kidney is normal a nephrectomy is usually the simplest (and correct) procedure.

Stenosis

Post-operative stenosis at the site of the reimplantation is rare if the state of the ureter and the reimplantation technique were originally satisfactory.

Urinary Infection

Pre-operative urinary tract infection usually subsides rapidly when any obstructive element has been dealt with at the reimplantation. Should renal infection recur and persist after reimplantation, stenosis at the site should be suspected and this will, of course, be demonstrated on an intravenous urogram. The decision between repeating the reimplantation and performing a nephrectomy depends on the factors previously discussed.

Reflux

Ureteric reflux is very frequent if the mucosal tunnel is absent or short. There may be slight loin discomfort on full bladder distension and/or on micturition, and a minor degree of ureteric dilatation, but usually the symptoms subside and the ureteric dilatation does not progress. After reimplantation by means of a Boari flap, ureteric reflux is usually absent. As could be expected, a technically satisfactory reimplanted ureter has the same high success rate as operations primarily for ureteric reflux.

Ureteroureteric reflux after transureteral ureterostomy must obviously be the rule but no complications due to it have been reported.

Late Recurrence of Ureterovaginal Fistula

Recurrence of leakage of urine through the vault of the vagina more than 3 months after reimplantation of the ureter in malignant cases usually indicates a recurrence of growth in the pelvis.

Summary

In the vast majority of cases of ureterovaginal fistula where the renal function on that side is worth preserving, the urinary tract can be reconstructed with very satisfactory results.

Results of procedures to reimplant the ureter into the urinary tract could be expected to vary with a number of factors: variations in the individual ureteric blood supply, infection, irradiation, the diameter of the ureter, the degree of tension accepted by the operator, and variations in the details of technique. It is therefore difficult to present a very accurate prognosis of these procedures. Obviously, lower injuries could be expected to have a better prognosis than higher ones, particularly as many of the latter are no doubt treated as if they were lower than they really are, with resulting tension at the anastomosis.

Personal experience and a review of the literature suggest that unless there are particularly adverse factors an early success rate of around 90% can be expected; later follow-up intravenous urograms show normal upper urinary tracts in about 50% of patients and no more than a moderate degree of dilatation of the ureter in most of the remainder.

Reference

Ockerblad NF (1947) Re-implantation of the ureter into the bladder by a flap method. J Urol 57:845–847

16 Pharmacology of the Bladder and Urethra

Alan J. Wein

Introduction

As a result of the renewed interest in the neuropharmacology and neurophysiology of the urinary bladder and its outlet, pharmacological therapy now exists which is effective in the management of many types of voiding dysfunction. It is the intention of this chapter to summarise briefly the pharmacological principles on which this drug therapy is based, and to show how pharmacological treatment fits into a functional scheme of therapy for disorders of micturition, specifically related to the female patient with urinary incontinence.

Pharmacology of the Lower Urinary Tract

The smooth muscle of the urinary bladder and its outlet is innervated by both the parasympathetic and sympathetic divisions of the autonomic nervous system, while the striated musculature of the external urethral sphincter receives only somatic innervation (Bradley et al. 1974; Kuru 1965; Ruch 1974; Wein and Raezer 1979). The sympathetic division of the autonomic nervous system consists of the fibres originating in the thoracic and lumbar regions of the spinal cord, whereas the parasympathetic division consists of those fibres originating in the cranial and sacral spinal nerves. The terms "sympathetic" and "parasympathetic" thus refer to anatomical divisions of the autonomic nervous system. In both subsystems and in the somatic nervous system other adjectives are used to describe the nature of the chemical transmitter involved in the transmission of impulses from pre-ganglionic to post-ganglionic nerves and from nerves to muscle (Fig. 16.1). "Cholinergic" refers to those receptor sites where acetylcholine is the neurotransmitter. Peripheral cholinergic fibres include somatic motor fibres, pre-ganglionic autonomic fibres and post-ganglionic parasympathetic fibres. Cholinergic receptor sites are further classified as "muscarinic" or "nicotinic" (Koelle 1975a; Mayer 1980). The effects of cholinergic stimulation at peripheral autonomic effector cells, such as bladder smooth-muscle cells, are referred to as muscarinic actions, since the alkaloid muscarine

Neurohumoral transmission

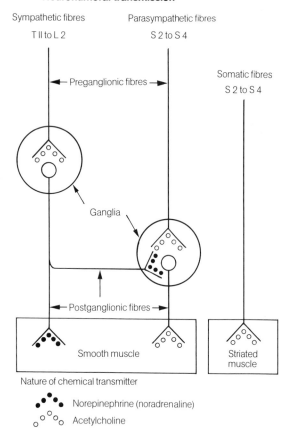

Fig. 16.1. Neuroanatomical and neuropharmacological details of the innervation of the smooth muscle of the bladder and urethra and the striated muscle of the external urethral sphincter. Note the termination of some post-ganglionic sympathetic (adrenergic) fibres on parasympathetic ganglion cells, providing the morphological substrate for sympathetic inhibition of parasympathetic ganglion cell transmission.

also activates these receptors. Atropine generally exhibits a more or less complete blocking action at these receptor sites (Weiner 1980a). Nicotinic effects refer to the low-dose stimulation and high-dose blockade of autonomic ganglia and of the motor end plates of skeletal muscle; such effects are produced by acetylcholine, nicotine and various other agents. The nicotinic receptors of autonomic ganglia and skeletal muscle are not identical, since they respond differently to certain stimulating and blocking agents. However, curare blocks transmission at all nicotinic sites, though more effectively at motor end plates. Receptor sites where noradrenaline is the neurotransmitter are termed "adrenergic", and include most post-ganglionic sympathetic fibres and probably the fibres of certain

tracts in the central nervous system (Koelle 1975a). The term "adrenergic" also technically applies to those receptor sites where other catecholamines may function as transmitters.

Adrenergic receptor sites are classified as "alpha" or "beta" on the basis of the effects elicited by a series of catecholamines (Koelle 1975a; Wein and Raezer 1979; Mayer 1980). Alpha-mediated effects, such as vasoconstriction and contraction of the smooth musculature of the lower urinary tract, are stimulated most potently by noradrenaline and adrenaline and cannot be elicited by isoprenaline. These effects are inhibited by phentolamine and phenoxybenzamine. Recently, there has been a great deal of attention paid to the identification and sub-classification of adrenergic receptors (Hoffman and Lefkowitz 1980; Weinshiebaum 1980; Weiner, 1980b,c). At the present time, the generally accepted convention is that alpha-1 receptors include typical post-synaptic alpha receptors which mediate smooth muscle contraction. Alpha-2 receptors include a group of pre-synaptic (located in the post-ganglionic fibre), autoregulatory receptors whose function is that of a negative feedback mechanism for the release of noradrenaline in response to post-ganglionic neural stimulation. Alpha-2 receptors also include some less typical adrenergic receptors such as those which exist on human platelets. Beta-adrenergic effects, such as cardiac stimulation, vasodilation and smooth muscle relaxation are stimulated most potently by isoprenaline and less so by adrenaline and noradrenaline. These beta effects are antagonised by propranolol. Beta-adrenergic responses can be further subdivided into "beta-1" and "beta-2" types. Beta-1 receptors are located chiefly at cardiac sites, produce inotropy when stimulated, are stimulated more potently by isoprenaline than adrenaline and noradrenaline (equipotent) and are preferentially inhibited by metoprolol. Beta-2 receptors are present primarily in smooth muscle and gland cells. They cause inhibition of smooth muscle contractility when stimulated, are stimulated most potently by isoprenaline, but more so by adrenaline than by noradrenaline, and are somewhat selectively inhibited by butoxamine. In general, the effect of activation of alpha-1 receptors in smooth muscle is excitatory, while that of beta-2 receptors is inhibitory. Activation of alpha-2 receptors inhibits the neural release of noradrenaline (and therefore may decrease an alpha-1 effect caused by neural stimulation).

In addition, specific receptors for dopamine exist which are most potently stimulated by dopamine or dopaminergic agonists, such as apomorphine and bromocriptine, and blocked by dopaminergic antagonists, including phenothiazines, butyrophenones, metoclopramide and sulpiride (Thorner 1975). Specific dopamine receptors have been identified in the mesenteric and renal vascular beds and the central nervous system, and may exist at other sites as well. Although specific cholinergic and alpha- and beta-adrenergic receptor sites exist in abundance in the lower urinary tract, there is at present no published evidence of the existence of specific dopamine receptors in the bladder or urethra. The effect of dopamine on smooth muscle is generally inhibitory (Thorner 1975). Benson et al. (1976b) found that, in vitro, dopamine caused contraction in smooth-muscle strips from the dog proximal urethra, bladder base and bladder body; these responses were, however, all blocked with phentolamine.

Anatomically and embryologically, the bladder has been classically separated into the trigone and the detrusor muscle. Neuroanatomically and neuropharmacologically, however, the bladder is more appropriately divided into base and body (El Badawi and Schenk 1966, 1968, 1971; Raezer et al. 1973). The base is that area lying circumferentially distal to the level at which the ureters enter the detrusor muscle on its posterior aspect, and the body is the area proximal to this level. The posterior base, therefore, consists of the trigone and the detrusor muscle beneath it.

The smooth muscle of the bladder and urethra in a variety of experimental animals and in man contains both alpha-adrenergic receptors (producing contraction) and beta-adrenergic receptors (producing relaxation). Beta receptors are distributed primarily in the bladder body, whereas alpha receptors predominate in the bladder base and the proximal urethra (Awad et al. 1974; Benson et al. 1976a; Donker et al. 1972; Edvardsen 1968a, 1968b, 1968c, 1968d; Raezer et al. 1973; Nergardh 1975; Wein and Levin 1979). Tanagho and his group (Tanagho and Meyers 1969; Tanagho et al. 1969) believe that the urethral adrenergic receptor sites are located in the smooth musculature of the vasculature, and it is stimulation and blockade of these receptors rather than receptors on the urethral smooth musculature itself that produce the changes in urethral resistance seen in response to sympathetic nerve stimulation or alpha-adrenergic agents. However, evidence has been provided by

others (Benson et al. 1976; Donker et al. 1972; Raz and Caine 1972; Raz et al. 1972; Tulloch 1974) that alpha-adrenergic receptor sites are abundant in the urethral smooth musculature itself.

Adrenergic agonists therefore have the potential to facilitate urine storage at a peripheral level in at least two ways (Wein and Raezer 1979). Firstly, the stimulation of contractile alpha-adrenergic receptors in the bladder base and proximal urethral would facilitate functional closure of this area, and secondly activation of the inhibitory beta receptors in the bladder body would directly inhibit bladder muscle contractility in this area. In addition, De Groat (De Groat and Saum 1972, 1976; De Groat and Theobald 1976) has described a further adrenergic mechanism by which bladder contractility can be inhibited: sympathetic nerve-induced depression of transmission in vesical parasympathetic ganglia (Fig. 16.1). This effect, although inhibitory, has been found to be mediated by alpha-adrenergic receptors.

The smooth muscle of the bladder and urethra in a variety of experimental animals and in man has been shown to contain typical atropine-sensitive muscarinic receptor sites (Todd and Mack 1969; Raezer et al. 1973; Nergardh 1975; Khanna 1976; Benson et al. 1976a,c). Quantitation of these receptor sites, using a specific radioligand assay, shows quite clearly that muscarinic receptor sites are more common in the bladder body than in the bladder base (Levin et al. 1980a). A sustained bladder contraction is generally produced by stimulation of the parasympathetic pelvic nerves (Wein and Raezer 1979; De Groat and Booth 1984). The potent muscarinic blocking agent atropine only partially antagonises the bladder response to this or to direct electrical stimulation of bladder smooth muscle strips, although it does completely antagonise the response of bladder smooth muscle strips to exogenously administered acetylcholine. The most attractive explanation for this relative "atropine resistance" phenomenon is that a portion of the neurotransmitter released by pelvic nerve stimulation is non-cholinergic in nature (see Wein and Raezer 1979, for a complete discussion). Burnstock (1979) has proposed that this "missing" contractile neurotransmitter is purinergic, i.e. that the non-cholinergic induced portion of the bladder contraction is secondary to the neural liberation of adenosine triphosphate (ATP). There are a number of other substances which have been theorised to be released upon pelvic nerve stimulation, and which have been proposed as alternate excitatory neurotransmitter or neuromodulators, notably histamine, various prostaglandins and serotonin.

Pelvic nerve stimulation and stimulation by acetylcholine or acetylcholine-like agents have been noted in some in vivo experiments to cause an increase in urethral resistance (Khanna et al. 1975; Tanagho et al. 1969). However, in this type of experimental preparation it is difficult to differentiate functional changes in the components of urethral resistance that occur as a result of detrusor contraction from changes that result from the direct stimulation of receptors in the urethral smooth musculature. Adaptive changes in the musculature of the bladder outlet during voiding would tend to decrease urethral resistance, while transmission of the intravesical pressure head during micturition would tend to increase it. Nergardh and Boreus (1973) found that urethral resistance to flow in the cat was increased by endogenous or exogenous acetylcholine, and proposed that this effect was mediated via short intramural ganglion cells belonging to the sympathetic system. According to their theory, noradrenaline, not acetylcholine, is released at this neuroeffector site. This type of analysis would also explain the atropine resistance of this effect. However, in vitro studies of human urethral strips performed by Ek et al. (1977) demonstrated a low sensitivity to acetylcholine, and the contractile responses that did occur were blocked with atropine. Similar data presented by Persson and Andersson (1976) for the cat and the guinea pig suggest that the effect on the urethra of pelvic nerve stimulation or exogenous acetylcholine is mediated by muscarinic cholinergic receptors rather than by the short adrenergic neuron system.

Most of the agents which alter the urodynamics of the lower urinary tract affect (a) synthesis, transport, storage or release of neurotransmitter, or (b) the combination of the neurotransmitter with post-junctional receptors, or (c) the inactivation, degradation or reuptake of neurotransmitter. It is obvious that the complex metabolic changes which occur after receptor activation are also potential sites of pharmacological stimulation, inhibition or modulation. Calcium plays an important role in excitation–contraction coupling in striated, cardiac and smooth muscle cells (Andersson 1978). The dependence of contractile activity on the inflow of calcium from extracellular sources or on its release from intracellular stores varies from tissue to tissue, but interference with these processes, interference

with intracellular calcium utilising mechanisms or acceleration of calcium extrusion from the cells are all potential mechanisms for the mediation of at least vascular smooth muscle relaxation (Movsesian 1982). Such mechanisms which are "metabolically distal" to the membrane receptor sites, whether concerned with calcium metabolism or other as yet unexplored factors influencing contractility, are also obvious potential sites of pharmacological stimulation, inhibition or modulation. Finally, the recent knowledge "explosion" in the field of neuropeptide physiology has also provided potentially new insights into lower urinary tract function and its pharmacological alteration. Endogenous encephalins are thought to exert a tonic inhibitory effect on the micturition reflex (Roppolo et al. 1983; De Groat and Booth 1984), and agents such as narcotic antagonists offer a new possibility for stimulating reflex bladder activity (Vaidyanathan et al. 1981; Thor et al. 1983). Vasoactive intestinal polypeptide (VIP) is inhibitory in vitro to bladder smooth muscle activity and a decreased concentration of this in bladder tissue may be associated with the unstable bladder syndrome (Mundy 1984), raising another possibility for future therapeutic alterations to influence bladder contractility.

Principles of Pharmacological Therapy

Most pharmacological agents produce their effects by combining with specialised functional components of cells. The cell component directly involved in the initial action of a drug is known as its receptor. The drug-receptor interaction alters the function of the cell component involved, and initiates the series of biochemical and physiological changes that characterise the effects produced by the agent. The agents discussed here either affect a step in neurohumoral transmission, each representing a potential point of pharmacological stimulation, inhibition or modulation, or have a direct effect on the smooth muscle itself.

In considering any description of drug effects, one must remember that: (a) pharmacological agents may act at more than one site and even at several sites within a neural pathway or a muscle; (b) they may have different effects at different concentrations; (c) species differences in pharmacological responses may exist; and (d) the type, location and physiological state of a neural pathway or muscle may influence its response to a particular drug.

It should be remembered that the acute effects of a drug may differ from its long-term effects. Also, multiple effects can occur at any of the levels of action, each within a different time scale. The sensitivity, number and type of receptors in a particular tissue can be affected by its physiological state (denervation, distention, hypertrophy, inflammation, ischaemia) and by the drug itself.

Specific Methods of Pharmacological Therapy

The lower urinary tract performs two basic functions: the storage and the emptying of urine. All varieties of voiding dysfunction and their therapy can be very simply classified according to how well the bladder performs these two functions (Table 16.1) (Wein et al. 1976; Wein 1981). Table 16.1 clearly shows in what situations the various types of pharmacological therapy are potentially applicable. The ensuing discussion about the use of specific agents will follow this basic outline. Generally speaking, the simplest and least hazardous form of treatment should be tried first. A combination of therapeutic manoeuvres or pharmacological agents can sometimes be used to achieve a particular effect, especially if their mechanisms of action are different and their side-effects are not synergistic. It should be noted that, in our experience, although great improvement often occurs with rational pharmacological therapy, a perfect result (restoration to normal status) is seldom achieved.

Therapy to Facilitate Bladder Emptying

Inadequate bladder emptying may cause the type of urinary incontinence generally referred to as retention with overflow. A complete or relative failure to empty the bladder may coexist with any of the various kinds of urinary incontinence seen in the female (Stanton 1977) or may follow corrective surgery for this dysfunction (Stanton et al. 1978). The causes of this inability to empty may be

a permanent or temporary impairment of nerve function, anatomical or functional bladder outlet obstruction or a permanent or temporary impairment of bladder contractility (e.g. smooth-muscle hypotonia). Whatever the aetiology, potential pharmacological treatment includes measures to increase intravesical pressure by increasing bladder contractility, measures to decrease outlet resistance, or both (see Table 16.1).

Increasing Intravesical Pressure

Acetylcholine itself cannot be used for therapeutic purposes because of its diffuse actions (nicotinic and central, as well as muscarinic) and because of its rapid hydrolysis by acetylcholinesterase and non-specific cholinesterase (Koelle 1975b; Taylor 1980). Many acetylcholine-like drugs exist—methacholine, carbachol, bethanechol chloride, pilocarpine, muscarine and arecoline. However, only bethanechol chloride (Myotonechol, Myotonine, Duvoid, Urecholine) exhibits a relatively selective action on the urinary bladder and gut, with little or no action at therapeutic dosages on ganglia or on the cardiovascular system (Koelle 1975b; Ursillo 1967). Bethanechol chloride is cholinesterase resistant and causes a contraction in vitro of smooth muscle from all areas of the bladder (Raezer et al. 1973). It has been recommended in a subcutaneous dose of 5–10 mg for the treatment of post-operative or post-partum urinary retention. It should be used in this instance only if the patient is awake and alert and there is no outlet obstruction. Lapides, Diokno and Sonda (Diokno and Koppenhoeffer 1976; Diokno and Lapides 1977; Lapides 1964, 1974; Sonda et al. 1979) have reported its usefulness in "rehabilitating" atonic or hypotonic bladders; the drug is administered subcutaneously in a dosage of 5–10 mg every 4–6 h and the patient is asked to try to void by the clock (optimally, 10–20 min after a subcutaneous dose). This regimen may be initiated with an indwelling catheter in place and the catheter removed after a few doses have been administered, or with the patient on intermittent catheterisation. When the residual urine has decreased to an acceptable level, the subcutaneous dosage is decreased to 5 mg q.i.d. and then changed to an oral dose of 50–100 mg q.i.d. Subsequently, the drug can sometimes be discontinued altogether. In cases of partial but incomplete bladder emptying, a therapeutic trial of the oral agent in a dosage of

Table 16.1. Functional classification of therapy for disorders of micturition

I. Therapy to facilitate bladder emptying
A. Increase intravesical pressure
  1. External compression
  2. Promotion of initiation of reflex contractions
    a) Trigger zones or manoeuvres
    b) Bladder training, tidal drainage
  3. Pharmacological manipulation
    a) Parasympathomimetic agents (acetylcholine-like agents, anti-cholinesterases)
    b) Blockers of inhibition (alpha-adrenergic blockade; opioid antagonists?)
  4. Electrical stimulation
    a) Directly to the bladder
    b) To the spinal cord or nerve roots
B. Decrease outlet resistance
  1. At the level of the bladder neck
    a) Incision or resection
    b) Y–V plasty of the bladder neck
    c) Pharmacological manipulation (alpha-adrenergic blockade, beta-adrenergic stimulation?)
  2. At the level of distal mechanism[a]
    a) External spincterotomy
    b) Urethral over-dilatation
    c) Pudendal nerve interruption
    d) Pharmacological inhibition
      i) External sphincter/pelvic floor (striated muscle relaxant, mono- and polysynaptic spinal cord reflex inhibition)
      ii) Proximal urethra (alpha-adrenergic blockade, beta-adrenergic stimulation?)
    e) Psychotherapy, biofeedback
C. Circumvent problem
  1. Intermittent catheterisation
  2. Urinary diversion
	II. Therapy to facilitate urine storage
	A. Inhibit bladder contractility
	  1. Pharmacological manipulation
	    a) Anticholinergic agents
	    b) Beta-adrenergic stimulation
	    c) Musculotropic relaxants
	    d) Polysynaptic inhibitors
	    e) Calcium antagonists
	    f) Prostaglandin inhibitors
	  2. Interruption of innervation
	    a) Subarachnoid block
	    b) Sacral rhizotomy
	    c) Peripheral bladder denervation
	  3. Bladder distension
	  4. Electrical stimulation (reflex inhibition)
	  5. Augmentation cystoplasty[b]
	B. Increase outlet resistance
	  1. At the level of the bladder neck
	    a) Alpha-adrenergic stimulation, beta-adrenergic blockade?
	    b) Vesicourethral suspension
	    c) Mechanical compression
	  2. At the level of the distal mechanism
	    a) Alpha-adrenergic stimulation (smooth muscle), beta-adrenergic blockade?
	    b) Mechanical compression
	    c) Electrical stimulation of the pelvic floor
	C. Circumvent problem
	  1. Intermittent catheterisation
	  2. Urinary diversion

[a] Includes the smooth muscle of the proximal urethra and the striated musculature of the external and intramural urethral sphincter.
[b] Augments bladder capacity and secondarily inhibits bladder contractility by raising volume thresholds for sensation and distension.

25–100 mg q.i.d. can be used in conjunction with timed voiding every 4 h with the Credé manoeuvre.

Our own experience with bethanechol chloride in the treatment of patients with inadequate bladder emptying has been disappointing. Similar views have been expressed by Gibbon (1965), Merrill and Rotta (1974), Yalla et al. (1977a) and Light and Scott (1982) with respect to its use in neurogenic bladder dysfunction. Although a subcutaneous dose of 5 mg does increase the intravesical pressure at all points along the accommodation curve of the cystometrogram and does decrease the bladder capacity threshold (Lapides et al. 1963; Yalla et al. 1977b; Sonda et al. 1979), its ability to stimulate a physiological bladder contraction in a patient who cannot normally initiate one is questionable. Our own evidence suggests that this generally does not occur. What does seem to occur is an increase in tension in all areas of the bladder smooth muscle,

such as one would expect from in vitro studies. Although augmentation of "weak" detrusor contractions may occur, documentation of this phenomenon is difficult. In addition, urethral resistance may actually be increased by parenteral bethanechol chloride, an observation made originally by Tanagho's group (Tanagho et al. 1969). We tried a pharmacologically active subcutaneous dose (5 mg) but could not demonstrate significant changes in flow parameters or residual urine, either in women with a residual urine volume equal to or greater than 20% of bladder capacity but with no evidence of neurological disease or outlet obstruction, or in a group of 27 "normal" women of approximately the same mean age (Wein et al. 1980b). A similar dose also failed to produce urodynamic evidence of improved emptying in patients with a positive bethanechol supersensitivity test (Wein et al. 1980a). This dosage, however, did increase the intravesical pressure at all points along the filling limb of the cystometrogram and also decreased the bladder capacity threshold, consistent with findings previously described by others. The effectiveness of oral bethanechol chloride is even more questionable. In a double-blind study we failed to demonstrate any significant dose-related cystometric or subjective response in a group of men who received up to 100 mg orally (Wein et al. 1978). Diokno and Lapides (1977) did demonstrate a statistically significant increase in intravesical pressure at 100 ml volume 2 h after the oral administration of 100 mg bethanechol chloride to a group of patients with hypotonic bladders, but this pressure increase amounted to only 5 cmH$_2$O. They, too, found that a single 50-mg dose had no effect.

Philip et al. (1980) reported that a 4 mg oral dose of carbachol, a cholinergic agonist which possesses also some ganglionic stimulating properties, had a much greater effect on urodynamic parameters than a 50-mg dose of bethanechol, without an apparent increase in side effects. This agent is available only as an optic solution in the United States. Anticholinesterase agents, which inhibit the enzymatic degradation of acetylcholine, also have the net effect of producing or enhancing cholinergic stimulation. Cameron (1966) reported that distigmine bromide, a long-acting anticholinesterase, was effective in preventing post-operative urinary retention. Philip and Thomas (1980) have reported that parenteral, but not oral, distigmine improved voiding efficiency in patients with neurogenic bladder dysfunction with reflex detrusor activity. They recommended an intramuscular dose of 0.5 mg of this agent per day. It is also available as a 5-mg oral preparation.

Can repeated oral or subcutaneous doses of a cholinergic agonist achieve an effect that a single dose cannot? The mechanisms involved in such an effect might conceivably include a change in the number or sensitivity of cholinergic receptors, a desensitisation of some tonic inhibitory effect on the bladder muscle cell or a facilitation of the micturition reflex arc. However, no evidence, in our opinion, exists at present to substantiate any such effects. Studies purporting to show long-term rather than acute effects must totally exclude the effects of other manoeuvres such as surgical procedures, timed voiding with Credé and bladder decompression. As far as the "rehabilitative" effect of the agent on hypotonic detrusor is concerned, no pharmacological basis for such an action has been demonstra-

ted and such reported effects must be carefully distinguished from the benefits of other simultaneous manoeuvres. Can a cholinergic agonist be combined with agents to decrease outlet resistance and thereby facilitate voiding? Khanna (1976) gave patients with atonic bladders and functional outlet obstruction a daily dose of 50–100 mg oral bethanechol chloride combined with 20–30 mg phenoxybenzamine and reported satisfactory results. Our own experience in this situation with such combined pharmacological therapy, utilising even 200 mg of oral bethanechol daily, has been extremely disappointing. Certainly, most would agree that a daily dose of 50–100 mg rarely affects any urodynamic parameter at all (Lapides et al. 1963; Diokno and Lapides 1977; Wein et al. 1978; Philip et al. 1980; Barrett 1981).

The potential side-effects of the cholinergic agonists and the anticholinesterase agents are similar, and include flushing, nausea, vomiting, diarrhoea, gastrointestinal cramps, bronchospasm, headache, salivation, sweating and difficulty with visual accommodation (Taylor 1980). Intramuscular or intravenous use of bethanechol is contraindicated, as such use can precipitate acute and severe side-effects resulting in acute circulatory failure and cardiac arrest. Contraindications to the use of these general categories of drug include bronchial asthma, peptic ulcer, bowel obstruction, enteritis, history of recent gastrointestinal surgery, cardiac arrhythmia, hyperthyroidism and any type of bladder outlet obstruction.

Other agents have been shown to have direct stimulatory effects on bladder smooth muscle. Of these, only the prostaglandins have been tried clinically. Bultitude et al. (1976) hypothesised that both prostaglandins and acetylcholine were necessary for the maintenance of bladder tone and spontaneous bladder activity. They summarised their supporting evidence as follows: (a) prostaglandins were produced by the bladder; (b) PGE$_2$ and PGF$_{2a}$ caused a dose-related contraction in in vitro bladder strips; and (c) inhibitors of prostaglandin synthesis caused a decrease in bladder tone and spontaneous activity. Other experiments have suggested that prostaglandins may contribute to purinergic excitation of rabbit and guinea pig bladder (Andersson et al. 1980; Anderson 1982). Instillation of 0.5 mg PGE$_2$ into the bladders of females with varying degrees of urinary retention was reported to result in acute emptying and to improve long-term emptying in two-thirds of the patients studied (Bultitude et al.

1976). Desmond et al. (1980) also reported favourable results with this agent in patients whose bladders exhibited no contractile activity or in whom bladder contractility was relatively impaired. A 1.5-mg dose of PGE_2 in diluent was infused intravesically and left for 1 h. Twenty of 36 patients showed a strongly positive and six a weakly positive immediate response. Fourteen patients showed prolonged beneficial effects, all but one of whom had shown a strongly positive immediate response. Stratification of the data revealed that an intact sacral reflex arc was a prequisite for any type of positive response. The authors also noted that the effects of PGE_2 appeared to be additive or synergistic with cholinergic stimulation in some patients. Other reliable investigators, including Stanton (1978) and Delaere et al. (1981), have reported no success with this type of treatment. Prostaglandins have a relatively short half-life and it is difficult to understand how any effects after a single application can last up to even several months. If such an effect does occur, it must be the result of a "triggering effect" on some as yet unknown physiological or metabolic mechanism. Potential side-effects of prostaglandin usage include bronchospasm, chills, hypotension, tachycardia, cardiac arrhythmia, convulsions, hypocalcaemia and diarrhoea (Moncada et al. 1980).

If the sympathetic nervous system promotes urine storage by exerting an inhibitory effect on parasympathetic ganglionic transmission, by directly inhibiting bladder-body muscle contractility via beta-adrenergic receptors and by stimulating the contractile alpha-adrenergic receptors in the bladder neck and proximal urethra, a theoretical basis exists for the use of adrenergic blocking agents to increase bladder contractility and at the same time decrease outlet resistance. Guanethidine (Hartviksen 1966) and methyldopa (Raz et al. 1977) have been used with this rationale, but subsequent reports of their efficacy have not appeared. Raz (Raz and Smith 1976) advocated a trial of alpha-adrenolytic therapy (phenoxybenzamine in doses of 10–40 mg per day) for the treatment of non-obstructive urinary retention. Theoretically, at least, a doubly beneficial effect occurs: urethral resistance is decreased and, at the same time, pelvic parasympathetic ganglionic transmission is facilitated. We have had some anecdotal success using this approach, but would caution that this mechanism of clinical facilitation of bladder contractility has been inferred from De Groat's work

with cats (De Groat and Saum 1972, 1976; De Groat and Theobald 1976) and has not yet been shown to exist in humans. Clearly, similar neurophysiological studies in other species are necessary, as well as a double-blind clinical trial.

Decreasing Outlet Resistance

Functional outlet obstruction may occur at the level of the smooth musculature of the bladder neck, the proximal urethra or both. This diagnosis should be considered when inadequate emptying occurs despite an adequate bladder contraction in a patient without anatomical obstruction or external sphincter dyssynergy. It may also be confirmed by a successful therapeutic trial with an alpha-adrenergic blocking agent (Johnston and Farkas 1975; Khanna 1976; Krane and Olsson 1973; Mobley 1976; Stockamp 1975; Stockamp and Schreiter 1975; Whitfield et al. 1976). A successful result can often be correlated with an objective change in the urethral pressure profile (a decrease in pressure along the profile curve and a decrease in the area under the functional urethral length). The effectiveness of such therapy can often be predicted by measuring the urinary flow rate before and after an intravenous dose of 5 mg phenotolamine (Regitine) and plotting the results on a normogram relating the flow rate to volume voided (Olsson et al. 1977). Many of the studies that report successful results with such therapy have been poorly controlled, and at least some of the favourable results are probably due to simultaneous changes in other variables. It is obvious, however, that such drugs are pharmacologically active and capable of improving voiding in selected cases.

There is also a rationale for the addition of alpha-adrenolytic therapy in the patient with inadequate emptying secondary to neuropathic voiding dysfunction, after conventional pharmacological treatment has failed, such as after radical pelvic surgery. It has been reported that parasympathetic decentralisation leads to a marked increase in adrenergic innervation of the bladder, with a resultant conversion in response to sympathetic stimulation of the usual beta response of the bladder body to an alpha effect (Norlen et al. 1976; Sundin et al. 1977). Although the alterations in innervation have been disputed (Nordling et al. 1980), the alteration in receptor function has not. Koyanagi

(1978, 1979) showed supersensitivity of the urethra to alpha-adrenergic stimulation in a group of patients with autonomous neuropathic bladders. This implies a similar change in adrenergic receptor function in the urethra with parasympathetic decentralisation. Parsons and Turton (1980) provide a different pharmacological explanation for a similar type of neuropathic urethra. They ascribe the cause to adrenergic supersensitivity of the urethral smooth muscle caused by sympathetic decentralisation, resulting in an inappropriately high sensitivity to alterations in circulating catecholamine levels brought about as a part of normal cardiovascular homeostasis. Nordling et al. (1981) describe a similar phenomenon in females after radical hysterectomy and attribute this change to damage to the sympathetic innervation of the lower urinary tract. In addition to the effect on smooth muscle, it has been suggested that alpha-adrenergic blocking agents may decrease perineal striated muscle activity and that this action may contribute to their effect in decreasing outlet resistance (Nanninga et al. 1977). If this is so, it would seem that such a mechanism must be a central one, or must be mediated by non-innervated receptors, as adrenergic innervation of the striated urethral sphincter seems lacking (Wein et al. 1979; Rossier et al. 1982).

Phenoxybenzamine is the alpha-adrenolytic agent which was most commonly used in the treatment of voiding dysfunction (Wein 1980). The initial adult dosage of this agent is 10 mg daily. The dose may be increased by 10 mg every 4–5 days to a recommended maximum of 60 mg daily. Daily doses larger than 10 mg are generally divided and given every 8–12 h. The maximum effect of a particular dose usually becomes apparent only after a week following the initiation of, or a change in, therapy. After discontinuation, the effects of daily administration persist for about the same period of time. We found that patients who responded favourably to this agent generally did so at doses less than 30 mg and did not respond to dose increases with incremental improvement. Some patients who responded to 10 mg daily could be maintained on an even lower dose. Potential side-effects include orthostatic hypotension, reflex tachycardia, nasal congestion, diarrhoea, miosis, sedation and nausea and vomiting (secondary to local irritation) (Weiner 1980c). Those who still use phenoxybenzamine for long-term therapy should be aware of the recently reported adverse in vitro and in vivo mutagenicity

studies with this agent (McNally 1982). These reports indicate that phenoxybenzamine produced increases in gene mutation in in vitro systems employing Salmonella bacteria and mouse lymphoma cells, but it did not increase the frequency of micronuclei in mouse bone marrow cells in vivo. Further, a more recent letter from the manufacturer indicated a dose-related incidence of gastrointestinal tumours in rats (Tannenbaum 1984). Although this agent has been in use for some 30 years in humans without any adverse epidemiological associations, it is obvious that one must now carefully consider the potential medicolegal ramifications of long-term phenoxybenzamine therapy, especially in younger individuals.

Prazosin hydrochloride (Minipress) is a new antihypertensive agent with an affinity for post-synaptic alpha-1 receptors, at least in vascular smooth muscle (Graham and Pettinger 1979; Weiner 1980c). It has little affinity for alpha-2 receptors, in contrast to phentolamine and phenoxybenzamine, both of which have blocking properties at both alpha-1 and alpha-2 receptor sites. Prazosin causes alpha-1 blockade in the smooth muscle of the canine and human urethra (MacGregor and Diokno 1981; Andersson et al. 1981) and has also been used successfully and safely to lower outlet resistance in some patients (Andersson et al. 1981). In this respect, it is theoretically preferable to phenoxybenzamine because of its relatively selective blockade of post-synaptic receptor sites. It also produces less tachycardia because of a lesser increase in plasma noradrenaline. Therapy with prazosin is generally begun in daily divided doses of 2–3 mg. The dose may be very gradually increased to a maximum of 20 mg daily, although we seldom use more than 12–15 mg daily in three divided doses. The exact daily dose which is equivalent to the "standard" 10 mg dose of phenoxybenzamine for voiding dysfunction is as yet unknown, but seems to us to be 9–12 mg in most patients. The potential side-effects of prazosin are due to its alpha-1 blockade. Additionally, the "first dose phenomenon" occurs occasionally: a symptom complex of faintness, dizziness, palpitation, and (infrequently) syncope, thought to be due to acute postural hypotension. The incidence of this phenomenon can be minimised by restricting the initial dose of the drug to 1 mg and by administering this dosage at bedtime. Other side-effects associated with chronic prazosin therapy are generally mild and rarely necessitate withdrawal of the drug (Graham and Pettinger 1979).

Beta-adrenergic stimulation has been shown experimentally to decrease the urethral pressure profile and by inference urethral resistance (Raz and Caine 1971). This accounts for the decrease in urethral closure pressure after administration of terbutaline, a relatively specific beta-2 agonist (Vaidyanathan et al. 1980). Whether this drug or other pharmacologically similar agents will prove useful to facilitate bladder emptying by decreasing outlet resistance is still unanswered.

Functional obstruction can occur also at the level of the striated musculature which comprises the external and intramural urethral sphincter. Although this entity is usually seen only in patients with overt neurological damage between the sacral spinal cord and the brain stem, it can be seen in patients without a demonstrable neurological deficit (Allen 1977; Raz and Smith 1976). Unfortunately, there is no pharmacological agent that will selectively relax the striated musculature of the pelvic floor. Various drugs do exist that are classified as "centrally acting muscle relaxants" (Bianchine 1980). These include diazepam (Valium), chlordiazepoxide hydrochloride (Librium), methocarbamol (Robaxin) and orphenadrine citrate (Norflex). Diazepam is the most widely used drug of this group. Recommended dosages range as high as 10–15 mg q.i.d. in adults. The primary side-effect of all members of this group of agents is noticeable sedation, which many feel is largely responsible for its muscle relaxing effect when administered orally. Some controlled studies of the efficacy of diazepam as a muscle relaxant exist, but only a few show any advantage over a placebo or aspirin (Byck 1975). Although free of autonomic side-effects, diazepam can have undesirable adverse reactions, most commonly drowsiness, ataxia and fatigue. If the aetiology of incomplete emptying is obscure and the patient has what appears to be inadequate relaxation of the pelvic floor, a trial of diazepam may be worthwhile. Beneficial results which occasionally occur under these conditions, however, may be due to the drug's anti-anxiety effect, or to the modified biofeedback therapy which consciously or unconsciously accompanies such therapy in these patients. Dantrolene sodium (Dantrium) is a relatively new skeletal muscle relaxant that directly affects skeletal muscle by acting upon excitation-contraction coupling (Bianchine 1980). The drug has no autonomic side-effects, but especially at higher doses it may induce generalised weakness severe enough to compromise its therapeutic bene-

fits. Other potential side-effects include transient euphoria and dizziness, diarrhoea and severe hepatotoxicity (which should be checked with frequent liver function studies). The drug has been used with success in some patients with classical detrusor-external sphincter dyssynergy (Murdock et al. 1976), but our results and those of others (Teague and Merrill 1978) have been suboptimal. We do not recommend the routine use of this agent in the patient with presumed external sphincter dyssynergy but no other neurological findings.

Baclofen (Lioresal), a derivative of γ-aminobutyric acid, is an agent which inhibits the transmission of monosynaptic and polysynaptic spinal cord reflexes and has been found to be useful in the treatment of skeletal spasticity due to a variety of causes (Duncan et al. 1976; Kiesswetter and Schober 1975; Bianchine 1980). It may prove to be the pharmacological treatment of choice for external sphincter dyssynergy associated with a spinal cord lesion, and may also depress uninhibited bladder contractions secondary to a spinal cord lesion (Kiesswetter and Schober 1975). Side-effects may include drowsiness, insomnia, rash, pruritus, dizziness and weakness. Treatment should be started at a dosage of 5 mg t.i.d. and the dose doubled every 3 days until a total daily dose of 60 mg is reached. The manufacturer recommends that the maximum dose does not exceed 20 mg q.i.d. The drug should be discontinued gradually to prevent the hallucinations that sometimes occur after abrupt withdrawal (Abromowicz 1978). This agent should be used only in those with an obvious neurological deficit and should not be used empirically for the patient with a failure to empty.

Therapy to Facilitate Urine Storage

Classical (genuine) stress urinary incontinence is primarily a sphincter dysfunction and is, by definition, not associated with involuntary bladder contractions or decreased compliance. Pharmacological therapy directed primarily at increasing outlet resistance by stimulating adrenergic receptor sites in the smooth musculature of the bladder neck and proximal urethra may be effective in controlling or significantly improving such incontinence in many patients. A trial of this therapy may be offered as an alternative to surgical therapy or used in an attempt to supplement surgical therapy where the latter has produced only marginal or only temporary improvement.

Incontinence with or without urgency may result also from involuntary bladder contractions, which may be secondary to neurological disease, bladder outlet obstruction, or inflammatory disease (in our experience), or may be idiopathic. This type of incontinence may exist alone, together with classical stress incontinence, or may develop after corrective bladder or urethral surgery. Pharmacological attempts at treatment utilise agents that decrease bladder smooth muscle contractility.

The symptom of urgency, a term applied to both a strong desire to void or the feeling of imminent micturition, is one of the most distressing and problematical complaints with which the urologist and gynecologist must deal. This complaint may exist alone, with sphincteric (stress) incontinence or detrusor (involuntary bladder contraction or decreased compliance) incontinence, or may develop after surgery on the lower urinary tract. The treatment of this symptom is, initially at least, usually empirical and consists of using one or a combination of the agents used to inhibit bladder contractility. Often, however, this symptom is not associated with involuntary bladder activity, which most probably accounts for the generally less than optimal results achieved with this type of treatment. Urodynamic evaluation of these patients may show marked variations in urethral pressure or may be entirely normal. Whether attempts at pharmacological correction of urethral urodynamic abnormalities would significantly alter symptomatology is as yet unknown, but they offer some promise for future attempts at therapy. Certainly it would seem that the ideal treatment for this type of urgency, which seems to be more sensory than motor in origin, would be an agent that produces topical anaesthesia or hypoaesthesia of the bladder and urethral mucosa. Although there are agents that are reported to have this action as their primary effect (e.g. Pyridium), in our hands the clinical results obtained with such compounds have been poor. There is no doubt that, in at least some of these patients, the symptom of urgency exists on a psychosomatic basis. However, in many there may indeed exist an as yet undetected abnormality which may ultimately prove to be correctable by pharmacological or surgical means.

Inhibiting Bladder Contractility

Atropine and atropine-like agents produce a competitive blockade of acetylcholine receptors, primarily at post-ganglionic autonomic receptor sites (Weiner 1980a). In general, these agents (known as antimuscarinic agents, since they antagonise the muscarinic effects of acetylcholine) have little effect at nicotinic receptor sites, such as autonomic ganglia. They will depress involuntary bladder contractions of any aetiology. In patients with this urodynamic finding and a resultant inadequacy of urine storage, bladder capacity will often be increased and attendant symptoms reduced (Diokno et al. 1972; Pedersen and Grynderup 1966; Wein et al. 1976; Blaivas et al. 1980; Jensen 1981). Involuntary bladder contractions, whatever their aetiology, can generally be only partly inhibited, however, because of the previously mentioned relative insensitivity to atropine or atropine derivatives of bladder contractions mediated through the pelvic nerve. Interestingly, bladder compliance in normal individuals and in those with detrusor hyperreflexia, where the initial slope of the filling curve on cystometry is normal prior to the involuntary contraction, does not seem to be significantly altered (Jensen 1981) by antimuscarinic therapy. The effect of these agents on intravesical pressure during filling in patients who exhibit only decreased compliance has not been well studied.

Propantheline bromide (Pro Banthine) is the agent most commonly used clinically to produce this antimuscarinic effect. In adults it is given orally in dosages of 15–30 mg every 4–6 h. Clinical efficacy can often be predicted by observation of the effect of a 15–30 mg intravenous dose on the cystometrogram, a manoeuvre that may also be useful in the differential diagnosis of the aetiology of a small capacity bladder. The parenteral preparation is no longer available (at least in many hospitals in the United States) and atropine or glycopyrrolate may be used instead. For such studies we generally give 0.2 mg glycopyrrolate (available as a 1-cc single-dose vial) (Mirakhur and Dundee 1980). The side-effects of antimuscarinic agents may include drying of salivary secretions, blurred vision, mydriasis, increased heart rate, drowsiness and constipation. As propantheline possesses some ganglionic blocking activity, it may also cause orthostatic hypotension and impotence in men. It should not be given to patients with narrow angle glaucoma and should be used with caution in patients with significant bladder outlet obstruction, as it may significantly worsen urinary emptying, even to the point of precipitating complete urinary retention. There seems to be little difference between the antimuscarinic effects of propantheline and those of other antimuscarinic compounds such as hyoscyamine (Cystospaz), glycopyrrolate (Robinul), isopropamide iodide (Darbid) and anisotropine methylbromide (Valpin) (Weiner 1980a). Although there are obviously many other considerations which account for the activity of a given dose of a drug at its site of action, there is no oral drug available whose direct antimuscarinic binding potential, at least in vitro, approximates that of atropine better than the long available and relatively inexpensive propantheline bromide (Levin et al. 1982). Methantheline (Banthine) has a higher ratio of ganglionic blocking to antimuscarinic activity, but propantheline is more potent in each respect, dose for dose.

Emepronium bromide (Cetiprin) is classified as an anticholinergic agent with both antimuscarinic and ganglionic blocking (antinicotinic) effects (Stanton 1973; Hebjorn and Walter 1978). It, too, can increase bladder capacity in patients with involuntary bladder contractions, while decreasing intravesical pressure and urinary flow (Ekeland and Sander 1976). The recommended oral dosage ranges from 100 to 200 mg three to four times daily. However, there are significant doubts as to its effectiveness when administered orally (because of poor absorption) (Ritch et al. 1977), and it seems most effective when given intramuscularly in dosages of 25–50 mg (Ekeland and Sander 1976; Ritch et al. 1977; Cardozo and Stanton 1979). Bladder responses to an intramuscular dose of 0.3 mg per kg, however, were found to be insignificant by Perera et al. (1982). In elderly patients with urinary incontinence and involuntary bladder contractions, Hansen et al. (1982) found no difference between the effects of oral emepronium 200 mg t.i.d. and placebo, although there was a significant overall subjective cure or improvement rate (both groups) of 79%. Potential side-effects of this agent are predominantly antimuscarinic, but they also include mucosal alteration, sometimes leading to oral ulcers and oesophagitis. This agent is not available for use in the United States.

Other drugs used to inhibit bladder contractility are classified as musculotropic relaxants (antispasmodics). They purport to act directly on smooth muscle at a site distal to the cholinergic receptor mechanism (Finkbeiner et al. 1978; Wein 1979).

Although in the laboratory all three of the agents to be discussed do relax smooth muscle by a papavarine-like activity, all have been found, additionally, to possess variable antimuscarinic and local anaesthetic properties. There is still some question as to how much of their clinical efficacy is due simply to their atropine-like effect. If in fact any of these agents do exert a clinically significant inhibitory effect which is independent of an antimuscarinic action, there exists a therapeutic rationale for combining their use with that of a relatively pure antimuscarinic agent.

Oxybutynin chloride (Ditropan) has been described as a moderately potent anticholinergic agent with both strong independent musculotropic relaxant activity and local anaesthetic activity (Lish et al. 1965; Fredericks et al. 1975; Finkbeiner et al. 1977; Fredericks et al. 1978). This agent has been successfully used to relieve urinary discomfort and "bladder spasm" following endoscopic resection (Diokno and Lapides 1972; Paulson 1978), and to depress detrusor hyperreflexia in patients with neurogenic bladder dysfunction (Thompson and Lauvetz 1976). A randomised double-blind control study in 30 patients with detrusor instability comparing oxybutynin 5 mg t.i.d. and placebo was carried out by Moisey et al. (1980). Of 23 patients who completed the study with oxybutynin, 17 had symptomatic improvement and 9 had evidence of urodynamic improvement, mainly an increase in bladder volume at first contraction and an increase in total bladder capacity. The recommended adult dose is 5 mg 3 or 4 times daily; the potential side-effects and contraindications are the same as for propantheline.

Dicyclomine hydrochloride (Bentyl) is another agent with at least a direct in vitro relaxant effect on smooth muscle, in addition to an antimuscarinic action (Johns et al. 1976; Downie et al. 1977; Awad et al. 1977; Khanna et al. 1979). An oral dose of 20 mg t.i.d. in adults has been reported to increase bladder capacity in patients with detrusor hyperreflexia (Fischer et al. 1978). Our own experience suggests that the individual dose must often be raised to at least 30 mg to achieve a good clinical effect. The potential side-effects are antimuscarinic ones. Flavoxate hydrochloride (Urispas) is another compound reported to have a direct inhibitory action on smooth muscle, in addition to anticholinergic and local analgesic properties (Kohler and Morales 1968; Bradley and Cazort 1970). Favourable clinical effects have been noted in patients with frequency, urgency and incontinence and in patients with urodynamically documented detrusor hyperreflexia (Stanton 1973; Delaere et al. 1977; Jonas et al. 1979a). However, Briggs et al. (1980) reported essentially no effect of this agent on detrusor hyperreflexia in an elderly population, an experience that would coincide with our own subjective impression of limited clinical efficacy in situations where other less expensive agents have failed (Benson et al. 1977). The recommended adult dose is 100–200 mg 3 or 4 times daily. Reported side-effects are rare and primarily antimuscarinic in nature.

Attempts have been made to increase bladder capacity with beta-adrenergic stimulation. Such stimulation can cause significant increases in the capacity of animal bladders which contain a moderate density of beta receptors (Larsen and Mortensen 1978). Terbutaline (Brethine) in oral doses of 5 mg t.i.d. has been reported to have a "good clinical effect" in some patients with urgency and urgency incontinence, but no significant effect on the bladders of neurologically normal humans without voiding difficulty (Norlen et al. 1978). Although these results may be compatible with those in other organ systems (beta-adrenergic stimulation has no acute effect on total lung capacity in normal humans while it does favourably affect patients with bronchial asthma), few if any adequate studies are available on the effects of beta-adrenergic stimulation in patients with detrusor hyperactivity.

Multiple mechanisms exist whereby inhibitors of prostaglandin synthesis might decrease bladder contractility. Cardozo et al. (1980) reported beneficial effects in a double-blind placebo study of 30 women with detrusor instability utilising the prostaglandin synthetase inhibitor flurbiprofen in an oral dose of 50 mg t.i.d. Abnormal bladder activity, however, was not abolished in significantly more drug-treated than placebo-treated patients, and actual bladder capacity likewise showed no change. It was concluded that the drug did not abolish detrusor hyperreflexia but delayed the intravesical pressure rise to a greater level of distension. Forty-three per cent of the patients experienced side-effects from the drug, primarily nausea, vomiting, headache, indigestion, gastric distress, constipation and rash. Cardozo and Stanton (1980) reported symptomatic improvement in patients with detrusor instability given indomethacin in oral doses of 50–200 mg daily. However, this was a short-term study with no cystometric data, and the drug was compared only with bromocriptine. Although the incidence of side-effects was high, no patient had to stop treatment because of these.

The rationale underlying the potential use of calcium antagonists for the inhibition of bladder contractility has been described previously. Nifedipine has been shown to effectively inhibit contraction induced by several mechanisms in human and guinea pig bladder muscle (Forman et al. 1978; Sjogren and Andersson 1979) and to be capable of completely blocking the non-cholinergic portion of the contraction produced by electrical field stimulation in rabbit bladder (Husted, Sjogren and Andersson, cited by Husted et al. 1980). Terodiline, an agent with both calcium blocking and anticholinergic properties, caused a complete inhibition of the response of rabbit bladder to electrical field stimulation (Husted et al. 1980). At low concentrations, terodiline seemed to have a mainly antimuscarinic action, whereas at higher concentrations the calcium antagonist effect became evident. These two effects seemed at least additive in vitro with regard to inhibition of bladder contractility. Whether the drug is in vivo actually more effective than standard antimuscarinic agents alone remains to be established. Rud et al. (1980), however, reported that, in oral doses of 12.5 mg 2 or 3 times daily, it produced a marked decrease in the number of hyperreflexic contractions in a group of seven women with urgency incontinence and in two with nocturnal enuresis. Bladder capacity was approximately doubled and the amplitude of the contractions was decreased. Similarly, Ekman et al. (1980) reported an increase in bladder capacity and in the volume at which the sensation of urgency was experienced in all but one of 12 patients with motor urge incontinence treated in a double-blind study with terodiline, whereas placebo treatment had no effect on either objective or subjective parameters. Palmer et al. (1981) reported a double-blind placebo trial with a single 20 mg daily dose of flunarizine in 14 females with urinary frequency, incontinence and urodynamically proven detrusor instability. A statistically significant decrease in urgency was produced in the flunarizine-treated group, but there was no change in urinary frequency. There was no statistically significant improvement in cystometric parameters, although there was a positive trend. The side-effects produced in patients who have been treated with calcium antagonists for voiding dysfunction have been small in number, but it should be noted that the potential side-effects of these agents can be of considerable magnitude and consist of hypotension, facial flushing, headache, dizziness, abdominal discomfort, constipation, nausea, skin rash, weakness, palpitations and heart block. This class of agents may yet prove to be a promising alternative or adjunct to existing therapy for the inhibition of bladder contractility.

Increasing Outlet Resistance

Stimulation of the alpha-adrenergic receptors of the smooth musculature of the bladder neck and proximal urethra can increase outlet resistance sufficiently to improve many cases of mild to moderate sphincteric incontinence. Improvement has been correlated with changes in objective urodynamic parameters, most commonly an increase in maximum urethral closure pressure. Ephedrine is a non-catecholamine sympathomimetic agent that directly stimulates both alpha- and beta-adrenergic receptors (Weiner 1980b) and causes a peripheral release of noradrenaline. It is used in an adult dosage of 25–50 mg q.i.d. Theoretically, at least, any beta-adrenergic effect that the drug has should simultaneously depress bladder contractility, but we have not been impressed that this latter mechanism is operative at doses used clinically.

Potential side-effects of all agents that produce a peripheral sympathetic effect include blood pressure elevation and anxiety and insomnia caused by central nervous system stimulation. All of these agents should be used with caution in patients with hypertension, cardiovascular disease and hyperthyroidism. Pseudoephedrine hydrochloride (Sudafed) is a stereoisomer of ephedrine that is used for similar indications with similar precautions (Wein 1979). The adult dosage is 30–60 mg q.i.d. Tachyphylaxis seems to be a problem with the long-term usage of both ephedrine and pseudoephedrine.

Phenylpropanolamine hydrochloride shares the pharmacological potencies of ephedrine and is approximately equal in peripheral potency, while causing less central stimulation (Weiner 1980b). In doses of 50 mg t.i.d., this agent has been shown to be effective in some cases of stress incontinence. Utilising this dose, Awad et al. (1978) found that, after 4 weeks of therapy, 11 of 13 females and 6 of 7 males with stress incontinence (severity not noted) were significantly improved. Maximum urethral closure pressure (MUCP) was increased

from a mean of 47 to 72 cmH$_2$O in the empty bladder and from 43 to 58 cmH$_2$O with a full bladder. Fifty milligrams of phenylpropanolamine was combined with 8 mg chlorpheniramine (an antihistamine) and 2.5 mg isopropamide (an antimuscarinic) as a sustained release capsule called Ornade, used primarily for the relief of symptoms of allergic rhinitis. Using one capsule twice daily, Stewart et al. (1976) found that of 77 women with urinary stress incontinence, 18 were completely cured, 28 were much better, 6 were slightly better and 25 were no better. Subsequently, Montague and Stewart (1979) carried out urethral profilometry in 12 women with moderate to marked stress incontinence and 6 women with no history of incontinence. The maximum urethral pressure (MUP) increased more than 20% in 11 of the incontinent women and only 1% in the continent group. The formulation of Ornade has now been changed, so that each capsule contains 75 mg phenylpropanolamine and 12 mg chlorpheniramine; it is also available as a liquid. Midodrine is a long-acting alpha-adrenergic stimulator reported to be useful in the treatment of seminal emission and ejaculation disorders following retroperitoneal lymphadenectomy (Jonas et al. 1979b). Treatment with 5 mg b.i.d. for 4 weeks in women with stress incontinence produced a cure in 1 and improvement in 14 (Kiesswetter et al. 1983). The mean MUCP rose by 8.3% and the planimetric index of the continence area on profilometry increased by 9%. This agent is not yet available for general use in the United States.

Although some clinicians report spectacular cure and improvement rates with alpha-adrenergic agonists in females with stress urinary incontinence, our own experience coincides with those who report that treatment with such agents often produces improvement but rarely total dryness in cases of severe or even moderate stress incontinence. A clinical trial is certainly worthwhile, however, and will at least assure the patient that the possibility of one type of non-surgical therapy has been explored.

Theoretically, beta-adrenergic blocking agents might be expected to "unmask" or potentiate an alpha-adrenergic effect in the bladder outlet, thereby increasing resistance. Gleason et al. (1974) reported success in treating stress urinary incontinence with propranolol, a beta-adrenergic blocking agent, in oral doses of 10 mg q.i.d. The beneficial effect, however, became manifest only after 4–10 weeks of treatment, a fact which is difficult to explain on a pharmacological basis as the cardiac effects occur rather promptly after administration. However, the hypotensive effects of propranolol do not usually appear as rapidly (Weiner 1980b). Such treatment has been suggested as an alternative method (to alpha-adrenergic stimulation) of pharmacological therapy of stress incontinence in patients with hypertension. Few, if any, subsequent reports have appeared to support this approach, however, and it should be noted that others have been unable to show significant increases in urethral profilometry pressures in normal women after administration of a beta-adrenergic blocking agent (Donker and VanderSluis 1976). Although 10 mg q.i.d. is a relatively small dose of propranolol, it should be remembered that the major potential side-effects are related to the drug's therapeutic beta-adrenergic blocking effects. Heart failure may develop, as well as an increase in airway resistance, and asthma is a contraindication to the use of this drug. Abrupt discontinuation may precipitate an exacerbation of anginal attacks and rebound hypertension (Weiner 1980b).

Caine and Raz (1973) reported that a daily dose of 2.5 mg Premarin improved stress incontinence and increased urethral pressures in post-menopausal patients, effects which they attributed to mucosal proliferation with a consequently improved "mucosal seal effect" and to enhancement of the alpha-adrenergic contractile response of urethral smooth musculature to endogenous catecholamines. The first use of oestrogen to treat stress incontinence was actually reported by Salmon et al. (1941). Schreiter et al. (1976) reported similar benefits after 10 days of treatment with daily divided doses of 6 mg oestriol. They also showed that the effects of oestrogen and of exogenous alpha-adrenergic stimulation were additive. Hodgson et al. (1978) reported that the sensitivity of the rabbit urethra to alpha-adrenergic stimulation was oestrogen dependent, as castration caused a decreased sensitivity which treatment with low levels of oestrogen reversed. Rud (1980a) studied the effects of 4 mg daily doses of oestradiol and 9 mg daily doses of oestriol on 30 women with an average age of 61 years, 24 of whom had stress urinary incontinence. Profilometry parameters were recorded at a bladder volume of 200 cc with a microtransducer technique. Small but statistically significant changes occurred in the MUP, the functional urethral length and the actual urethral length. No statistically significant change occurred

in urethral closure pressure. Eight of the 24 incontinent patients experienced subjective and objective improvement, nine experienced subjective improvement only and seven experienced neither subjective nor objective improvement. There was no correlation between subjective or objective improvement and the previously mentioned urodynamic parameters. However, in 18 patients pressure transmission to the urethra was recorded during cough, and in seven of these, this improved. All of these patients had subjective improvement and five were shown to be objectively dry. Rud points out that it is hard to believe that the small changes in urodynamic parameters, even though statistically significant, are directly related to resumption of continence. He pointed out also that the increased pressure transmission ratio might be due to factors outside the urethra—either in the pelvic floor striated musculature or in the periurethral vasculature or supporting tissues. Interestingly, he found no changes in urodynamic parameters in five continent and three stress incontinent women with cystic glandular hyperplasia treated with a single injection of 1000 mg of intramuscular progesterone, except that the pressure transmission ratio was lower in the three patients in whom this parameter was measured. Rud (1980b) also recorded profilometric parameters during the menstrual cycle in six females. There was no change in any profilometric parameter during the menstrual cycle and no correlation between oestrogen levels and MUP. It may be, as he suggests, that at physiological levels oestrogens have little influence on urodynamic parameters related to continence and that only pharmacological doses cause urodynamically significant change. Further, pharmacological doses may alter responses to other exogenous autonomic stimulation, particularly alpha-adrenergic, as the previously described laboratory experiments by Hodgson et al. (1978) would suggest.

Parenteral oestrogen administration can change the alpha-adrenergic receptor content and the autonomic innervation of the lower urinary tract of immature female rabbits (Levin et al. 1980b; Levin et al. 1981). Whether these experiments have any clinical significance is unknown. Oestrogen therapy seems capable of facilitating urinary storage in some women by increasing outlet resistance and by an augmentative or perhaps additive effect to alpha-adrenergic therapy in this regard. Whether the levels achieved by commonly utilised oral or parenteral oestrogen preparations or by oestrogen vaginal creams (which simply provide a convenient vehicle for systemic absorption) actually increase the alpha-adrenergic receptor content of the smooth muscle of the bladder outlet or the "mucosal seal effect" is still a matter for speculation. The potential long-term effects of such treatment must be carefully considered, however, in the light of the current controversy over whether oestrogen therapy predisposes to the development of endometrial carcinoma in menopausal and post-menopausal women.

Effect of Tricyclic Antidepressants

Some authors have found tricyclic antidepressants, especially imipramine hydrochloride, to be particularly useful agents for facilitating urinary storage (Milner and Hills, 1968; Peterson et al. 1974; Raezer et al. 1977; Castleden et al. 1981). All these agents possess varying degrees of at least three major pharmacological actions (Hollister 1978; Richelson 1983): (a) central and peripheral anticholinergic actions at some, but not all, sites; (b) blockade of the active transport system in the presynaptic nerve ending which is responsible for the re-uptake of the released amine neurotransmitters serotonin and noradrenaline; and (c) a sedative effect, which occurs presumably on a central basis, but is perhaps related to their antihistaminic properties. There is also evidence that they desensitise alpha-2 receptors on central noradrenergic neurons (Crews and Smith 1978; Spyraki and Fibiger 1980).

Imipramine has prominent systemic anticholinergic effects (Baldessarini 1980). However, it appears to have only a weak such effect on bladder smooth muscle (Diokno et al. 1972; Dhattiwalla 1976; Olubadewo 1980). A strong direct inhibitory effect on bladder smooth muscle does exist, however, which is neither anticholinergic nor adrenergic (Dhattiwalla 1976; Benson et al. 1977; Fredericks et al. 1978; Tulloch and Creed 1979; Olubadewo 1980). This may be due to a local anaesthetic-like action at the nerve terminals in the adjacent effector membrane, an effect that seems to occur also in cardiac muscle (Bigger et al. 1977), or to an inhibition of the participation of calcium in the excitation–contraction coupling process (Olubadewo 1980). Clinically, the drug seems effective in decreasing bladder contractility and in

increasing outlet resistance (Cole and Fried 1972; Mahony et al. 1973; Raezer et al. 1977; Tulloch and Creed 1979; Castleden et al. 1981). One might hypothesise that the increase in outlet resistance is due to a peripheral blockade of noradrenaline re-uptake, which would tend to produce or enhance an alpha-adrenergic effect in the smooth muscle of the bladder base and proximal urethra. Theoretically, at least, this latter action, if indeed it occurs in the lower urinary tract as it does centrally, might also tend to stimulate predominantly beta-adrenergic receptors in bladder body smooth musculature, an action which would further facilitate urine storage by decreasing the excitability of smooth muscle in that area.

Castleden et al. (1981) began imipramine therapy in elderly patients with detrusor instability using a single 25-mg night-time dose which was increased every third day by 25 mg until the patient was continent, side-effects occurred or the dosage reached 150 mg. Six of ten patients became continent and, in those who underwent repeat cystometry, bladder capacity increased by a mean of 105 cc and bladder pressure at capacity decreased by a mean of 18 cmH$_2$O. MUP increased by a mean of 30 cmH$_2$O. Our usual adult dose of imipramine for voiding dysfunction is 25 mg q.i.d., and half that dose in elderly patients. In our experience, the effects of imipramine on the lower urinary tract are often additive to those of the atropine-like agents. Consequently, a combination of imipramine and propantheline is sometimes especially useful to decrease bladder contractility (Raezer et al. 1977). If imipramine is to be used in conjunction with an atropine-like agent, it should be noted that the anticholinergic side-effects of the drugs may be additive.

When used in the generally larger doses employed for antidepressant activity, the most frequent side-effects of this group of agents are those attributable to their systemic anticholinergic activity. Allergic phenomena, including rash, elevated liver function studies, obstructive jaundice and agranulocytosis may also occur, but rarely. Side-effects on the central nervous system may include weakness, fatigue, a parkinsonian effect, a fine tremor (most noted in the upper extremities) and a manic or schizophrenic picture. Sedation may also result from an antihistaminic effect. Postural hypotension may be seen, presumably on the basis of alpha-1 receptor blockade. Antidepressants can be shown electrophysiologically and haemodynamically to have a depressant effect upon the myocardium shortly after their institution (Burgess and Turner 1980; Muller and Schulze 1980). Whether cardiotoxicity will prove to be a legitimate concern in patients receiving somewhat smaller doses for lower urinary tract dysfunction remains to be seen. The onset of significant side-effects (severe abdominal distress, nausea, vomiting, headache, lethargy and irritability) following abrupt cessation of high dose imipramine in children (Petti and Law 1981) would suggest that the drug should be discontinued gradually, especially in patients receiving high doses. Tricyclic antidepressants can also cause excess sweating of obscure aetiology and a delay of orgasm and orgasmic impotence, whose cause is likewise unclear (Baldessarini 1980). The use of imipramine is contraindicated in patients receiving monamine oxidase inhibitors, as severe central nervous system toxicity (hyperpyrexia, seizures and coma) can be precipitated.

Effects of Other Pharmacological Agents

It is obvious from the foregoing discussion that any one of a number of agents prescribed for reasons unrelated to voiding dysfunction can affect autonomic nervous system and receptor function, and can thereby influence urine storage, urine emptying or both.

Agents which decrease outlet resistance may predispose a patient to sphincteric incontinence or worsen an already existing condition. Agents which increase intravesical pressure by increasing bladder muscle contractility may decrease functional bladder capacity since the threshold pressure at which the sensation of distention is perceived will be reached at a lower intravesical volume. An increase in urinary frequency and perhaps a feeling of

Table 16.2. Acknowledged and potential effects of various pharmacological agents on urine storage and emptying

Agent	Facilitate emptying		Facilitate storage	
	Increase bladder contractility	Decrease outlet resistance	Inhibit bladder contractility	Increase outlet resistance
Acetylcholine-like agents	+ +			
Anticholinesterases	+ +			
Prostaglandins E_2 and F_{2a}	+ +			
Digitalis	+			
a-Adrenergic antagonists	+	+ +	+	
β-Adrenergic agonists		+	+	
Centrally acting muscle relaxants[a]		+ +	+	
Polysynaptic inhibitors		+ +	+	
Direct-acting skeletal muscle relaxants		+ +	+	
Atropine-like agents			+ +	
Ganglionic blocking agents			+ +	
Musculotropic relaxants			+ +	
Calcium antagonists			+ +	
Antihistamines			+ +	
Theophylline			+ +	
Phenothiazines		+	+ +	
Phenytoin		+	+ +	
Prostaglandin inhibitors			+ +	
Narcotics			+ +	
Tricyclic antidepressants			+ +	+ +
a-Adrenergic agonists			+	+ +
L-dopa				+ +
Amphetamines				+ +
β-Adrenergic antagonists				+

+, theoretical or laboratory effects that are not widely clinically acknowledged.
+ +, accepted, widely acknowledged clinical effects.
[a] These act primarily through central effects and may cause decreased emptying on the basis of oversedation or bladder inhibition.

urgency may occur. Agents which inhibit bladder contractility may decrease the urinary flow rate and may cause relative or even, in some cases, complete urinary retention. If emptying is inhibited, an increase in residual urine could well occur and an increase in urinary frequency (because of a decreased functional capacity) may result. Compounds that increase outlet resistance can cause the same end-effects on voiding efficiency as those that decrease bladder contractility. It is obvious that adverse and unwanted pharmacological effects on voiding do not occur in the great majority of patients treated with agents that can potentially cause them. Such effects are usually most manifest in those patients whose pre-treatment voiding status already borders on being pathological. For the sake of completeness, some of these agents and their potential effects are listed in Table 16.2.

References

Abromowicz A (ed) (1978) Baclofen (Lioresal). Med Lett Drugs Ther 20:43–44

Allen TD (1977) The non-neurogenic neurogenic bladder. J Urol 117:232–238

Anderson G (1982) Evidence for a prostaglandin link in the purinergic activation of rabbit bladder smooth muscle. J Pharmacol Exp Ther 220:347–351

Andersson K (1978) Effects of calcium and calcium antagonists on the excitation contraction coupling in striated and smooth muscle. Acta Pharmacol Toxicol (Copenh) 43 (1):5–14

Andersson K, Husted S, Sjogren C (1980) Contribution of prostaglandins to the adenosine triphosphate induced contraction of rabbit urinary bladder. Br J Pharmacol 70:443–448

Andersson K, Ek A, Hedlung H, Mattiasson A (1981) Effects of prazosin on isolated human urethra and in patients with lower motor neuron lesions. Invest Urol 19:39–42

Awad SA, Bruce AW, Carro-Ciampi G, Downie JW, Lin M (1974) Distribution of alpha and beta adrenoreceptors in human urinary bladder. Br J Pharmacol 50:525–529

Awad SA, Bryniak S, Downie JW, Bruce A (1977) The treatment of the uninhibited bladder with dicyclomine. J Urol 117:161–163

Awad SA, Downie JW, Kiruluta HG (1978) Alpha adrenergic agents in urinary disorders of the proximal urethra. Part I. Sphincteric incontinence. Br J Urol 50:332–335

Baldessarini R (1980) Drugs and the treatment of psychiatric disorders. In: Gilman AG, Goodman LS, Gilman A (eds) The pharmacological basis of therapeutics, Macmillan, New York, pp 391–447

Barrett D (1981) The effect of oral bethanechol chloride on voiding in female patients with excessive residual urine: a randomized double-blind study. J Urol 126:640–646

Benson GS, Jacobowitz D, Raezer DM, Corriere JN Jr, Wein AJ (1976a) Adrenergic innervation and stimulation of canine urethra. Urology 7:337–340

Benson GS, Raezer DM, Anderson JR, Saunders CD, Corriere JN Jr (1976b) Effect of levodopa on urinary bladder. Urology 7:24–28

Benson GS, Wein AJ, Raezer DM, Corriere JN Jr (1976c) Adrenergic and cholinergic stimulation and blockade of the human bladder base. J Urol 116:174–175

Benson GS, Sarshik SA, Raezer DM, Wein AJ (1977) Comparative effects and mechanisms of action of atropine, propantheline, favoxate, and imipramine on bladder muscle contractility. Urology 9:31–35

Bianchine J (1980) Drugs for Parkinson's disease: centrally acting muscle relaxants. In: Gilman AG, Goodman LS, Gilman A (eds) The pharmacological basis of therapeutics. Macmillan, New York, pp 475–493

Bigger JT, Giardina EGV, Perel JM, Kantor SJ, Glassman AH (1977) Cardiac antiarrhythmic effect of imipramine hydrochloride. N Engl J Med 296:206–207

Blaivas J, Labib K, Michalik S, Zayed A (1980) Cystometric response to propantheline in detrusor hyperreflexia: therapeutic implications. J Urol 124:259–262

Bradley D, Cazort R (1970) Relief of bladder spasm by flavoxate: a comparative study. J Clin Pharmacol 10:65–68

Bradley WE, Timm GW, Scott FS (1974) Innervation of the detrusor muscle and urethra. Urol Clin North Am 1:3–27

Briggs R, Castleden C, Asher M (1980) The effect of flavoxate on uninhibited detrusor contractions and urinary incontinence in the elderly. J Urol 123:665–666

Bultitude MI, Hills NH, Shuttleworth KED (1976) Clinical and experimental studies on the action of prostaglandins and their synthesis inhibitors on detrusor muscle in vitro and in vivo. Br J Urol 48:531–637

Burgess C, Turner R (1980) Cardiotoxicity of antidepressant drugs. Neuropharmacology 19:1195–1199

Burnstock G (1979) Past and current evidence for the purinergic nerve hypothesis. In: Baer HP, Drummond GI (eds) Physiological and regulatory functions of adenosine and adenine nucleotides. Raven, New York, pp 3–32

Byck R (1975) Drugs and the treatment of psychiatric disorders. In: Goodman LS, Gilman A (eds) The pharmacological basis of therapeutics, 5th edn. Macmillan, New York, pp 152–200

Caine M, Raz S (1973) The role of female hormones in stress incontinence. In: Proceedings of the 16th Congress of Société Internationale d'Urologie, Amsterdam

Cameron MD (1966) Distigmine bromide (ubretid) in the prevention of post-operative retention of urine. J Obstet Gynaecol Br Commonw 73:847–849

Cardozo L, Stanton SL (1979) An objective comparison of the effects of parenterally administered drugs in patients suffering from detrusor instability. J Urol 122:58–59

Cardozo L, Stanton S, Robinson H, Hole D (1980) Evaluation of flurbiprofen in detrusor instability. Br Med J 280:281–283

Castleden C, George C, Renwick A, Asher M (1981) Imipramine—a possible alternative to current therapy for urinary incontinence in the elderly. J Urol 125:318–320

Cole A, Fried F (1972) Favorable experiences with imipramine in the treatment of neurogenic bladder. J Urol 107:44–47

Crews F, Smith C (1978) Presynaptic alpha receptor subsensitivity after long-term antidepressant treatment. Science 202:322–325

De Groat WC, Booth A (1984) Autonomic systems to the urinary bladder and sexual organs. In: Dyck P, Thomas P, Lambert E, Bunge E (eds) Peripheral neuropathy. Saunders, Philadelphia, pp 285–299

De Groat WB, Saum WR (1972) Sympathetic inhibition of the urinary bladder and of pelvic ganglionic transmission in the cat. J Physiol 220:297–314

De Groat WC, Saum WR (1976) Synaptic transmission in parasympathetic ganglia in the urinary bladder of the cat. J Physiol 256:137–158

De Groat WC, Theobald RJ (1976) Reflex activation of sympathetic pathways to vesical smooth muscle and parasympathetic ganglia by electrical stimulation of vesical afferents. J Physiol 259:223–237

Delaere K, Michiels H, Debruyne F, Moonen W (1977) Flavoxate hydrochloride in the treatment of detrusor instability. Urol Int 32:377–381

Delaere K, Thomas C, Moonen T, Debruyne F (1981) The value of prostaglandin E_2 and F_{2a} in women with abnormalities of bladder emptying. Br J Urol 53:306–309

Desmond A, Bultitude M, Hills N, Suttleworth K (1980) Clinical experience with intravesical prostaglandin E_2. A prospective study of 36 patients. Br J Urol 53:357–366

Dhattiwalla AS (1976) The effect of imipramine on isolated and innervated guinea pig and rat urinary bladder preparations. J Pharm Pharmacol 28:453–455

Diokno AC, Koppenhoeffer R (1976) Bethanechol chloride in neurogenic bladder dysfunction. Urology 8:455–458

Diokno AC, Lapides J (1972) Oxygutynin: a new drug with analgesic and anticholinergic properties. J Urol 108:307–309

Diokno AC, Charles W, Hyndman D, Hardy A, Lapides J (1972) Comparison of action of imipramine (Fotranil) and propantheline (Probanthine) on detrusor contraction. J Urol 107:42–43

Diokno AC, Lapides J (1977) Action of oral and parenteral bethanechol on decompensated bladder. Urology 10:23–24

Donker P, VanderSluis C (1976) Action of beta adrenergic blocking agents on the urethral pressure profile. Urol Int 31:6–12

Donker PJ, Ivanovici F, Noach EL (1972) Analyses of the urethra pressure profile by means of electromyography and the administration of drugs. Br J Urol 44:180–193

Downie JW, Twiddy DAS, Awad SA (1977) Antimuscarinic and noncompetitive antagonist properties of dicyclomine hydrochloride in isolated human and rabbit bladder muscle. J Pharmacol Exp Ther 201:662–668

Duncan GW, Shahani BT, Young RR (1976) An evaluation of baclofen treatment for certain symptoms in patients with spinal cord lesions. Neurology (NY) 26:441–446

Edvardsen P (1968a) Nervous control of the urinary bladder in cats. 1. The collecting phase. Acta Physiol Scand 72:157–171

Edvardsen P (1968b) Nervous control of the urinary bladder in cats. 2. The expulsion phase. Acta Physiol Scand 72:172–182

Edvardsen P (1968c) Nervous control of the urinary bladder in cats. 3. Effects of autonomic blocking agents in the intact animal. Acta Physiol Scand 72:183–193

Edvardsen P (1968d) Nervous control of the urinary bladder in cats. 4. Effects of autonomic blocking agents on responses to peripheral nerve stimulation. Acta Physiol Scand 72:234–247

Ek A, Alm P, Andersson KE, Persson CGA (1977) Adrenoreceptor and cholinoceptor mediated responses of the isolated human urethra. Scand J Urol Nephrol 11:97–102

Ekeland A, Sander S (1976) An urodynamic study of emepronium bromide in bladder dysfunction. Scand J Urol Nephrol 10:195–199

Ekman G, Andersson K, Rud T, Ulmsten U (1980) A double-blind crossover study of the effects of terodoline in women with unstable bladder. Acta Pharmacol Toxicol 46(1):39–43

El Badawi A, Schenk EA (1966) Dual innervation of the mammalian urinary bladder: a histochemical study of the distribution of cholinergic and adrenergic nerves. Am J Anat 119:405–427

El Badawi A, Schenk EA (1968) A new theory of the innervation of bladder musculature. 1. Morphology of the intrinsic vesical innervation apparatus. J Urol 99:585–587

El Badawi A, Schenk EA (1971) A new theory of the innervation of bladder musculature. 2. The innervation apparatus of the ureterovesical junction. J Urol 105:368–371

Finkbeiner A, Bissada N, Welch L (1977) Uropharmacology IV. Parasympathetic depressants. Urology 10:503–510

Finkbeiner A, Welch L, Bissada N (1978) Uropharmacology IX. Direct acting smooth muscle stimulants and depressants. Urology 12:231–235

Fischer CP, Diokno A, Lapides J (1978) The anticholinergic effects of dicyclomine hydrochloride in uninhibited neurogenic bladder dysfunction. J Urol 120:328–329

Forman A, Andersson K, Henriksson L, Rud T, Ulmsten U (1978) Effects of nifedipine on the smooth muscle of the human urinary tract in-vitro and in-vivo. Acta Pharmacol Toxicol 43:111–116

Fredericks C, Anderson G, Kreulen D (1975) A study of the anticholinergic and antispasmodic activity of oxygutynin (Ditropan) on rabbit detrusor. Invest Urol 12:317–319

Fredericks C, Green R, Anderson G (1978) Comparative in-vitro effects of imipramine, oxybutynin and flavoxate on rabbit detrusor. Urology 12:487–491

Gibbon NOK (1965) Urinary incontinence in disorders of the nervous system. Br J Urol 37:624–629

Gleason DM, Reilly RJ, Bottaccini MR, Pierce MJ (1974) The urethral continence zone and its relation to stress incontinence. J Urol 112:81–88

Graham R, Pettinger W (1979) Prazosin. N Engl J Med 200:232–234

Hansen W, Hansen L, Maegaard E, Mayhoff H, Nordling J (1982) Urinary incontinence in old age. A controlled clinical trial of emepronium bromide. Br J Urol 54:249–253

Hartviksen K (1966) Discussion. Acta Neurol Scand [Suppl] 42:180–181

Hebjorn S, Walter S (1978) Treatment of female incontinence with emepronium bromide. Urol Int 33:120–122

Hodgson B, Dumas S, Bolling D, Heesch D (1978) Effect of estrogen on sensitivity of rabbit bladder and urethra to phenylephrine. Invest Urol 16:67–72

Hoffman B, Lefkowitz R (1980) Alpha adrenergic receptor subtypes. N Engl J Med 302:1390–1396

Hollister L (1978) Tricyclic antidepressants. N Engl J Med 299:1106–1109

Husted S, Andersson K, Sommer L, Ostergaard J (1980) Anticholinergic and calcium antagonistic effects of terodiline in rabbit urinary bladder. Acta Pharmacol Toxicol 46(1):20–30

Jensen D Jr (1981) Pharmacological studies of the uninhibited neurogenic bladder. Acta Neurol Scand 64:175–179

Johns A, Tasker JJ, Johnson CE, Theman MA, Paton DM (1976) The mechanism of action of dicyclomine hydrochloride on rabbit detrusor muscle and vas deferens. Arch Int Pharmacodyn Ther 224:109–117

Johnston JH, Farkas A (1975) Congenital neuropathic bladder: practicalities and possibilities of conservational management. urology 5:719–727

Jonas U, Petri E, Kissal J (1979a) Effect of flavoxate on hyperactive detrusor muscle. Eur Urol 5:106–111

Jonas D, Linzbach P, Weber W (1979b) The use of midodrine in the treatment of ejaculation disorders following retroperitoneal lymphadenectomy. Eur Urol 5:184–187

Khanna OP (1976) Disorders of micturition: neuropharmacological basis and results of drug therapy. Urology 8:316–328

Khanna OP, Heber D, Gonick P (1975) Cholinergic and adrenergic neuroreceptors in urinary tract of female dogs: evaluation of function with pharmacodynamics. Urology 5:616–623

Khanna O, DiGregorio C, Barbieri E, McMichael R, Ruch E (1979) In-vitro study of antispasmodic effects of dicyclomine hydrochloride on vesicourethral smooth muscle of guinea pig and rabbit. Urology 13:457–462

Kiesswetter H, Schober W (1975) Lioresal in the treatment of neurogenic bladder dysfunction. Urol Int 30:63–71

Keisswetter H, Hennrich F, Englisch M (1983) Clinical and urodynamic assessment of pharmacologic therapy of stress incontinence. Urol Int 38:58–64

Koelle GB (1975a) Neurohumoral transmission and the auto-nomic nervous system. In: Goodman LS, Gilman A (eds) The pharmacological basis of therapeutics, 5th edn. Macmillan, New York, pp 404–444

Koelle GB (1975b) Parasympathomimetic agents. In: Goodman LS, Gilman A (eds) The pharmacological basis of therapeutics, 5th edn. Macmillan, New York, pp 467–476

Kohler RP, Morales PA (1968) Cystometric evaluation of flavox-ate hydrochloride in normal and neurogenic bladder. J Urol 100:729–730

Koyanagi T (1978) Denervation supersensitivity of the urethra to alpha adrenergics in the chronic neurogenic bladder. Urol Res 6:89–92

Koyanagi T (1979) Further observation on the denervation supersensitivity of the urethra in patients with chronic neuro-genic bladders. J Urol 122:348–352

Krane RJ, Olsson CA (1973) Phenoxybenzamine in neurogenic bladder dysfunction. II. Clinical considerations. J Urol 110:653–656

Kuru M (1965) Nervous control of micturition. Physiol Rev 45:425–594

Lapides J (1964) Urecholine regimen for rehabilitating the atonic bladder. J Urol 91:658–659

Lapides J (1974) Neurogenic bladder: principles of treatment. Urol Clin North Am 1:81–97

Lapides J, Friend CR, Ajémian E, Sonda LP (1963) Comparison of action of oral and parenteral bethanechol chloride upon the urinary bladder. Invest Urol 1:94–99

Larsen J, Mortensen S (1978) Effect of ritodrine on the bladder capacity in unanesthetized pigs. Acta Pharmacol Toxicol 43:405–408

Levin R, Jacobowitz D, Wein A (1981) Autonomic innervation of the rabbit urinary bladder following estrogen administra-tion. Urology 17:449–453

Levin R, Shofer F, Wein A (1980a) Cholinergic, adrenergic and purinergic response of sequential strips of rabbit urinary blad-der. J Pharmacol Exp Therap 212:536–542

Levin R, Shofer F, Wein A (1980b) Estrogen induced alteration in the autonomic responses of the rabbit urinary bladder. J Pharm Exp Ther 215:614–619

Levin R, Staskin D, Wein A (1982) The muscarinic cholinergic binding kinetics of the human urinary bladder. Neurourology Urodynamics 1:221–226

Light J, Scott F (1982) Bethanechol chloride and the traumatic cord bladder. J Urol 128:85–89

Lish PM, Labbude JA, Peters EL, Robbins SI (1965) Oxybutynin: a musculotropic antispasmodic drug with moderate anti-cholinergic action. Arch Int Pharmacodyn Ther 156:467–488

MacGregor R, Diokno A (1981) The alpha adrenergic blocking action of prazosin hydrochloride on the canine urethra. Invest Urol 18:426–429

Mahony DT, Laferte RO, Mahoney JE (1973) Observations on sphincter augmenting effect of imipramine in children with urinary incontinence. Urology 1:317–323

Mayer S (1980) Neurohumoral transmission and the autonomic nervous system. In: Gilman AG, Goodman LS, Gilman A (eds) The pharmacological basis of therapeutics. Macmillan, New York, pp 56–90

Merrill DC, Rotta J (1974) A clinical evaluation of detrusor denervation supersensitivity using air cystometry. J Urol 111:27–30

Milner G, Hills N (1968) A double-blind assessment of antidepres-sants in the treatment of 212 neurotic patients. Med J Aust 1:943–948

Mirakhur R, Dundee J (1980) Comparison of the effects of atropine and glycopyrrolate on various end organs. J Soc Med 73:727–731

Mobley DF (1976) Phenoxybenzamine in the management of

neurogenic vesical dysfunction. J Urol 116:737–738

Moisey C, Stephenson T, Brendler C (1980) The urodynamic and subjective results of treatment of detrusor instability with oxybutynin chloride. Br J Urol 52:472–477

Moncada S, Flower R, Vane J (1980) Prostaglandins, prostacyclin and thromboxane A$_2$. In: Gilman AG, Goodman LS, Gilman AG (eds) The pharmacological basis of therapeutics. Macmil-lan, New York, pp 668–681

Montague D, Stewart B (1979) Urethral pressure profiles before and after Ornade administration in patients with stress incon-tinence. J Urol 122:198–204

Movsesian M (1982) Calcium physiology in smooth muscle. Prog Cardiovasc Dis 25:211–214

Muller J, Schulze S (1980) Imipramine cardiotoxicity: an electri-cardiographic and hemodynamic study in rabbits. Acta Pharmacol Toxicol 46:191–196

Mundy A (1984) Neuropeptides in lower urinary tract function. World J Urol 2:211–216

Murdock MM, Sax D, Krane RJ (1976) Use of dantrolene sodium in external sphincter spasm. Urology 8:133–137

Nanninga J, Kaplan P, Lal S (1977) Effect of phentolamine on perineal muscle EMG activity in paraplegia. Br J Urol 49:537–542

Nergardh A (1975) Autonomic receptor functions in lower uri-nary tract: a survey of recent experimental results. J Urol 113:180–185

Nergardh A, Boreus LO (1973) The functional role of cholinergic receptors in the outlet region of the urinary bladder: an in vitro study in the cat. Acta Pharmacol Toxicol 32:467–480

Nordling J, Christensen B, Gosling J (1980) Noradrenergic innervation of the human bladder in neurogenic dysfunction. Urol Int 35:188–193

Nordling J, Meyhoff H, Hald T, Gerstenberg T, Walter S, Christen-sen N (1981) Urethral denervation supersensitivity to noradrenaline after radical hysterectomy. Scand J Urol Nephrol 15:21–27

Norlen L, Dahlstrom A, Sundin T, Svedmyr N (1976) The adrenergic innervation and adrenergic receptor activity of the feline urinary bladder and urethra in the normal state and after hypogastric and/or parasympathetic denervation. Scand J Urol Nephrol 10:177–181

Norlen L, Sundin T, Waagstein F (1978) Beta-adrenoceptor stimulation of the human urinary bladder in-vivo. Acta Pharmacol Toxicol (Copenh) 43 (11):26–30

Olsson C, Siroky M, Krane RJ (1977) The phentolamine test in neurogenic bladder dysfunction. J Urol 117:481–485

Olubadewo J (1980) The effect of imipramine on rat detrusor muscle contractility. Arch Int Pharmacodyn Ther 245:84–94

Palmer J, Worth P, Exton-Smith A (1981) Flunarizine: a once daily therapy for urinary incontinence. Lancet, Aug 8, 279–281

Parsons K, Turton M (1980) Urethral supersensitivity and occult urethral neuropathy. Br J Urol 52:131–137

Paulson DF (1978) Oxybutynin chloride in control of post tran-surethral vesical pain and spasm. Urology 11:237–238

Pedersen E, Grynderup V (1966) Clinical pharmacology of the neurogenic bladder. Acta Neurol Scand 42 [Suppl 20]

Perera L, Ritch A, Hall M (1982) The lack of effect of intramuscular emepronium bromide for urinary incontinence. Br J Urol 54:259–262

Persson CGA, Andersson KE (1976) Adrenoceptor and cholino-ceptor mediated effects in the isolated urethra of cat and guinea pig. Clin Exp Pharmacol Physiol 3:415–426

Peterson K, Anderson O, Hansen T (1974) Mode of action and relative value of imipramine and similar drugs in the treatment of nocturnal enuresis. Eur J Clin Pharmacol 7:187–194

Petti T, Law W (1981) Abrupt cessation of high dose imipramine therapy treatment in children. JAMA 246:768–770

Philip NH, Thomas D (1980) The effect of distigmine bromide

on voiding in male paraplegic patients with reflex micturition. Br J Urol 52:492–496

Philip N, Thomas D, Clarke S (1980) Drug effects on the voiding cystometrogram: a comparison of oral bethanechol and carbachol. Br J Urol 52: 484–487

Raezer DM, Wein AJ, Jacobowitz D, Corriere JN Jr (1973) Autonomic innervation of canine urinary bladder: cholinergic and adrenergic contributions and interaction of sympathetic and parasympathetic systems in bladder function. Urology 2:211–221

Raezer D, Benson G, Wein A, Duckett J (1977) The functional approach to the management of the pediatric neuropathic bladder. J Urol 117: 649–654

Raz S, Caine M (1971) Adrenergic receptors in the female canine urethra. Invest Urol 9:319–323

Raz S, Smith RB (1976) External sphincter spasticity syndrome in female patients. J Urol 115:443–446

Raz S, Caine M, Zeigler M (1972) The vascular component in the production of intraurethral pressure. J Urol 108:93–96

Raz S, Kaufman JJ, Ellison GW, Mayers L (1977) Methyldopa in treatment of neurogenic bladder disorders. Urology 9:188–190

Richelson E (1983) Antimuscarinic acid and other receptor blocking properties of antidepressants. Mayo Clin Proc 58:40–45

Ritch AES, George CF, Castleden CM, Hall MRP (1977) A second look at emepronium bromide in urinary incontinence. Lancet I:504–506

Roppolo J, Booth A, DeGroat W (1983) The effects of naloxone on the neural control of the urinary bladder of the cat. Brain Res 204:355–359

Rossier A, Fa B, Lee I, Sarkarati M, Evans D (1982) Role of striated and smooth muscle components in the urethral pressure profile in traumatic neurogenic bladders: a neuropharmacological and urodynamic study. A preliminary report. J Urol 128:529–533

Ruch TC (1974) The urinary bladder: Physiology and biophysics. In: Ruch TC, Patton HD (eds) Circulation, respiration and fluid balance. Saunders, Philadelphia, pp 525–546

Rud T (1980a) The effects of estrogens and gestagens on the urethral pressure profile in urinary incontinent and stress incontinent women. Acta Obstet Gynecol Scand 59:265–270

Rud T (1980b) Urethral pressure profile in continent women from childhood to old age. Acta Obstet Gynecol Scand 59:331–336

Rud T, Andersson K, Boye N, Ulmsten U (1980) Terodiline inhibition of human bladder contraction. Effects in vitro and in women with unstable bladder Acta Pharmacol Toxicol 46 (1):31–38

Salmon UJ, Walter RI, Gerst SH (1941) The use of estrogen in the treatment of dysuria and incontinence in post-menopausal women. Am J Obstet Gynecol 42:845–849

Schreiter F, Fuchs P, Stockamp K (1976) Estrogenic sensitivity of alpha receptors in the urethral musculature. Urol Int 31:13–19

Sjogren C, Andersson K (1979) Effects of cholinoceptor blocking drugs, adrenoceptor stimulants and calcium antagonists on the transmurally stimulated guinea pig urinary bladder in-vitro and in-vivo. Acta Pharmacol Toxicol 44:228–234

Sonda L, Gershon C, Diokno A, Lapides J (1979) Further observations on the cystometric and uroflowmetric effects of bethanechol chloride on the human bladder. J Urol 122:775–777

Spyraki C, Fibiger H (1980) Functional evidence for subsensitivity of noradrenergic a-2 receptors after chronic desipramine treatment. Life Sci 27:1863–1867

Stanton SL (1973) A comparison of emepronium bromide and flavoxate hydrochloride in the treatment of urinary incontinence. J Urol 110:529–532

Stanton SL (1977) Female urinary incontinence. Lloyd-Luke, London, pp 11–12, 69–70

Stanton SL (1978) Diseases of the urinary system. Drugs acting on the bladder and urethra. Br Med J I:1607–1608

Stanton SL, Cardozo L, Chaudhury N (1978) Spontaneous voiding after surgery for urinary incontinence. Br J Obstet Gynaecol 85:149–152

Stewart BH, Banowsky LHW, Montague DK (1976) Stress incontinence: conservative therapy with sympathomimetic drugs. J Urol 115:558–559

Stockamp K (1975) Treatment with phenoxygenzamine of upper urinary tract complications caused by intravesical obstruction. J Urol 113:128–131

Stockamp K, Schreiter F (1975) Alpha adrenolytic treatment of the congenital neuropathic bladder. Urol Int 30:33–36

Sundin T, Dahlstrom A, Norlen L, Svedmyr N (1977) The sympathetic innervation and adrenoreceptor function of the human lower urinary tract in the normal state and after parasympathetic denervation. Invest Urol 14:322–328

Tanagho EA, Meyers FH (1969) The "internal sphincter": is it under sympathetic control? Invest Urol 7:79–89

Tanagho EA, Meyers FH, Smith DR (1969) Urethral resistance: its components and implications. 1. Smooth muscle component. Invest Urol 7:136–149

Taylor P (1980) Cholinergic agonists. In: Goodman L, Gilman A (eds) Pharmacological bases of therapeutics, 6th edn. Macmillan, New York, pp 91–100

Teague CT, Merrill DC (1978) Effect of baclofen and dantrolene on bladder stimulator induced detrusor sphincter dyssynergia in dogs. Urology 11:531–535

Thompson IM, Lauvetz R (1976) Oxygutynin in bladder spasm, neurogenic bladder and enuresis. Urology 8:452–454

Thor K, Roppolo J, De Groat W (1983) Naloxone induced micturition in unanesthetized paraplegic cats. J Urol 129:202–207

Thorner MO (1975) Dopamine is an important transmitter in the autonomic nervous system. Lancet I:662–664

Todd JK, Mack AJ (1969) A study of human bladder detrusor muscle. Br J Urol 41 [Suppl]:448–452

Tulloch AGS (1974) The vascular contribution to intraurethral pressure. Br J Urol 46:659–664

Tulloch A, Creed K (1979) A comparison between propantheline and imipramine on bladder and salivary gland function. Br J Urol 51:359–362

Ursillo RC (1967) Rationale for drug therapy in bladder dysfunction. In: Boyarsky S (ed) The neurogenic bladder. Williams & Wilkins, Baltimore, pp 187–190

Vaidyanathan S, Rao M, Bapna B, Chary K, Palaniswamy R (1980) Beta adrenergic activity in human proximal urethra: a study with terbutaline. J Urol 124:869–872

Vaidyanathan S, Rao M, Charry K, Sharma P, Das N (1981) Enhancement of detrusor reflex activity by naloxone in patients with chronic neurogenic bladder dysfunction. Preliminary report. J Urol 126:500–504

Wein AJ (1979) Pharmacological approach to the management of neurogenic bladder dysfunction. J Cont Ed Urol 18:17

Wein A (1980) Pharmacology of the bladder and urethra. In: Stanton SL, Tanagho EA (eds) Surgery of female incontinence, 1st edn. Springer, Berlin, Heidelberg, New York, pp 185–199

Wein AJ (1981) Classification of neurogenic voiding dysfunction: overview. J Urol 125: 605–609

Wein A, Levin R (1979) Adrenergic receptor density in the human urinary bladder as compared to that of the dog and rabbit. Surg Forum 30:576–580

Wein AJ, Raezer DM (1979) Physiology of micturition. In: Krane R, Siroky M (eds) Clinical neurourology. Little Brown, Boston, pp 1–33

Wein AJ, Raezer DM, Benson GS (1976) Management of neurogenic bladder dysfunction in the adult. Urology 8:432–443

Wein AJ, Hanno PM, Dixon DO, Raezer DM, Benson GS (1978)

The effect of oral bethanechol chloride on the cystometrogram of the normal adult male. J Urol 120:330–331

Wein A, Benson G, Jacobowitz D (1979) Lack of evidence for adrenergic innervation of external urethral sphincter. J Urol 121:324–326

Wein A, Raezer D, Malloy T (1980a) Failure of the bethanechol supersensitivity test to predict improved voiding after subcutaneous bethanechol administration. J Urol 123:202–204

Wein A, Malloy T, Shofer F, Raezer D (1980b) The effects of bethanechol chloride on urodynamic parameters in normal women and in women with significant residual urine volumes. J Urol 124:397–405

Weiner N (1980a) Aropine, scopolamine and related antimuscarinic drugs. In: Gilman AG, Goodman LS, Gilman A (eds) The pharmacological basis of therapeutics. Macmillan, New York, pp 120–137

Weiner N (1980b) Norepinephrine, epinephrine and the sympathomimetic amines. In: Gilman AG, Goodman LS, Gilman A (eds) The pharmacological basis of therapeutics. Macmillan, New York, pp 138–175

Weiner N (1980c) Drugs that inhibit adrenergic nerves and block adrenergic receptors. In: Gilman AG, Goodman LS, Gilman A (eds) The pharmacological basis of therapeutics. Macmillan, New York, pp 176–210

Weinshiebaum R (1980) Antihypertensive drugs that alter adrenergic function. Mayo Clin Proc 55:390–402

Whitfield HN, Doyle PT, Mayo ME, Poopalasingham N (1976) The effect of adrenergic blocking drugs on outflow resistance. Br J Urol 47:823–827

Yalla SV, Blunt KJ, Fam BA, Constantinople NL, Gittes RF (1977a) Detrusor-sphincter dyssynergia. J Urol 118:1026–1029

Yalla SV, Rossier AB, Fam BA, Gabilondo FB, DiBenedetto M, Gittes RF (1977b) Functional contribution of autonomic innervation to urethral striated sphincter: studies with parasympathetic, parasympatholytic and alpha adrenergic blocking agents in spinal cord injury and control male subjects. J Urol 117:494–499

17 Electrostimulation*

Emil A. Tanagho

Introduction

More than 1.5 million persons in the United States suffer from various forms of neuropathic bladder dysfunction. Although a high percentage of these patients have spinal cord injuries, with either partial or complete lesions, they by no means represent the entire affected population. Among the estimated 20 million diabetics in the United States, 10% will develop sequelae involving the peripheral nerves and the autonomic nervous system, with resultant impairment of bladder function. Many other disorders, including multiple sclerosis, cerebral strokes, myelomeningocele and Parkinson's disease, also have associated detrusor neuropathic dysfunction.

Deterioration of the urinary tract is responsible for a high incidence of morbidity and mortality among these patients. Dysfunction of the urinary bladder is the underlying cause of this morbidity: it precipitates urinary tract infection and urinary incontinence and creates back pressure on the kidney, leading to kidney infections and pyelonephritis, kidney stones and progressive renal damage, which, if left untreated, ends in renal failure. Incomplete bladder emptying and a concomitant large volume of residual urine are at the heart of these problems.

Current methods of treatment have their limitations as well as their own morbidity. The common means of management is limited to three main modalities: (a) intermittent catheterisation, mainly self-catheterisation, with all its complications; (b) pharmacological manipulation, either to inhibit detrusor hyperreflexia or to initiate bladder contraction, again with limitations; and (c) sphincterotomy and the elimination of bladder outlet resistance to permit complete bladder emptying, but with the sacrifice of continence.

Although some or all of these modalities achieve a certain degree of success, none really offers the ideal answer to the basic problem, or actually corrects or replaces the loss of neural control in the urinary bladder.

---

* The bibliography at the end of this chapter is intended as a guide to further reading, not as a comprehensive set of references to the original literature

Neurostimulation, however, has been proved to be a scientifically feasible means of attaining complete control of bladder evacuation. As such, it promises to eliminate most, if not all, of the urinary problems associated with neuropathic dysfunction.

Sacral Root Stimulation

Background

Over the last 20 years, several investigators have used various techniques of electrical stimulation of the denervated bladder; direct pelvic nerve stimulation has also been tried. The results, however, have not been very satisfactory. Direct detrusor stimulation by implanted electrode over the bladder base has been attempted, but with limited success. More recently, stimulation of the spinal cord micturition centre in a small number of patients has produced some favourable results.

This prompted us to evaluate such a method, hoping to achieve complete reproducible control of bladder function. Accordingly, we explored the possibility of direct spinal cord stimulation. This, too, proved unsuccessful: it provoked a higher rise in outflow resistance (sphincteric mechanism), which resulted in unsatisfactory, insufficient voiding. When emptying did take place, it was only what we have labelled post-stimulus voiding—a spurt of urine at the end of stimulation.

We then concentrated our efforts on isolating a detrusor centre from a sphincteric centre in the spinal cord, hoping that we could stimulate one centre separately from the other. It became clear after repeated testing that the two centres overlap and that there is no way of stimulating one at the level of the spinal cord without stimulating the other. It was then that the possibility of stimulating the sacral roots was explored, with the hope that there might be one particular sacral root destined to innervate the detrusor primarily and another to innervate the sphincter.

Animal Studies

In comparing the anatomy of the canine and human roots, it was found that the gross anatomy of the human sacral nerves is very similar to that of the dog. The ventral root is distinct and separated from the dorsal root by a prominent sheet of epineurium. The sacral roots have a long course within the dura, yet they also have a relatively long course extradurally but within the spinal canal. We elected to apply the stimulus on the extradural intraspinal segment of the sacral root.

In the dog, it was clear that S_2 is the preferable root for stimulation. This conclusion was based on urodynamic testing—simultaneous monitoring of bladder pressure, of two urethral sphincter pressures (one for the smooth sphincteric element, the second for the striated sphincter) and of anal sphincter activity (as another parameter to measure the responses of the entire pelvic floor musculature). Being able to quantify the response to stimulation at various levels in the lower urinary tract permitted selection of the sacral roots most suitable for stimulation to initiate detrusor contraction with the least possible sphincteric involvement.

Individual sacral roots were stimulated under various conditions (Fig. 17.1):

1. Intact sacral root
2. Ventral component of the sacral root
3. Dorsal component of the sacral root
4, 5. Proximal and distal cut ends of the motor ventral component
6, 7. Proximal and distal cut ends of the dorsal component of the sacral root.

After these extensive and variable means of stimulation were completed, it became clear that (a) stimulation of the intact root is the least effective, and (b) stimulation of the ventral component of the root is most effective.

Results of stimulation of the dorsal component were very close to those of stimulation of the ventral component. Our explanation was that neurostimulation resulted in synaptic activation of multiple ventral roots. This was confirmed by stimulating both proximal and distal ends of the cut dorsal component. Stimulation of the sacral root was compared between the two sides and there proved to be no difference between left and right root stimulation.

Unilateral stimulation was compared with bilateral stimulation at the same level; again, the responses were identical, except for the cumulative effect of bilateral stimulation when compared with

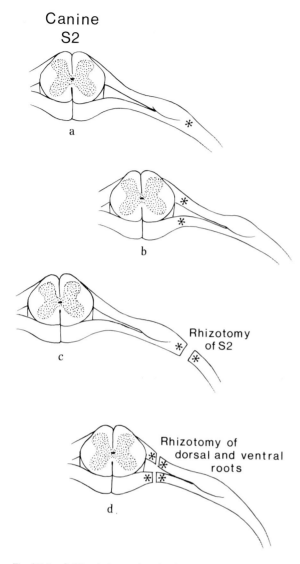

Canine
S2

a

b

Rhizotomy
of S2

c

Rhizotomy of
dorsal and ventral
roots

d

Fig. 17.1a–d. Stimulation with pudendal nerves intact in the dog. **a** Stimulation of intact nerve; **b** stimulation of intact dorsal and ventral roots; **c** stimulation of proximal and distal ends of divided S2; **d** stimulation of divided dorsal and ventral roots. *, points of stimulation.

unilateral stimulation. The outcome of these studies was that, to achieve the maximal detrusor response, it is preferable to isolate the ventral from the dorsal component of the root and to limit stimulation to the ventral component; to this end we sectioned the dorsal element completely. The advantage of such an approach was quite clear—to eliminate pain and any synaptic activation of multiple ventral roots. It also is more selective in that the ventral root sends the impulses towards the bladder, thus initiating detrusor contraction.

We found, however, that stimulation of the ventral component of the selected sacral root, while inducing detrusor contraction, also induced some degree of sphincter contraction because the ventral component carries both autonomic and somatic fibres to the pelvic floor musculature. A further refined set of experiments was then designed that allowed us to become more selective in these parameters of stimulation (Fig. 17.2). The ventral components were stimulated after:

1. Total unilateral pudendal neurotomy
2. Selective sectioning of somatic fibres of the stimulated sacral root before they join the rest of the components of the other sacral roots to form the pudendal nerve (Fig. 17.2).

It was found that selective somatic neurotomy was as effective as total pudendal neurotomy. This series of experiments (Fig. 17.3) showed that to achieve maximally specific detrusor stimulation with minimal sphincter activation, one must (a) separate the dorsal component from the ventral component, and (b) isolate and selectively section the somatic fibres of the sacral root to be stimulated. Anatomical study in the dog proved that this is feasible and quite practical surgically and technically.

Human Studies

Comparative anatomical study in the human showed that the entire procedure can be done from the back by separating the dorsal from the ventral component; then, through an opening into the sacral bone over the sacral canal, one can readily gain access to the somatic subdivision of that sacral root (one has to follow that particular root through the sacral foramen), which can be easily sectioned. We have done this repeatedly in the cadaver and the technical feasibility has been proved.

Electrode Implantation

During the past 2 years, six patients (five quadriplegics and one paraplegic) have undergone multiple sacral root electrode implantation without complication. All patients were evaluated

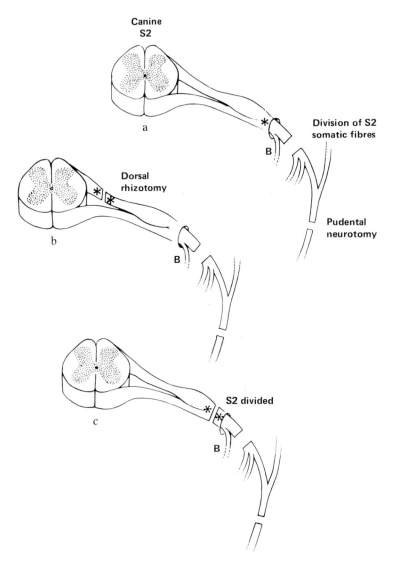

Fig. 17.2a–c. Stimulation after pudendal neurotomy in the dog. **a** Stimulation of S2. **b** Dorsal rhizotomy, proximal and distal stimulation. **c** S2 divided, proximal and distal stimulation. *, points of stimulation; *B*, ventral root.

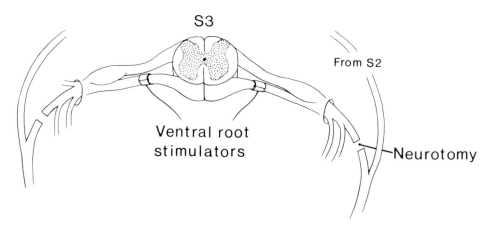

Fig. 17.3. Selective somatic neurotomy of the third sacral root with ventral root stimulators in place.

urodynamically for graphic demonstration of their behaviour disturbance, and each was found to have uniquely disrupted coordination between the bladder and the urethral sphincter.

Pre-operative Evaluation

With the patient in the prone position an insulated needle was passed into at least two sacral foramina, usually S_3 bilaterally and one S_2 as well. Responses of the bladder, urethral and anal sphincters and rectum were monitored graphically during test stimulation. The effects of neurostimulation on storage were assessed by filling the bladder during stimulation and comparing its storage capability to that without stimulation. The ability to produce a bladder contraction was assessed after both unilateral and bilateral selective pudendal nerve blockage. Voiding was accomplished in all patients, but only after bilateral pudendal block. Such blocks remove most meaningful activity within the urethral sphincter induced by stimulation but do not totally denervate the pelvic floor musculature. This indicates that a rather extensive selective division of the pudendal nerves may be carried out for voiding, but not risk incontinence. Significantly, bladder spasticity or excitability decreased greatly after bilateral pudendal block, and as a result bladder storage ability improved markedly. None of the patients experienced stress incontinence after the block, which remained effective for 3–6 h owing to the use of Marcaine with adrenaline.

Method

The method of electrode implant was as follows:

Under general anaesthesia, the patients were positioned in the operating room prone but with the hips and knees flexed. Recording catheters were then placed anally and urethrally and fixed in place. An S-shaped incision was made over the sacrum to avoid the bony prominence and resultant post-operative decubitus ulcer. In the last three patients, the sacral roots were exposed and monopolar cuff electrodes were placed on the ventral or entire roots. The incision was then extended into the buttock unilaterally. The sacrotuberous spinous ligament was identified and used, along with electrical stimulation, to locate the pudendal nerve. Once

identified, the pudendal nerve and its various branches could be traced towards the sacral canal. Test stimulation at the S_2 and S_3 levels and stimulation of the various nerve components of the main pudendal nerve were then used to effect, as completely as possible, a division of all somatic nerves from the S_3 level contributing to the pudendal nerve. The wounds were then closed. Post-operative evaluation was carried out at 1 and 6 weeks. Without exception, the patients demonstrated a marked decline in peripheral spasticity immediately post-operatively. The bladder could be contracted but no meaningful voiding was elicited, indicating that the contralateral side of the pelvic floor was responding to the stimulus because of the spread of current to adjacent nerves, either directly or reflexively. Although voiding could be produced at 1 week, it was not seen at 6 weeks as bladder contraction greatly declined in response to stimulation. There was no change in the reflex behaviour of the bladder or in continence as a result of these implants.

Accomplishments from Human Implantations

1. Demonstration of bladder evacuation via percutaneous sacral root stimulation and pudendal block.
2. Suppression of peripheral spasticity (i.e. a decrease in spontaneous bowel evacuation and in spontaneous spasms of the limbs, etc.) for a transient 2–3 week period after implant. During this time, bladder contraction could be induced by stimulation; after 4–6 weeks, peripheral spasticity gradually returned to pre-operative levels and the ability to induce bladder contractions became much reduced, necessitating higher current densities. This suggests some intrinsic inhibition of the bladder associated with the return of spasticity. (Spontaneous evacuation of the bladder, however, does take place in a pattern similar to that before implant.) Our present feeling is that the detrusor is suppressed or inhibited by the spastic tightness of the pelvic floor; with future pudendal neurectomies, minimising the tone of the pelvic floor, the bladder will be more amenable to evacuation. This was suggested by the voiding seen after bilateral block of the pudendal nerves (Fig. 17.2). Although pharmacological blockade approaches 100%, it never achieves it, and this is what we would hope to accomplish via selective surgical division of the S_3 contribution to the pudendal nerve.

3. Confirmation of the principle defined in the spinalised animal, wherein evacuation of the bladder was accomplished by means of sacral root stimulation after elimination of the pelvic floor response to stimulation. (There must be no pelvic floor contractile activity initiated by electrical stimulation; if possible, intrinsic behaviour within the pelvic floor must be minimised through step-sectioning of various components of the pudendal nerve.)

4. Elucidation of the changes in reflex bladder behaviour after selective pudendal block. Such changes might be expected after permanent sectioning of various components of the pudendal nerve unilaterally and bilaterally.

5. Demonstration of unchanged reflex behaviour from electrode implants. The ventral and dorsal roots of both the S_3 and S_2 nerves were separated and the S_3 contribution to the pudendal nerve was selectively divided on one side, yet no change in spontaneous detrusor behaviour from that seen post-operatively was found.

6. Demonstration that the S_3 nerve can be traced surgically in the buttock from its origin in the sacral canal to its branch contributions in the sciatic plexus and then the pudendal nerve. Neuroanatomy is quite complex and varies considerably among individuals. In only one of the patients was it possible to identify the contribution of the S_3 nerve directly to the pudendal nerve. In the remaining patients, the S_3 nerve blended with the sacral plexus, and branches from this plexus formed the pudendal nerve. However, by stimulation at the S_2 and S_3 levels via the implanted electrodes, along with stimulation of various nerve bundles contributing to the pudendal nerve, it was possible to stage-section the contributions to the pudendal nerve, leaving the S_2 sections intact but eliminating the contributions from the S_3 nerve. At no time were the autonomic contributions to the pelvis at risk because of their ventral orientation to the S_3 nerve. All surgical exposure of the sciatic plexus and pudendal nerve was dorsal and lateral to the point of separation between the somatics and the autonomics.

7. Measurement of current densities required to trigger sphincter and bladder behaviour. A graphic record of approximate current densities achieved at various settings on the transmitter is possible for each patient, should the settings differ post-operatively from those recorded intra-operatively.

The charge densities for stimulation proved to be quite high and were associated with current spread to adjacent dorsal roots as well as to adjacent nerves.

8. Safe separation of the dorsal and ventral roots at the S_3 level was accomplished without any apparent change in the reflex behaviour of the bladder.

9. Completion of the experimental animal model in the last human implant resulted in an ideal bladder pacemaker as the patient is catheter and infection free, continent and has no residual urine.

Other Applications of Percutaneous Sacral Root Implantation

Five patients underwent implantation of electrodes to correct voiding dysfunction resulting from neurological injury. A single electrode was implanted percutaneously within the S_3 foramen for the sole purpose of modulating reflex behaviour to improve bladder function.

The degree of symptomatically significant urinary incontinence from neurological disease or injury varies. If the mechanism of urinary leakage results in precipitate voiding (i.e. there is a sudden spontaneous reflex bladder contraction or reflex sphincter relaxation triggering the bladder contraction), control may be restored via a simple free-floating S_3 electrode. Electrical stimulation inhibits muscle behaviour and suppresses spontaneous bladder contractions and/or sphincter neurological deficits with their associated hyperreflexive changes that affect control of micturition.

Ideally, the bladder function should be predominantly that of emptying without residual urine. If there is sufficient sphincter tone to offset stress-induced leakage, a more appropriate balance can be obtained between bladder storage and bladder evacuation.

If patients are unable to void completely because of sphincter dyssynergia, it is possible to combine electrical stimulation of the sphincter with intermittent self-catheterisation. Thus, a patient will be able to empty the bladder effectively but will still be secured from the social embarrassment of urine leakage.

These five patients represent good examples of these principles. They were all significantly symptomatic from overfacilitated behaviour of the pelvic floor, the bladder or both. They underwent a successful trial implant of an S_3 foramen electrode with dramatic results that justified the permanent insertion of such a device.

Summary

Neurostimulation of selected sacral roots has proved to be scientifically feasible. The results presented above offer a new approach to the control of micturition and suggest that the same principles might be applied in the future for the control of sphincteric mechanisms—the urinary sphincter as well as the anal sphincter.

Achieving complete control of bladder function from storage to emptying will eliminate most, if not all, urinary problems associated with neuropathic dysfunction. As such, it will have a tremendous impact on the patient's overall well-being.

References

Bazeed MA, Thuroff JW, Schmidt RA, Wiggin DW, Tanagho EA (1982) Effect of chronic electrostimulation of the sacral roots on the striated urethral sphincter. J Urol 128:1357–1362

Boyced WN, Lathem E, Hunt LD (1964) Research related to the development of artificial electrical stimulator for the paralyzed human bladder. J Urol 91:41–51

Graber P, Tanagho EA (1975) Urethral response to autonomic nerve stimulation. Urology 6:52–58

Habib HN (1967) Experience and recent contributions in sacral nerve stimulation for voiding in both human and animal. Br J Urol 39:73–83

Hald T, Agarwal G, Kantrowitz A (1966) Studies in stimulation of the bladder and its motor nerves. Surgery 60:848–856

Heine JP, Schmidt RA, Tanagho EA (1977) Intraspinal sacral root stimulation for controlled micturition. Invest Urol 15:78–82

Holmquist B (1968) Electromicturition by pelvic nerve stimulation in dogs. Scand J Urol Nephrol 2 [Suppl 2]:7–27

Janez J, Plevnik S, Suhel P (1979) Urethral and bladder responses to anal electrical stimulation. J Urol 122:192–194

Jonas U, Heine JP, Tanagho EA (1975) Studies on the feasibility of urinary bladder evacuation by direct spinal cord stimulation. I. Parameters of most effective stimulation. Invest Urol 13:143–150

Jonas U, Jones LW, Tanagho EA (1975) Spinal cord stimulation versus detrusor stimulation. A comparative study in six acute dogs. Invest Urol 13:171–174

Jonas U, Tanagho EA (1975) Studies on the feasibility of urinary bladder evacuation by direct stimulation of the spinal cord. II. Post stimulus voiding: a way to overcome outflow resistance. Invest Urol 13:151–153

Jones LW, Jonas U, Tanagho EA, Heine JP (1976) Urodynamic evaluation of a chronically implanted bladder pacemaker. Invest Urol 13:375–379

Nashold BS, Friedman H, Glenn JF, Grimes JH, Barry WF, Avery R (1972) Electromicturition in paraplegia. Arch Surg 104:195–202

Rossier AB (1974) Neurogenic bladder in spinal cord injury. Urol Clin North Am 1:125–138

Schmidt RA (1983) Neural prostheses and bladder control. Engineering in Medicine and Biology 2:31–36

Schmidt RA, Bruschini H, Tanagho EA (1978) Feasibility of inducing micturition through stimulation of sacral roots. MB Wesson Essay, Western Section, AUA, 1977, Urology 12:471–477

Schmidt RA, Bruschini H, Tanagho EA (1979) Sacral root stimulation in controlled micturition: Peripheral somatic neurotomy and stimulated voiding. Invest Urol 17:130–134

Schmidt RA, Bruschini H, Tanagho EA (1979) Urinary bladder and sphincter responses to stimulation of dorsal and ventral sacral roots. Invest Urol 16:300–304

Schmidt RA, Tanagho EA (1979) Feasibility of controlled micturition through electric stimulation. Urol Int 32:199–230

Stenberg CC, Burnett HW, Bunts RC (1967) Electrical stimulation of human neurogenic bladders. Experience with 4 patients. J Urol 97:79–84

Tanagho EA (1973) Vesicourethral dynamics. In: Lutzeyer W and Melchior H (eds) Urodynamics, Springer, Berlin Heidelberg New York, pp 215–236

Tanagho EA, Schmidt RA (1982) Bladder pacemaker: Scientific basis and clinical future. Urology 20:614–619

Tanagho EA, Schmidt RA, deAraujo CG (1982) Urinary striated sphincter: What is its nerve supply? Urology 20:415–417

Tanagho EA, Smith DR (1966) The anatomy and function of the bladder neck. Br J Urol 38:54–71

Teaque CT, Merrill DC (1977) Electric pelvic floor stimulation: Mechanism of action. Invest Urol 15:65–69

Thuroff JW, Bazeed MA, Schmidt RA, Lue TF, Tanagho EA (1982) Regional topography of spinal cord neurons innervating pelvic floor muscles and bladder neck in the body. Urol Int 37:110–120

Thuroff JW, Bazeed MA, Schmidt RA, Tanagho EA (1982) Mechanisms of urinary continence: Animal model to study urethral responses to stress conditions. J Urol 127:1202–1206

Thuroff JW, Bazeed MA, Schmidt RA, Wiggin DM, Tanagho EA (1982) Functional pattern of sacral root stimulation in dogs. I. Micturition. J Urol 127:1031–1033

Thuroff JW, Bazeed MA, Schmidt RA, Wiggin DM, Tanagho EA (1982) Functional pattern of sacral root stimulation in dogs. II. Urethral closure. J Urol 127:1034–1038

Thuroff JW, Schmidt RA, Bazeed MA, Tanagho EA (1983) Chronic stimulation of the sacral roots in dogs. Eur Urol 9:102–108

Timm G, Bradley W (1969) Electrostimulation of the urinary detrusor to effect contraction and evacuation. Invest Urol 6:562–568

Woodside JR, McGuire EJ (1979) Urethral hypotonicity after suprasacral spinal cord injury. J Urol 121:783–785

18 Post-operative Voiding Dysfunction

Richard A. Schmidt

As pre-operative assessments of urinary incontinence have become more sophisticated, so more factors contributing to the loss of sphincteric efficiency have become apparent. We must now assess not just whether leakage occurs with depression of the bladder on straining, but also the intrinsic capabilities of the voluntary sphincter components within the urethra itself and the pelvic floor, the presence or absence of urethral versus detrusor instability, voiding dyssynergia, rectal behaviour and tonus, perineal sensation, urethral sensitivity and tissue compliance. Simple anatomical decensus will give the best surgical results. However, the more causative urodynamic factors present, the more difficult it will be to obtain a satisfactory surgical cure. Perhaps more important than failing surgically is to avoid aggravating a patient's problems.

One of the more significant advances in understanding has been the appreciation that the pelvic floor is composed of both slow- and fast-twitch muscles. Muscle behaviour within the pelvis should thus be understood in terms of the physiological behaviour of these muscle fibre types. Because behaviour of the sphincteric muscles of the pelvic floor has a pivotal influence on the nature of bladder activity, the two principal functions of the bladder—storage and evacuation—can be viewed as the natural consequence of neuromuscular reflexes controlling the pelvic floor musculature. Although this is a simplified characterisation of complex neuronal interactions, it serves as a practical standard by which dysfunctional voiding states can be understood and managed.

Pathophysiology

The efficiency of coordination between the bladder and sphincter will have a significant impact upon the results of continence surgery. Certainly, many patients present with mixed complaints involving not only stress-induced urinary leakage but also associated irritative voiding symptoms. It is important to assess these irritative symptoms carefully to determine whether they will reflect significantly on the patient's ability to void after continence surgery. Stress incontinence in its purest form will be based purely on weakness within the striated muscles forming the external sphincter. On occasion, however, weakness may be less relevant than spontaneously occurring dyssynergic activities of the external sphincter, which can cause leakage through an inappropriate, brief loss of the outlet resistance. The clinician should be careful to screen these patients before submitting them to any type of incontinence surgery. The importance of identifying dyssynergic tendencies within the external sphincter is that these patients are prone to have persisting problems post-operatively. Voiding dysfunction may even be aggravated by surgery. This is especially true if surgery is performed vaginally.

It is not uncommon to find during pre-operative urodynamic evaluations that patients void by abdominal straining without any real awareness of the need to initiate a void through pelvic floor relaxation. These patients, on straining, are able to push their pelvic floor down with the bladder and urethra, thus minimising outlet resistance intrinsic to the urethra as well as the participation of the pelvic floor muscles. Voiding is possible in this situation because of relatively little intrinsic urethral resistance and an open bladder neck due to the decensus of the bladder. After surgery, following replacement of the bladder neck within the pelvis, all the resistance becomes much more efficient and there is correction of the funnelling of the bladder neck. Simple straining does not work well in this situation. Active contraction of the detrusor is required to open up the proximal urethra. These patients thus need to be re-educated pre-operatively to relax their pelvic muscles properly in order to permit a natural physiological void. Without relaxation of the pelvic muscles, the detrusor remains neurologically suppressed and the active contraction required to open the proximal urethra along with the natural relaxation of the external sphincter does not occur.

Problems of Inhibition—the Large Bladder

Usually an efficient bladder contraction is preceded by sphincteric relaxation. Normal relaxation of sphincter tone before voiding is a slow event, as is its return after voiding. Spontaneous contractions that briefly interrupt urine flow occur much faster. These differences can be ascribed to slow- and fast-twitch muscle behaviour of the pelvic floor and urethral sphincter. Both can be dyssynergic (Fig. 18.1) and associated with inhibition of the detrusor—one on a more sustained basis, one very briefly. They may occur together or separately:

for example, spastic contractions of the urethral sphincter can be superimposed on a non-relaxed or relaxed basal tone. The neurological basis for such altered striated muscle behaviour in the pelvis is not understood, but generally has its origin in organically based neuropathies, local inflammations or psychological influences.

Poor sphincteric relaxation will suppress detrusor contractility via peripheral reflex arcs, involving just the pudendal nerve, spinal micturition centre and pelvic nerves. However, higher CNS centres in addition to local sphincter factors may be responsible for failure of the sphincter to relax. In either case, once sphincteric relaxation occurs, bladder contractions will almost invariably follow with a resulting void.

Clinically, the physician may find an acontractile bladder on CMG. By implication, there will almost always be a failure of the sphincter to relax, although this may be very subtle. This failure to relax can be appreciated by careful observation of the perineum for movements of the levators. Infrequent voiding because of prolonged suppression of the urge to void leads to overstretching of the detrusor muscle. Subtle degrees of holding for many years can easily account for the large, thin-walled bladders not uncommonly seen in women of middle age or older. Incorrect voiding techniques or poor voiding habits from childhood or young adulthood can explain these findings. Mild inflammatory and traumatic insults or even hormonal influences, accumulated over many years, may lead to a change in the compliance of the tissue or to loss of its elasticity, contributing to the inability to open the urethra. Nerve endings concerned with exteroceptive and proprioceptive feedback to the spinal cord would be affected by these changes, with consequent alterations in the central nervous system's regulation of the micturition reflux.

Many female patients with large, poorly contractile bladders are seen at a stage when the altered dynamics of the voiding dysfunction may not be demonstrable. However, careful urodynamic monitoring can provide clues: the patient will characteristically be unable to tighten or relax her pelvic muscles voluntarily. Typically, such patients have habitually voided by straining more than by the properly coordinated relaxation of the pelvic muscles.

Personality factors can contribute greatly to the neurological imbalance which leads to the large inefficient bladder. Nervous individuals with high degrees of tension in all their skeletal muscles may

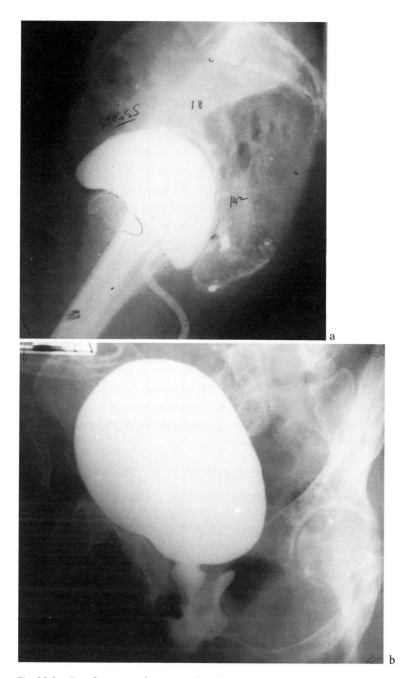

Fig. 18.1. a Female patient who presented with mixed symptoms of urgency, frequency and incontinence. The patient subsequently underwent a colpocysto-urethral suspension to correct a marked cystocele. **b** Post-operatively the patient was unable to empty her bladder completely because of external urethral sphincter dyssynergia. The patient performed self-catheterisation once a day to empty a residual of 200 cc

have particular difficulty in achieving relaxation of the bladder outlet. These patients have a generalised difficulty in the conscious relaxation of skeletal muscles, and experience even greater difficulty relaxing pelvic striated muscles, which operate for the most part on a subconscious level.

Urodynamic studies help in assessing the integrity of the detrusor and the sphincter. Large bladders associated with weak sphincters are compromised intrinsically by a deficiency in the muscle tissue itself; those associated with cystoceles but with effective voluntary augmentation of sphincter tone suggest healthy urethral muscle compromised by the urethral foreshortening which accompanies a cystocele. Inability to show an increase in sphincter tone urodynamically, either with a voluntary hold manoeuvre or on the urethral pressure profile performed with the bladder neck lifted per vaginam using an open ring forceps and in the vagina, suggests intrinsic weakness of urethral muscles.

Problems of Facilitation—the Unstable Bladder

Traditional provocative stimuli to diagnose unstable bladder contractions have included rapid cystometry, posture shift and triggering with an indwelling Foley catheter. However, it is our exper-

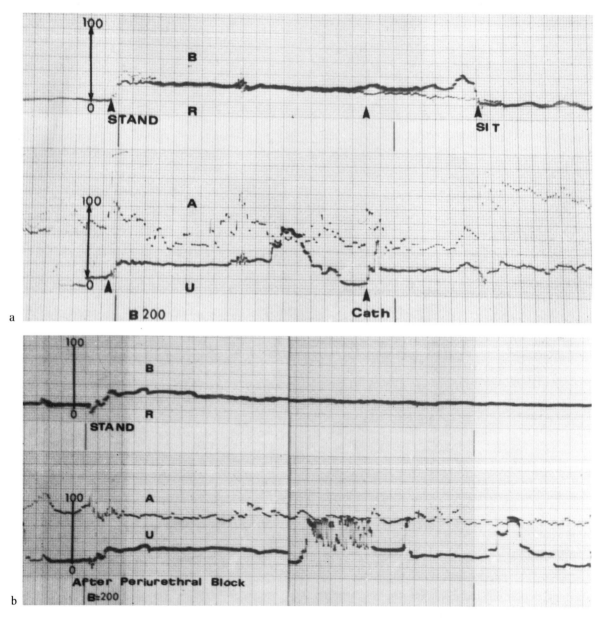

Fig. 18.2. a Female patient with urinary frequency and incontinence. The patient was found to have low resting urethral tone but voiding triggered by catheter friction in the external urethral sphincter zone. **b** After xylocaine 1% infiltration of the distal urethral wall, no further detrusor contractions could be triggered, even with rapid movement of the catheter within the zone of the urethral sphincter. Suspension surgery in this patient was not performed as the cause of the leakage was felt to be neurological rather than anatomical.

ience that mechanical stimulation in the zone of the external sphincter is the most provocative trigger of the unstable bladder contraction. This clearly indicates an afferent role of the pelvic floor and the pudendal nerves in contributing to this abnormal behaviour. Hyperreflexic activity of the bladder is always accompanied by a degree of reciprocal behavioural change within the urethra. Blocking these nerves by either peri-urethral infiltration of Xylocaine (lidocaine hydrochloride) or a pudenal block can change the excitablity of the detrusor (Fig. 18.2). The unstable bladder should be viewed as a composite problem encompassing the entire urethra and the pelvic floor and the pudendal nerves that control them.

The facilitation (and inhibition) of the detrusor is linked to higher centres within the central nervous system, but also to peripheral factors that we are not able to explain fully and document at present.

Hypersensitivity within the zone of urethral striated sphincter is often associated with an effect on the detrusor. It may or may not be associated with unstable spastic behaviour of the urethral sphincter, but it will always be associated with increased frequency of urination. Urodynamically, there may be an increase in sphincter tone, unstable detrusor behaviour, or detrusor sphincter dyssynergia on voiding. The important point is that irritation within the urethra can serve as a trigger for premature and dysfunctional voiding.

Injuries to the spine or disc disease, however mild, can account for a disturbance of the facilitatory and inhibitory reflex arcs controlling bladder behaviour. Such mild inflammations can indeed upset the delicate neurological balance influencing voiding and account for a mild voiding dysfunction.

Surgical Causes

There are a number of reasons for poor voiding subsequent to incontinence surgery. The most common and easiest pitfall are procedures which result in direct obstruction of the urethra. The reasons for the obstruction vary from case to case, depending upon the type of surgical procedure pursued. In a classic Marshall-Marchetti-Krantz procedure, where sutures are placed adjacent to the urethra between the meatus and bladder neck, the mechanism of obstruction lies in overstretching or over-correcting

the decensus. Pulling the vaginal tissues excessively so that the bladder neck comes to lie high behind the symphysis leads to obstruction through simple attenuation of lumen through overstretch of collagenous tissues of the urethra. Excessively lax pelvic tissues make this possible. There is a natural tendency to push the vaginal walls up towards the back of the symphysis via fingers of an assistant placed within the vagina as the sutures are tied. One should aim to bring the bladder neck up to the inferior margin of the symphysis or behind the lower third of the symphysis and avoid excessive over-correction. If the urethra is pulled too aggressively, tension is placed on the external sphincter and this can aggravate irritative symptoms intrinsic to this zone of the urethra. Over-correction leads to a loss of the normal compliance necessary for proper voiding (Fig. 18.3). Other procedures or techniques can result in direct compression of the urethra. The sling procedures are particularly prone to this, as are techniques which result in placement of sutures too close to the urethra. The obstruction in this situation is the result of direct compression of the urethral walls, or bladder neck fibrosis secondary to ischaemic injury of the bladder neck vascular pedicles.

It should be remembered that anatomically the urethra lies sandwiched between the anterior vaginal wall behind and the endopelvic fascia in front. Sutures placed into the vaginal wall and then directed such that they have a lateral pull on these tissues, as in the Burch procedure, in effect can compress the urethra by closing the sandwich—that is by tightening the anterior vaginal wall against the endopelvic fascia and thereby compressing the urethra. Sutures should be directed in as forward a direction as possible and tightened only to a modest degree so that the bladder neck is not brought excessively high up behind the symphysis. Generally a finger can be placed down between the symphysis and the bladder and the urethra when this is done correctly.

Prevention

The key to keeping post-voiding problems to a minimum is, of course, understanding all the physiological aspects which may have a bearing on the outcome of any one particular patient. It is

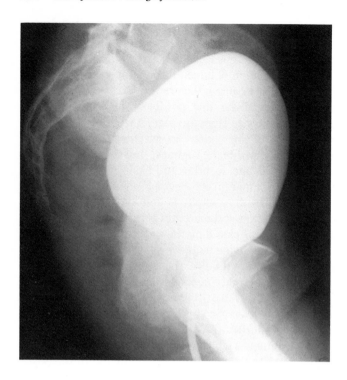

Fig. 18.3. Patient with obstructive voiding symptoms following a bladder suspension procedure. The bladder neck was high, above the mid-symphysial level, and adhered to the symphysis.

recommended that all patients undergo a thorough evaluation before surgical correction of incontinence. This will provide not only an insight into the subtleties of a patient's physiological problems, but also a baseline for difficulties which may develop in the post-operative period. All patients should have at the very least a lateral cystogram evaluation and a flow rate measurement. These techniques will allow for anatomical replacement of the bladder within the pelvis and an indication of spasticity and irritability. Such changes as trabeculation and an excessively large bladder suggest the possiblity of a neurological abnormality.

Urethral pressure profiles performed pre-operatively will provide an assessment of the intrinsic capabilities of the sphincter. The urethral pressure profile can be performed before and during a bladder neck elevation procedure using a ring forceps carefully placed in the vagina to lift the bladder neck back against the symphysis, and a profile taken in this circumstance will certainly provide insight as to the results can be obtained through a bladder suspension procedure. Patients who do not show a clear-cut improvement in their profile under these circumstances are more prone to failure, quite possibly due to intrinsic weakness of the urethral sphincter tissues. Concern regarding the success of surgery may very well be raised by other aspects of

the evaluation, e.g. X-ray and cystoscopy suggesting a very attenuated and thin bladder. These patients may have very poor detrusor contractility with inability of their bladders to overcome post-operative increase in urethral resistance. Such patients are also likely to have intrinsic weakness of the urethral sphincter and thus be more prone to surgical failure.

Hypersensitivity of the urethra with evidence of irritability behaviour may predispose to the unstable behaviour in the urethra and the bladder seen post-operatively (Fig. 18.3). With this pre-operative information one can deal with expected irritative symptoms in the post-operative interval. Without such information one cannot separate those patients who were predisposed to aggravation of irritative symptoms in the post-operative period from those patients in whom these symptoms were created by the surgery. Anatomically, it is difficult to explain the creation of irritative symptoms unless a procedure results in direct interference with the innervation of the bladder neck and/or external urethral sphincter. One must remember that a plexus of nerves and vessels enters the bladder between the 4 and 8 o'clock positions on either side of the urethra. Surgery in this area risks injury to these nerves or vessels with the possibility of either disruption of normal reflexive voiding mechanisms or fibrosis of the bladder neck secondary to ischaemic injury. Techniques which involve placement of sutures on either side of the urethra alone are less prone to result in irritative voiding difficulties.

The important point is to identify particular aspects of a patient's voiding that will allow careful pre-operative counselling as to the difficulties that may be encountered. One can certainly become suspicious of those individuals in whom all factors necessary for good operative results are absent.

When patients are identified as having an element of "irritation" within the external sphincter and dyssynergic tendencies are demonstrated in the urethra, or tissue factors suggest that the patient will have difficulty voiding post-operatively, then it is best to manage these patients post-operatively via a suprapubic catheter. This will avoid aggravating irritation of the trigone and urethral sphincter zone and allow time for the tissues to recover from the trauma of the surgery. The catheter should be left for 10 days or until the patient demonstrates the ability to void per urethram. In most patients, a suprapubic catheter is left for 5–7 days post-operatively. This time interval allows the patient to recover and become sufficiently mobile from surgery for voiding to occur. Patients generally void better after this lapse of time than if the catheter is removed earlier. Voiding improves with increasing ambulation, a gradual lessening of the oedema around the urethra and the bladder neck due to surgery, and recovery of voiding reflexes from the stress of surgery. Patients can be converted to use of clean self-catheterisation techniques if residuals persist beyond 2–3 weeks. This will allow for removal of the suprapubic catheter.

Treatment

After determining whether a patient's voiding dysfunction results from excessive facilitation or inhibition of either the detrusor, sphincter or both, one can apply appropriate therapy to this physiological dysfunctional activity. One should carefully separate these patients into a group in which dysfunctional voiding is responsible for difficulty in voiding, and a group in which obstruction through surgical technique is the pre-eminent cause. In the post-operative period, careful evaluation, again

urodynamically and via cystogram, will help one to categorise these patients. If on urodynamic evaluation the detrusor instability appears to be a factor, and generally this is a result of excessive afferent facilitation via pudendal nerves, then treatment should be channelled towards minimising these afferent influences on the behaviour. Urethral dilatation, diminishing the proprioceptive feedback assoiated with muscle spasm, will help not only to facilitate urethral relaxation but also to improve bladder evacuation. Treatment of infection by antibiotics and by improved voiding will help decrease the inflammation and irritation. a-Adrenergic blockers (prazosin and phenoxybenzamine) help to decrease the excitability of sacral spinal reflexes and also diminish sphincter tone via a direct influence on the smooth muscle within the region of the sphincters and its effect on the bladder neck. This medication works well in combination with a generalised muscle relaxant such as diazepam or Flexoril. The detrusor muscle itself can be suppressed by anticholinergic drugs, but these affect the smooth muscle directly and do not alter neurological responses which may be underlying the urge or frequency sensations arising from the zone of the external sphincter or the bladder neck. Nevertheless, such suppression can have a therapeutic benefit on the pelvic floor because of reciprocal relationships between the urethra and the bladder. Thus combinations of various classes of drugs— skeletal muscle relaxants, a-blockers, anticholinergic agents and even the smooth muscle relaxants—can play a role. The goal would be to achieve a combination of therapy that effectively releases motor dysfunction and symptoms but does not create intolerable side-effects. Also by changing the overfacilitating responses of the urethra and the pelvic floor, the detrusor responses should improve.

Long-term Management

Patients in whom there is urodynamic and radiological evidence of over-correction and compression of the urethra can be managed either by maintenance of the suprapubic catheter until voiding improves such that residuals are below 100 cc, or by instruction in intermittent self-catheterisation. Patients should be carefully followed for a minimum of 6 months before entertaining a subsequent surgical procedure. The only choice in cases where obstruction is evident, is to take down the original procedure and redo the operation in such a way that the urethral obstruction is no longer a factor. If however, there is urodynamic evidence of marked intrinsic weakness of the external urethral sphincter mechanism, it may be preferable for the patient to accept the presence of residual urine. Dependence on intermittent clean self-catheterisation is far preferable to persistent urinary leakage.

References

Cardozo L, Stanton SL, Hafner J, Allan V (1978) Biofeedback in the treatment of detrusor instability. Br J Urol 50:250–254

DeGroat WC, Saum WR (1976) Synaptic transmission in parasympathetic ganglia in the urinary bladder of the cat. J Physiol 256:137–158

DeGroat WC, Booth AM, Milne RJ, Roppolo JR (1982) Parasympathetic preganglionic neurons in the sacral spinal cord. J Auton Nerv Syst 5:23–43

Freiha FS, Stamey TA (1980) Cystolysis: A procedure for the selective denervation of the bladder. J Urol 123:360–363

Frewen WK (1978) An objective assessment of the unstable bladder of psychosomatic origin. Br J Urol 50:246–249

Glen E (1975) Control of incontinence by electrical devices. In: Caldwell KPS (ed) Urinary incontinence. Grune & Stratton, New York, pp 89–113

Godec C, Kralj B (1976) Selection of patients with urinary incontinence for application of functional electrical stimulation. Urol Int 31:124–128

Gosling JA, Dixon JS, Critchley HOD, Thompson SA (1981) A comparative study of the human external sphincter and periurethral levator ani muscles. Br J Urol 53:35–41

Griffiths DJ (1973) The mechanics of the urethra and of micturition. Br J Urol 45:497–507

Kiesswetter H, Flamm J (1978) The mucosal electrosensitivity threshold (MST): A test for use in conjunction with electronic stimulation in urinary incontinence in women. Br J Urol 50:262–263

Merrill DC, Conway C, DeWolf W (1975) Urinary incontinence. Treatment with electrical stimulation of the pelvic floor. Urology 5:67–72

Richardson FH, Stonington OG (1969) Urethrolysis and external urethroplasty in the female. Surg Clin North Am 49:1201–1208

Schmidt RA (1983) Neural prosthesis and bladder control. Eng Med Biol 2(2):31

Tanagho EA, Lyon RP (1971) Urethral dilatation versus internal ureterotomy. J Urol 105:242–244

Torrens M, Hald T (1979) Bladder denervation procedures. Urol Clin North Am 6:283–293

Zinner NR, Ritter RC, Sterling AM (1976) The mechanism of micturition. In: Williams DI, Chisholm GD (eds) Scientific foundations of urology, vol 20. William Heinemann, London, pp 39–51

Zufall R (1963) Treatment of the urethral syndrome in women. JAMA 184:894–895

19 Post-operative Catheter Drainage

Richard A. Schmidt

Introduction

The use of an indwelling Foley catheter for catheter drainage is a common practice following pelvic operations. The reasons for catheterisation generally focus on operative needs and the inability of patients to empty in the immediate post-operative period. Roughly 80% of patients undergoing a gynaecological procedure will require post-operative catheter drainage. However, most of these patients will have short-term needs for a catheter. Rarely, if ever, will the results of pelvic surgery, other than for removal of the rectum, lead to permanent paralysis of the bladder. Still, a number of patients will require catheter drainage for a varying time. Fortunately, for these patients, suprapubic drainage now rivals the transurethral approach; the former is safe and for the most part preferred. The purpose of this chapter is to review some of the subtleties of catheterisation, both advantageous and disadvantageous, and to provide some guidelines for the practising clinician.

Indications

A catheter should always be viewed as a foreign body attended by risks. Its use should therefore be justifiable from a risk–benefit ratio favourable to the patient. Fortunately the risks of catheterisation are low.

Pre-operative indications for catheterisation imply either a medical need pre-dating surgery or an underlying dysfunctinal–*neuropathic* or non-*neuropathic* voiding state. The ability of a patient to empty her bladder prior to surgery should be established. Borderline efficiency in bladder evacuation can be a warning to the clinician about bladder problems which can occur after surgery. A simple inquiry into the patient's voiding habits (especially of frequency, urgency, hesitancy, intermittent voiding and incontinence) should be documented and if abnormal, investigated urodynamically.

In situations where catheter dependency has been established, some attempt to sterilise the urine should be made prior to surgery. For the most part, this would include placing the patient on an appropriate antimicrobial and intermittent catheterisation programme.

When indicated, the usual or preferred time for catheter insertion is intra-operatively. The chief reasons for doing this are to provide a palpable landmark to identify the urethra as well as the bladder neck, to provide a record of urine output and to allow voiding during the procedure as well as in the immediate post-operative phase. Intra-operatively the urethral catheter, with its inflated balloon, is a useful anatomical landmark for the surgeon. Traction on the balloon delineates the vesicourethral junction and, of course, the urethra. Both are important to the vaginal and pelvic surgeon trying to avoid an injury to the bladder or to the plexus of nerves entering the bladder neck.

Historically, some patients have difficulty emptying their bladder in the immediate post-operative period and the catheter avoids the problems of urinary retention until the patient becomes adequately mobile, at which time the bladder will function appropriately. The reasons for acute retention, apart from the patient being sedated by anaesthesia and analgesia, include muscle spasm due to oedema and trauma in the region of the sphincter and neuropraxic injury to the pelvic plexus. However, in general the neuropraxic injury is self-reversing over a short time period and oedema, which has a stiffening effect on muscle and thus effects a compliance change, will settle and disappear so that the muscle function will return. Also, neurologically there may be a refractory period post-surgery in which the reflexes governing micturition do not operate effectively. Procedures designed to accomplish bladder suspension in the presence of a catheter allow the surgeon to appropriately place sutures for suspension of the vesicourethral junction. The bladder itself may be so decompensated after years of voiding against virtually no resistance that it is unable to overcome the increased resistance of the urethral outlet. The patients who have become so accustomed to voiding by straining may be unable to void post-operatively because of poor relaxation of the pelvic muscles. Patients in this category must retrain themselves to void with coordinated relaxation of the pelvic floor once they have an efficient urethral sphincter mechanism. Post-operatively, as patient activity is restricted by pain and sedation, it is difficult to achieve evacuation of the bladder conveniently. The presence of a

catheter provides the patient with the opportunity to rest, allowing appropriate sedation to work effectively and avoids soiling of fresh perineal wounds with urine. It is also an opportunity to monitor kidney function.

Technically, during surgery it is useful to use a somewhat larger catheter that is more easily palpable. Thus a 20 or 22 Foley catheter with a balloon inflated to 10 cc is recommended. After surgery, the prime purpose is to accomplish drainage of the bladder and this can be achieved satisfactorily with a smaller diameter and more compatible Foley catheter, such as a 14 or 16 French gauge with a 5 cc balloon. Patients are generally left on continuous drainage until ambulatory, after which time the catheter is removed. The patient is allowed a trial of voiding with daily observation of residual urines, to ensure that they are less than 100 cc and not increasing. Reinsertion of the catheter may be required if they exceed 100 cc. In this case, a retrial of voiding can be performed at weekly intervals until the patient can be satisfactorily weaned from dependence on the catheter. Incontinence following such surgery may be secondary to retention and overflow, or a result of temporary dysfunction of the urethral sphincter due to the irritation of the pelvic and urethral muscles. Such dysfunction generally corrects itself in 4–5 days if secondary to the catheter, or as wound healing progresses if it is secondary to surgery on or near the bladder or urethra. At any rate, an awareness of a patient's voiding performance should be maintained during the entire post-operative care period. Physicians should be aware that many female patients tend to have irritation in the region of the urethral sphincter. This irritation is accompanied by varying degrees of urethral sphincter dysfunction which can only be aggravated by long-term presence of a catheter. If a patient is known to have irritative voiding symptoms it is best to manage them using suprapubic rather than transurethral drainage.

As to the type of catheter, this should preferably be Silastic or Teflon coated: these are less irritating as a rule, produce minimal encrustation but are also more rigid. Usually, catheters are not left indwelling long enough for encrustation to be a problem. Latex catheters are more irritating and this is a consideration. The Latex catheter, over a short period of time, is acceptable particularly as it is a much softer catheter. Catheters impregnated with antibiotics or silver nitrate have not yet been found to provide any advantage over standard catheters. There is, however, ongoing interest in researching these techniques.

Suprapubic Versus Urethral Drainage

For most procedures, catheter drainage via the urethra is perfectly adequate. It is simple and usually well tolerated by patients. Many surgeons now prefer suprapubic to urethral drainage. The chief advantage to this approach is that it allows the physician to assess voiding before catheter removal. The suprapubic catheter can simply be clamped for a day or two and reopened periodically to monitor the residual urine after a void. It is also preferred in situations where voiding difficulties are expected for several weeks post-operatively. This may take place, for example, following a difficult hysterectomy, where stretching and retraction of tissues within the pelvis could result in a temporary neuropraxia, which interferes with the efficiency of the bladder contraction. Following suprapubic bladder suspensions, where the urethra has been stretched or tightened, there is often a prolonged period of difficulty in voiding. Suprapubic drainage is also useful following certain extensive vaginal procedures, simply because of the spasm and irritation of the pelvic floor muscles. It is a decision based upon the experience of individual surgeons with particular techniques and may also be based upon surgical exposure used at the time of the operation. Certainly if the suprapubic (or transabdominal) approach is performed, the bladder is readily accessible and a Malecot catheter is easily left exiting from the dome of the bladder to avoid irritation of the trigone and bladder neck. Vaginal approaches do not provide this ready accessibility and for this reason urethral drainage is usually adequate and preferable. The morbidity from the use of a suprapubic catheter is, of course, secondary to the trauma in the bladder wall creating bladder spasms. This is not an insignificant factor, as individual tolerance to the catheter can be rather poor. Anticholinergic drugs may be required to control the spasms and these, of course, have side-effects. The main decision at the time of surgery is whether or not to open the bladder. There is a risk of leakage and bleeding from the cystostomy site, albeit small.

The indwelling urethral catheter is not associated with these particular problems or risks and thus is much simpler. It is, however, associated with a rather early bacterial contamination. Its major disadvantage is that the catheter rests on the trigone and the sphincter, producing irritation and discomfort. Generally this is of an acceptable level if the catheter is removed within 5 days. Certain patients with long-standing histories of urgency may not tolerate a urethral catheter well and early removal may be preferable. If continued catheter drainage is required then intermittent catheter techniques are perfectly acceptable, as the indwelling Foley catheter is only needed for the first 24 h post-operatively. Following this, intermittent catheterisation can be performed by the ward nurse or by the patient. If such a circumstance can be anticipated, it is far less costly in the long run to insert a suprapubic silastic tube. Changes are far less frequent and the higher cost of insertion would be more than offset if a patient had to resort to intermittent self-catheterisation for any length of time.

Technique

Urethral

The early contamination of urine by bacteria following placement of an indwelling Foley catheter is a reasonably common problem in females. Ninety-six per cent of bladders will have bacteriuria by the 4th day. Bacteria can be demonstrated as soon as 24 h following insertion of the catheter unless efforts are made to avoid this. Irrigation of the bladder with antibiotic solutions or administration of oral antibiotics is not helpful in preventing contamination of the urine and only risks overgrowth of fungi in the vagina and/or the urine. The urine will be clear of fungus once the antibiotics are stopped, the catheter withdrawn and the patient voids on her own without significant residual urine. To avoid the above problems simple techniques can be used. After catheterisation, there is a tendency to deal with catheters in a matter-of-fact way. Small details, however, can make a big difference to the morbidity of a particular patient. Because the source of bacteria for urinary tract contamination is the urethral meatus in one-third of patients, the bacterial concentration of the vaginal introitus, the vaginal vault and the periurethral area must be attended to prior to insertion of the catheter. Careful cleansing of these areas, perhaps including a vaginal douche with Betadine solution, will minimise the risk of early contamination or early bacterial recovery from the urine. The catheter should be inserted preferably immediately prior to the surgery in the operating theatre. This allows for adequate perineal and skin preparation. Post-operatively, catheters should be kept on closed drainage. Meatal cleansing and application of antibiotics have not only failed to decrease bacteria, but actually increase the risk of contamination because of non-augmentation of the urethra. The introitus is a moist area and a very attractive site for bacteria. Good nursing care involves proper cleansing of this area on a daily basis. The catheter should be taped to the thigh with the patient supine to allow for independent drainage of urine from the bladder. Once ambulatory, fixation of the catheter to the lower abdomen in the suprapubic region will minimise frictional irritation of the urethra and urethral meatus. Intra-abdominal pressure will assure adequate drainage because it will overcome the slight gravity pressure provided by the curve of the catheter as it curls upwards towards the abdomen. The catheters themselves are irritating and the less catheter movement there is, the better they will be tolerated. The source of infection in the bladder in the female is as much around the catheter as it is retrograde. Thus techniques which minimise the chance of infection are not always warranted.

Eventual bacterial contamination of the bladder will occur over 3–5 days. This does not automatically imply infection, only contamination of the urine. Cystitis is unusual as long as the bladder is adequately drained. With the catheter in place and functioning there is a continuous low pressure situation within the bladder. Obstruction of the bladder leads to high pressures, relative ischaemia of the bladder wall and increased likelihood of bacteraemia and pyelonephritis. Following removal of a catheter, there is no need to send the catheter tip for culture. This can be very misleading as the catheter must be withdrawn to the introitus leading to contamination and perhaps an incorrect bacterial isolation. Bacteria present in the urine will clear very quickly following removal of the catheter as long as the patient is able to empty her bladder without residual urine. At this point 1 or 2 days administration of

an antimicrobial is not unreasonable. The patient should be seen and examined within a week and a urine culture taken to exclude persistent contamination or infection of the urine. The patient with a neuropathic bladder or a non-neuropathic voiding dysfunction will be unlikely to clear the bladder without assistance of antimicrobial therapy.

Suprapubic

There are basically three techniques used to insert a suprapubic catheter. All involve the same principles so nicely outlined by Hodgkinson in 1969. There were:

1. Always instil at least 400 ml of fluid into the bladder before inserting the trocar.
2. Never select a site of trocar insertion above 3 cm from the superior border of the midsymphysis.
3. Never insert the trocar in a vertical direction.
4. Always direct the trocar downward at an angle of 30 degrees from the vertical.
5. When in doubt about bladder location, insert a 4-inch needle for orientation.
6. Never insert the trocar much further than that necessary to obtain free flow of bladder fluid.
7. Remember, the pressure required to insert the trocar depresses the anterior abdominal wall to increase the danger of excessive insertion and bladder transfixion.
8. Do not allow bladder fluid to escape before inserting the catheter because this may cause the anterior bladder wall to fall away from the tip of the cannula, causing the catheter to be placed in the space of Retzius rather than in the bladder.
9. Remember, in the patient who has had a lower abdominal incision, the peritoneum may be fixed, thereby restricting its elevation as the bladder is filled, to sharply limit the safe area from trocar insertion.
10. Always remember, a trocar of the dimensions used for suprapubic trocar cystostomy has the characteristic capabilities of a lethal weapon, and its safe use deserves and requires the respect and art due to the most ancient and venerable operation of suprapubic cystostomy.

The open cystostomy is generally used as part of a transabdominal procedure. The bowel and peritoneum are freed from the dome of the bladder.

The bladder is then grasped between two Allis clamps and opened with a Bovie (diathermy) to control bleeding. A 20-gauge Malecot catheter is inserted and the detrusor closed with 00 chromic catgut. The author does not suture the catheter to the bladder wall as this would produce difficulties with early removal. The catheter should exit via a separate stab wound to allow complete closure of the abdominal wound with minimum risk of infection. The catheter is then taped to the abdomen to avoid accidental removal. Closed drainage should be the method relied upon to minimise the risk of infection. Hydrogen peroxide instillations in the drainage bag or outlet tube from the drainage bag have been shown to decrease its risk of bacterial contamination. If the catheter is to be left for less than 5 days, such precautions are neither necessary nor cost-effective.

Use of a trocar to insert a catheter into the bladder is acceptable, if performed pre-operatively. The trocar catheter kit is very useful in this regard. When choosing a kit, basic principles would suggest a Malecot catheter of soft consistency. The following kits are commonly available and satisfactory and can all be inserted under local anaesthesia:

1. Bonanno catheter (Fig. 19.1). This is a 6 French gauge catheter which is secured by sutures through two small tabs and it therefore can be inserted close to a suprapubic transverse incision. The catheter may be left in place for around 3 weeks and is ideal for post-operative use. The manufacturers are Becton–Dickinson and Company.

2. Cystocath (Fig. 19.2). An 8 or 12 French gauge catheter with a large adhesive flange for attachment to the skin. This is ideal for longer term drainage, but the catheter is less suitable for placing near to a recent abdominal incision. The manufacturers are Dow Corning Corporation.

3. Argyle Ingram trocar catheter (Fig. 19.3). This catheter is available in 12 or 16 French gauge and is more solid in construction than other designs but may be uncomfortable for a mobile patient. It is secured by intravesical balloon with a flange sutured to the skin. An irrigation channel is provided and this catheter is ideal if there is intravesical bleeding. It is manufactured by Sherwood Medical Inc.

4. Stamey percutaneous catheter (Fig. 19.4). This is a 10 French gauge catheter, secured by Malecot-type flanges and is not sutured to the skin. The manufacturers are Cook Urological Inc.

The technique suggested by Shute and MacKinnon (1972) has become standard especially for placement of suprapubic catheter of 18–20 French gauge. General anaesthesia is usually required. A perforated male sound is inserted transurethrally, to

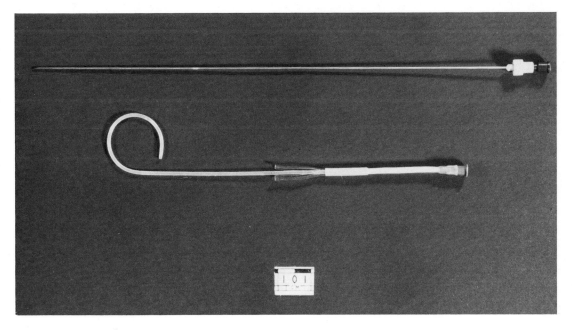

Fig. 19.1. Bonanno catheter.

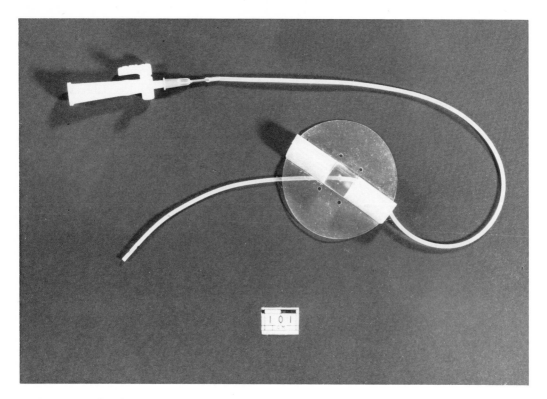

Fig. 19.2. Cystocath catheter.

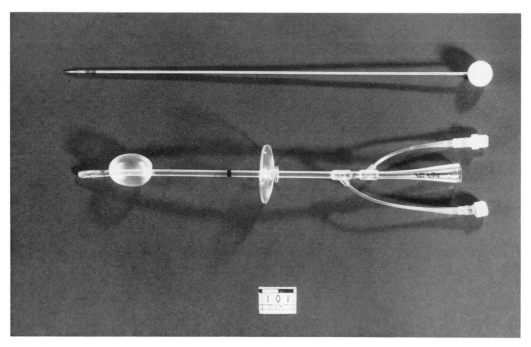

Fig. 19.3. Argyle Ingram trocar catheter. The intravesical balloon is inflated.

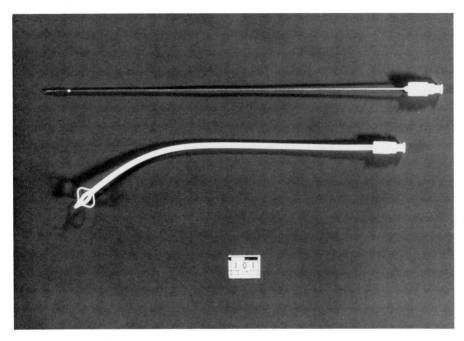

Fig. 19.4. Stamey catheter.

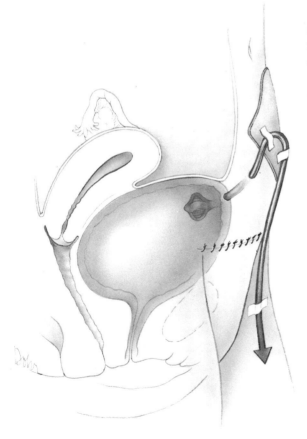

Fig. 19.5. Malecot suprapubic catheter in place.

elevate the dome of the bladder against the abdominal wall. A 1 cm incision is made over the tip of the sound and deepened down. When the tip of the sound exits through the abdominal wall, a Malecot catheter is tied to its tip. The sound is withdrawn, pulling the catheter into the bladder and then into the urethra. The suture is cut and the catheter is then pulled back into the bladder and fixed to the abdominal wall (Fig. 19.5).

Conclusion

As with all surgical procedures, no matter how minor, basic principles and good judgement must be used to avoid complications with the insertion of a suprapubic catheter. If there is any doubt about the safety of a closed insertion, either transurethral drainage should be used or an open cystostomy performed. Patients may be more comfortable with a suprapubic catheter, but safety should always prevail over convenience.

References

Bonanno PJ, Landers DE, Rock DE (1970) Bladder drainage with the suprapubic bladder needle. Obstet Gynecol 35:807–813

Brocklehurst JC (1978) The management of indwelling catheters. Br J Urol 50:102–105

Burke JP, Garibaldi RA, Britt MR, Jacobson JA, Conti M, Alling DW (1981) Prevention of catheter associated urinary tract infections. Efficacy of daily meatal care regimens. Am J Med 70:655–658

Cox CE, Hinman F Jr (1961) Experiments with induced bacteriuria, vesical emptying and bacterial growth on the mechanism of bladder defense to infection. J Urol 86:739–748

Desautels RE, Chibaro EA, Lang RJ (1982) Maintenance of sterility in urinary drainage bags. Surg Gynecol Obstet 154:838–840

Hodgkinson CP, Hodaii AA (1966) Trocar suprapubic cystostomy for post-operative bladder drainage. Am J Obstet Gynecol 96:773–783

Ingram JM (1977) Further experience with suprapubic drainage by Ingram catheter. Am J Obstet Gynecol 128:693

Koss EH, Schneiderman JJ (1957) Entry of bacteria in urinary tracts of patients with in-lying catheter. New Engl J Med 256:556–557

Lapides J (1981) Tips in self-catheterization. J Urol 126:223–225

Lapides J, Diokno AC, Silber SJ, Lowe BS (1972) Clean intermittent self-catheterization in treatment of urinary tract disease. J Urol 107:458–461

Maizels M, Schaeffer AJ (1980) Decreased incidence of bacteriuria associated with periodic instillation of hydrogen peroxide into the urethral catheter drainage. J Urol 123:841–845

Rassmussen OV, Kornen B, Moller-Sorenson P, Kromborg O (1977) Suprapubic vs. urethral bladder drainage following surgery for renal cancer. Acta Chir Scand 143:371–374

Schaefer AJ, Chmiel J (1983) Urethral meatal colonization in the pathogenesis of catheter associated bacteriuria. J Urol 130:1096–1099

Shapiro J et al. (1982) A comparison of suprapubic and transurethral drainage for post-operative urinary retention in general surgery patients. Acta Chir Scand 148:323–327

Shute WB, MacKinnon KJ (1972) Post-operative restoration of micturition and suprapubic catheterization. Am J Obstet Gynecol 113:849

Seski JC, Diokno AC (1977) Bladder dysfunction after radical abdominal hysterectomy. Am J Obstet Gynecol 128:643–651

Van Wagell JR Jr, Penny RM Jr, Roddick JW Jr (1972) Suprapubic bladder drainage following radical hysterectomy. Am J Obstet Gynecol 113:849–850

Wilson EA, Sprague AD, Van Wagell JR Jr (1973) Suprapubic cystostomy in gynecologic surgery: a comparison of two methods. Am J Obstet Gynecol 115:991–994

20 Choice of Surgery

Stuart L. Stanton and Emil A. Tanagho

PART I

Stuart L. Stanton

Introduction

According to the mechanism of continence (Chap. 1), the aims of continence surgery are elevation of the bladder neck, support for the urethra and occasionally increased urethral resistance. Urethral sphincter incompetence (genuine stress incontinence) may be due to one or several factors. With over 100 varieties of operations to choose from, it is important to select the correct procedure according to the cause of urethral sphincter incompetence, taking into account clinical and urodynamic characteristics of the patient.

Coexistent Gynaecological Conditions

Genital prolapse may coexist in up to 50% of patients and may be made worse by certain procedures, e.g. colposuspension. If symptomatic, the prolapse should be repaired at the same time. When a rectocele or enterocele is asymptomatic, it should be repaired if a colposuspension is to be performed.

However, I find no evidence to support a coincident hysterectomy in the absence of uterine pathology or descent.

Reduction in vaginal mobility and capacity (due to previous pelvic surgery or atrophic change) will determine whether it is technically feasible to perform certain procedures such as colposuspension or anterior colporrhaphy.

It is self-evident that when a patient is having sexual intercourse and already has some vaginal narrowing, this should not be compromised by operations which will further reduce the vaginal lumen, e.g. anterior or posterior colporrhaphy.

The elderly or physically frail are less likely to withstand a major abdominal than a minor vaginal procedure, and consideration should therefore be given to operations such as anterior colporrhaphy and the Stamey operation when appropriate.

Whilst coexistent frequency and urgency may sometimes be corrected by continence surgery, this is unpredictable and it is therefore unwise to offer an operation, such as an anterior colporrhaphy, to correct these symptoms per se.

Obesity certainly makes surgery technically more difficult and has a higher risk of postoperative deep vein thrombosis. I have never refused to operate because of this on its own. Occasionally stress incontinence is relieved by successful dieting, although conversely, I have not found that increasing obesity is a postoperative cause of failure (Stanton et al. 1978).

Urodynamic Contraindications

Voiding difficulties and detrusor instability are two conditions which are frequently made worse by most kinds of continence surgery. Therefore they need to be detected and evaluated beforehand. Consideration must be given to the relevant importance of the symptoms of stress incontinence due to urethral sphincter incompetence and of those due to voiding difficulty and detrusor instability.

With voiding difficulties, an acceptable balance can sometimes be achieved between the control of stress incontinence and only slight deterioration of symptoms of poor stream, incomplete emptying and straining to void. It has been shown that voiding difficulties following colposuspension are due to the amount of elevation and fixation of the bladder neck

within the pelvis (Dundas et al. 1982); unfortunately at present it is impossible to judge at operation how much elevation will secure continence but avoid the side-effects of voiding difficulty. Some clinicians, with the patient's agreement, will intentionally produce retention and encourage self-catheterisation. This is unphysiological, demands much patient compliance and is fraught with the hazards of urinary tract infection and upper tract dilatation. Prior management, according to urodynamic criteria, with drug therapy (Chap. 16) or urethrotomy (Chap. 13) may sufficiently improve the situation to permit continence surgery. Of all the procedures listed in Fig. 20.1, the anterior repair and Marshall-Marchetti-Krantz procedures are least prone to voiding difficulties.

Detrusor instability should be treated before surgery, because the cure of stress incontinence due to urethral sphincter incompetence is compromised by the presence of detrusor instability and urge incontinence is particularly likely to deteriorate. Only when a reasonable trial of medical treatment for detrusor instability (Chap. 16) has been attempted and the patient believes that stress incontinence is still a major symptom, should continence surgery be carried out.

Urodynamic Factors

Bladder Neck Elevation

The importance of bladder neck elevation has already been referred to. Most cases of urethral sphincter incompetence will have insufficient bladder neck elevation and this is the commonest factor to be corrected. It seems mechanically more effective to do this by "pulling up" from above via the suprapubic route, to "pushing up" from below via the vaginal route.

Urethral Alignment

Alignment of the proximal urethra and bladder neck to the postero-superior surface of the symphysis is probably responsible for transmission ratios of intra-abdominal pressure to intra-urethral pressure exceeding 100% as recorded during dynamic urethral pressure profiles after successful surgery (Hilton

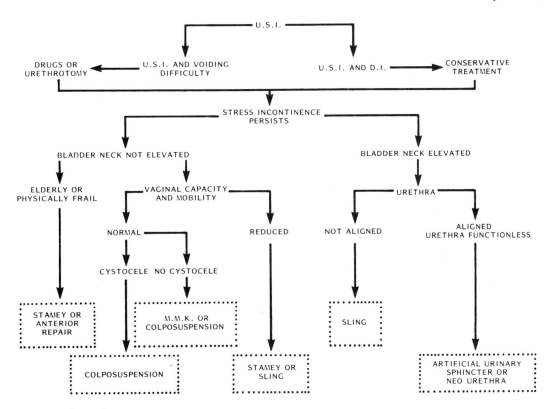

Fig. 20.1. Choice of continence surgery.

and Stanton 1983). Alignment is demonstrated using lateral bead chain urethrocystography on straining (Fig. 20.2). If the bladder neck is not elevated, a colposuspension or Marshall-Marchetti-Krantz procedure will produce elevation and alignment anteriorly to the symphysis. If the bladder neck is elevated and the proximal urethra is poorly aligned, or if an unsuccessful attempt has been made to elevate the bladder neck, a sling can be used to provide posterior support against which the proximal urethra can be compressed by anterior intraabdominal forces during strain. Minimal tension is required for the sling: excess tension may result in splendid bladder neck elevation, but unacceptable voiding difficulties and retention may occur. So far, no reliable scientific method exists for measuring sling tension. Attempts to measure intra-urethral pressure during surgery are usually without scientific proof or foundation and fail to take into account the effects of general anaesthesia and muscle relaxant therapy. A crude guide to correct tension is the clinical observation that on passing a urethral dilator, the urethral axis should be horizontal when the patient is in the horizontal lithotomy position.

Urethral Resistance

Present measurements of urethral function are imperfect and incomplete (Chap. 2). Intra-urethral pressure measurements, initially performed by the Brown and Wickham technique (1969) and later by single and twin microtip transducers (Asmussen 1976; Hilton and Stanton 1983), have significant clinical limitations in this area. Recent methods of detecting fluid within the urethra using a fluid bridge technique (Sutherst and Brown 1980) and modifications by measuring the change in electric impedance and deriving an electric conductance profile (Plevnik et al. 1983) and the measurement of urethral softness (Zinner et al. 1983) still await clinical evaluation.

At present the videocystourethrogram remains the most useful method of documenting voluntary and involuntary bladder neck opening, its movement under coughing and straining and its ability to close and remain competent.

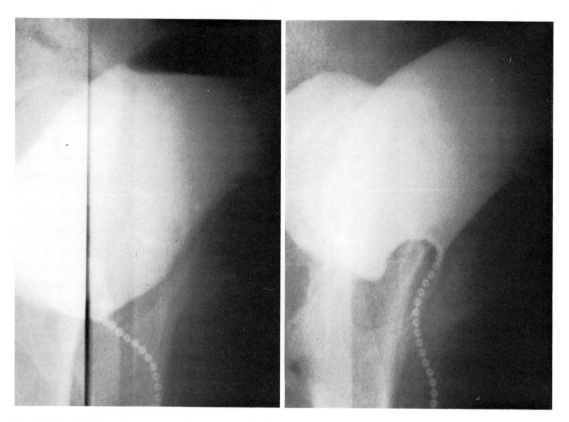

Fig. 20.2. Bead chain urethrocystogram. Lateral view with the patient standing erect and straining. *Left*, pre-operative; *right*, following successful colposuspension.

In the context of continence, the function of the urethra is to open at the commencement of voiding, to close and allow milkback of urine from the proximal urethra to the bladder at cessation of voiding and to maintain a higher intra-urethral pressure than intravesical pressure during bladder filling. The factors which allow for this are (1) hermetic sealing of urethral mucosa (urethral softness), (2) smooth and striated muscle of the urethral wall, (3) collagen and elastin tissue and blood vessel turgor within the urethral wall and (4) excursion and elevation of the bladder neck within the pelvis (controlled by the posterior pubo-urethral ligaments, pelvic floor muscles and pubocervical fascia). Urethral resistance and the ability to change it are an essential part of physiology. Function is compromised by childbirth (Snooks et al. 1984), previous bladder neck surgery with scarring and the menopause. Significant loss of urethral function is unlikely to be corrected by conventional continence surgery and may require treatment with either an artificial urinary sphincter (Chap. 11) or urethral reconstruction by a neourethra (Chap. 10).

Choice of Surgery (Fig. 20.1)

Hodgkinson (1970) stated that the first operation had the best chance of success and was the easiest to perform. This is true today and emphasises the importance of performing the best operation first time.

Whilst I believe from personal experience and from the literature, that suprapubic operations rather than anterior colporrhaphy offer the best and most permanent chance of cure, I think there is still a place for anterior colporrhaphy in the elderly and physically frail, where a short operating time and a pain-free post-operative course which will not limit mobilisation are important.

The commonest case presentation is the parous woman in her forties who has not had previous surgery. She will usually have descent of the bladder neck and normal vaginal capacity and mobility. She will be satisfactorily managed by a colposuspension or a Marshall-Marchetti-Krantz procedure. If there is an accompanying cystocele, colposuspension will correct that. My reasons for this choice are that the colposuspension offers a 95% cure of stress incontinence and is a technically simple operation to perform. The disadvantages are the incidence of postoperative voiding difficulty and detrusor instability.

Coincidental uterine descent can be corrected by an abdominal hysterectomy, and an enterocele by closure of the pouch of Douglas (Moschowitz procedure). If there is a rectocele, this will usually become more pronounced after a colposuspension and may need a posterior repair.

When vaginal capacity and mobility are reduced, a colposuspension may not be technically feasible and a Stamey or sling procedure is an alternative. I prefer a Stamey when the patient is elderly or physically frail, and a sling where it is likely that bladder neck elevation will not be achieved due to surrounding scar tissue and bladder neck immobility. Care should be taken to avoid excess sling tension in attempting to elevate the bladder neck for the reasons stated previously.

There are many tissues available, both organic and inorganic, for slings. I prefer medical grade Silastic (Stanton et al. 1985), which has the advantage of easy removal if the operation is not satisfactory. I usually insert the sling via a suprapubic route and create a sub-urethral tunnel. The sling is attached to each ileopectineal ligament. If the sling causes post-operative voiding difficulty, the sling can be released from the ileopectineal ligament or removed. If stress incontinence recurs, the sling may be cautiously tightened or if that fails, it can be removed and the cuff of an artificial urinary sphincter "railroaded" into its place with little additional dissection.

Satisfactory bladder neck elevation but failure of alignment of the proximal urethra may be treated by a sling procedure.

If the bladder neck or proximal urethra is found to be scarred and functionless yet with adequate bladder neck elevation, further conventional surgery is unlikely to succeed. My choice here would be an artificial urinary sphincter. Alternatively, I have used the neourethra operation in this situation, but have found it unpredictable in achieving success.

Finally, should these operations be inappropriate and non-surgical methods such as indwelling catheterisation be unacceptable and the patient wishes to be continent, a urinary diversion (Chap. 12) should be considered.

PART II
Emil A. Tanagho

Introduction

The key to success of the surgical approach for urinary incontinence lies in proper diagnosis. To limit the cause to one particular entity would be simplistic, as urinary incontinence has many variations: anatomical (genuine) stress incontinence, urge incontinence, neuropathic incontinence, congenital incontinence, false incontinence and iatrogenic or traumatic incontinence.

Differential Diagnosis

The first mentioned, *anatomical stress incontinence*, is the most common. Here, the sphincteric mechanism is intact; it is a weakness in the pelvic floor support that leads to incontinence. Fortunately, this is easy to recognise and cure: by restoring anatomy, one will restore function.

The urodynamic features of anatomical stress incontinence, essential to diagnosis, are quite basic: low closure pressure, a shortened functional length of the urethra and abnormal responses to stress. Should the first two not be immediately apparent, the last will establish the diagnosis. Upon further investigation, almost all patients will exhibit a drop in closure pressure with changes in position and/or bladder filling (e.g. when the hold manoeuvre or external sphincteric activity is being evaluated).

True *urge incontinence* is not associated with any anatomical abnormality, but is primarily detrusor hyperreflexia. There is no sphincteric weakness or dysfunction and, most importantly, no neuropathy. With urodynamic testing this entity can easily be distinguished from anatomical stress incontinence. However, the two commonly present in combination, and one must then quantify the relative contribution of each to determine which is primary and which secondary.

It is essential that the physician correctly identify *neuropathic incontinence* because what may be an appropriate treatment for other variants will never succeed with the neuropathic bladder. Although a neurological deficit is often evident, the manifestations of neuropathic incontinence can vary. Basically, there are two possible deficits: a flaccid sphincteric mechanism and a hyperreflexive bladder caused by the neuropathic lesion. Occasionally, these two varieties coexist.

Congenital incontinence presents a challenge. For example, although the ectopic ureter is probably the easiest anomaly to treat, it will often go undiagnosed for years. A typical patient referred to the urologist will be a young teenage girl who has been undergoing psychiatric therapy for bed-wetting when the problem is in fact congenital. In duplicated urinary systems, ectopy of the upper unit will be easily missed if the lower unit functions normally. In the single system, ectopy is rare; however, if it is bilateral the bladder will never fully develop and the patient will be wet all the time.

Female epispadias is not uncommon, but it is often missed. The characteristic bifid clitoris will be evident on careful examination of the external genitalia, as will the lack of formation of the anterior commissure. This entity will become quite clear on endoscopic examination.

False or overflow incontinence is rare in the female and may lead to mistaken diagnosis. The problem is often purely myogenic: defective detrusor activity will cause an increase in residual urine and, thus, the overflow. Iatrogenic obstruction is not uncommon, although congenital obstruction is.

Iatrogenic incontinence can result from surgery to the pelvis, ureter, bladder or urethra, and the site must be identified for appropriate treatment. A combined injury will present a problem: if the patient has both a vesical and a ureteric fistula, and one is left untreated, correction of the diagnosed fistula only will not cure the incontinence.

In the patient with a urethral fistula or diverticulum, its level will determine the extent of muscular involvement: the more proximal it is, the greater is the risk of sphincteric damage.

Traumatic incontinence most often results from surgical damage. The former practice of some urologists to undertake transurethral resection of the bladder neck or extensive internal urethrotomy with deep cuts to the entire length of the sphincter was largely responsible for the muscular damage. Now, urethral surgery is more commonly the cause. During fistula repair or excision of a urethral diverticulum, one must respect the delicate urethral musculature. The structure of the sphincter is so close and compact that, if one handles it indiscriminately, a scarred, fibrosed sphincteric segment beyond hope of repair will result.

Iatrogenic injury represents the most challenging manifestation of urinary incontinence because the sphincteric mechanism has already been damaged or lost. However, with an informed awareness of sphincteric anatomy and physiology, this can be successfully avoided.

Treatment

Anatomical repair should be uniformly successful. With adherence to basic surgical principles and careful patient selection, failure should never occur.

We prefer the suprapubic approach (colpocystourethropexy: Tanagho 1976) for correction of urinary stress incontinence and have found it to be uniformly successful in the virginal patient and in those who have suffered repeated surgical failures, in whom the prognosis is the least favourable.

The purpose of surgical repair in stress incontinence is to restore normal position and to provide adequate support to the vesico-urethral segment, yet to allow it limited mobility and to avoid any urethral compression or obstruction. In our technique, the anterior vaginal wall is actually used to act like a wide diffuse sling, supporting the bladder base and vesico-urethral segment after the latter is lifted to the normal position. The fact that the urethra is still free in a relatively wide retropubic space eliminates the possibility of post-operative obstruction or of false continence created by compression and obstruction.

If the sutures are placed too close to the urethra and pulled upward to the symphysis, urethral compression and strangulation against the back of the pubic bone are inevitable. Post-operative obstructive symptoms and variable volumes of residual urine are then commonly encountered.

Placement of heavy suture material in the urethral wall itself is extremely damaging and traumatising to its delicate muscular structure, which constitutes the main element of the sphincteric mechanism. If this is done, scarring of the urethral musculature is inevitable, with permanent intrinsic weakness of the sphincteric mechanism as the outcome.

Funneling of the internal meatus and vesiculation of the proximal urethral segment are results of the downward and posterior sagging of the vesical neck. Restoration of normal position permits the intact musculature to improve the closure of the proximal urethra and the internal meatus. No plication sutures are needed around the internal meatus anteriorly or posteriorly. The musculature of this segment should be left untouched. It will regain its tone and effectively close the internal meatus.

Restoration of the posterior vesico-urethral angle is not part of the repair. This angle corrects itself once the vesico-urethral segment is lifted to its normal position. Accordingly, vaginal repairs that are primarily aimed at correcting the posterior vesico-urethral angle are less than ideal for the treatment of urinary incontinence. Their effects are temporary at best. Except in cases of significant prolapse or cystocele, anterior vaginal repair should not be considered a procedure for the restoration of continence.

Colpocystourethropexy is similar in many respects to the techniques of Burch and Murnaghan. The use of Cooper's ligament as an anterior fixation point is well accepted and has proved successful. The main features of this method are the use of full thickness of the vaginal wall and placement of sutures far laterally from the urethra to avoid any compression of the latter, together with free mobilization.

Our technique has been uniformly successful in virginal cases. It has been highly successful after repeated previous failures. Actually, as physiological studies confirmed, the only cases of failure were those in which intrinsic damage had previously been inflicted to the sphincteric mechanism by surgical attempts that had traumatised and scarred the urethral musculature. The extent of the damage is usually dependent upon the technique or techniques used initially. We have encountered cases in which the urethra was nothing but a scarred fibrosed tube. No remedy is possible in these cases except creation of obstruction by compression or slings. It is the lesson we learned from such failures that led us to adopt the technique that will not damage the sphincteric elements.

The technique described is a rational approach to the surgical correction of urinary stress incontinence. If properly accomplished, it restores normal anatomical configuration and permits return of normal function without creating any obstruction or trauma.

In cases of urinary incontinence not amenable to anatomical repair, other modes of treatment should be explored.

Pharmacological manipulation directed at the bladder wall can reduce detrusor hyperreflexia. When given in an attempt to build up the tonus of the sphincteric element, however, the use of drugs has been disappointing in other than very mild, early cases.

Only when there is no intrinsic sphincteric element left should *reconstructive surgery* be considered. This is never as successful as anatomical repair, and it can be beneficial in 70%—80% of patients. It should be reserved for congenital anomalies, for severe trauma and complete disruption of the sphincteric mechanism, and for patients who have excessive scarring and fibrosis after ill-performed surgery. Either the anterior bladder wall technique or the trigonal and bladder base technique or their modifications may be used.

In patients with neuropathic incontinence, *neurostimulation* can be quite successful. It can act on both the bladder and sphincter; indeed, it can modulate the function of the entire lower urinary tract. With detrusor hyperreflexia, electrostimulation can alleviate both sensory and motor urge incontinence; with sphincteric weakness, repeated stimulation of the pudendal nerve or any sacral root can activate the external sphincter, converting striated muscle to tissue with attributes of both smooth and striated muscle that will resist fatigue and retain the tonus necessary for permanent sphincteric control. The potential of neurostimulation for bladder control is only now being recognised.

If reconstructive surgery is not feasible, if scarring and trauma leave one with no alternative but a mechanical device to attempt to maintain continence, then the *artificial sphincter* can be considered. Careful patient selection is of paramount importance, however, and the limitations of this device—especially in the female—are great.

Problems in Management

It cannot be stressed too strongly that the chief determinant of success or failure of any treatment for urinary incontinence is proper diagnosis. If one confuses the causes, mistaking one variant for another, then the surgical rationale will be unfounded and the operation will fail.

Never undertake a surgical approach simply because it is reportedly effective. Identify the site of incontinence. Only when one has determined the cause can one expect to effect a cure.

References

Asmussen M (1976) Intra-urethral pressure recording. Scand J Urol Nephrol 10:1–6

Brown M, Wickham J (1969) The urethral pressure profile. Br J Urol 41:211–217

Dundas D, Hilton P, Williams JE, Stanton SL (1982) Aetiology of voiding difficulties post colposuspension. Proceedings of the 12th Annual Meeting of the International Continence Society, Leiden, 132

Hilton P, Stanton SL (1983) Urethral pressure measurements by microtransducer: the results in symptom-free women and in those with genuine stress incontinence. Br J Obstet Gynaecol 90:919–933

Hodgkinson CP (1970) Stress urinary incontinence. Am J Obstet Gynecol 108:1141–1168

Plevnik S, Vrtacnik P, Janez J (1983) Detection of fluid entry into the urethra by electric impedance measurement: electric fluid bridge test. Clin Phys Physiol Meas 4:309–313

Snooks SJ, Swash M, Setchell M, Henry M (1984) Injury to innervation of pelvic floor sphincter musculature in childbirth. Lancet II:546–550

Stanton SL, Brindley G, Holmes D (1985) Silastic sling for urethral sphincter incompetence in the female. Br J Obstet Gynaecol 92:747–750

Stanton SL, Cardozo LD, Williams JE, Ritchie D, Allan V (1978) Clinical and urodynamic features of failed incontinence surgery in the female. Obstet Gynecol 51:515–520

Sutherst J, Brown M (1980) Detection of urethral incompetence in women using the fluid bridge test. Br J Urol 52:138–142

Tanagho E (1976) Colpocystourethropexy: the way we do it. J Urol 116:751–753

Zinner N, Sterling A. Ritter R (1983) Measuring softness of the inner female urethra. I and II. Urology 22:444–448

Subject Index